The depressed child and adolescent

In this new, thoroughly revised and updated edition an international, interdisciplinary team of mental health experts draws together the latest findings in the psychopathology of depression in young people. Combining theory and practice, the psychological, neurochemical and genetic causes are discussed and an account of the clinical characteristics and frequency of the condition is given. The key questions are fully addressed: the importance of life events and difficulties in the onset and continuation of depression; the efficacy of current psychological therapies and the role of medication; how depressed young people progress into adult life; and how depression arises and the effects it may ... ... pmental period.

T... ... ...ists and ... ...ologists, ...ntal psychologists, neuros... ... ...ical services.

'Ian Goodyer has assembled an internationally recognized group of researchers as authors . . . In the resulting tour de force, we are taken from an exposition of the development of emotional behavior and understanding, through the contributions of temperament, attachment and personality development, to depressive vulnerability . . . Each chapter contains a depth of information not found in usual textbooks and a subtlety of understanding that only experts of international standing who are reviewing the areas of their own research can provide . . . this book documents, with references, the great strides child and adolescent psychiatry and psychology have made in the past 30 years.'
From a review of the first edition in the *New England Journal of Medicine*.

Ian M. Goodyer is foundation Professor of Child and Adolescent Psychiatry at the University of Cambridge and Secretary-General of the International Association of Child and Adolescent Psychiatry and Allied Professions. He is widely published in the field of child and adolescent depression and the focus of his work is on the relations between social, emotional, cognitive and endocrine factors in the onset, course and outcome of major depression in young people.

Cambridge Child and Adolescent Psychiatry

Child and adolescent psychiatry is an important and growing area of clinical psychiatry. The last decade has seen a rapid expansion of scientific knowledge in this field and has provided a new understanding of the underlying pathology of mental disorders in these age groups. This series is aimed at practitioners and researchers both in child and adolescent mental health services and developmental and clinical neuroscience. Focusing on psychopathology, it highlights those topics where the growth of knowledge has had the greatest impact on clinical practice and on the treatment and understanding of mental illness. Individual volumes benefit both from the international expertise of their contributors and a coherence generated through a uniform style and structure for the series. Each volume provides firstly an historical overview and a clear descriptive account of the psychopathology of a specific disorder or group of related disorders. These features then form the basis for a thorough critical review of the etiology, natural history, management, prevention and impact on later adult adjustment. Whilst each volume is therefore complete in its own right, volumes also relate to each other to create a flexible and collectable series that should appeal to students as well as experienced scientists and practitioners.

Editorial board

Series editor Professor Ian M. Goodyer *University of Cambridge*

Associate editors

Professor Donald J. Cohen
Yale Child Study Center

Dr Robert N. Goodman
Institute of Psychiatry, London

Professor Barry Nurcombe
The University of Queensland

Professor Dr Helmut Remschmidt
Klinikum der Philipps-Universität, Germany

Professor Dr Herman van Engeland
Academisch Ziekenhuis Utrecht

Dr Fred R. Volkmar
Yale Child Study Center

Already published in this series:

The depressed child and adolescent

Second Edition

Edited by

Ian M. Goodyer
University of Cambridge

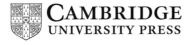

CAMBRIDGE
UNIVERSITY PRESS

PUBLISHED BY THE PRESS SYNDICATE OF THE UNIVERSITY OF CAMBRIDGE
The Pitt Building, Trumpington Street, Cambridge, United Kingdom

CAMBRIDGE UNIVERSITY PRESS
The Edinburgh Building, Cambridge CB2 2RU, UK
40 West 20th Street, New York, NY 10011-4211, USA
10 Stamford Road, Oakleigh, VIC 3166, Australia
Ruiz de Alarcón 13, 28014 Madrid, Spain
Dock House, The Waterfront, Cape Town 8001, South Africa

http:\\www.cambridge.org

First published 1995
Second edition published 2001

Printed in the United Kingdom at the University Press, Cambridge

Typeset in Dante MT 11/14pt [V N]

A catalogue record for this book is available from the British Library

Library of Congress Cataloguing in Publication data

The depressed child and adolescent by Ian M. Goodyer. – 2nd ed., rev. and updated.
      p. cm. – (Cambridge child and adolescent psychiatry)
   Includes bibliographical references and index.
   ISBN 0 521 79426 9
   1. Depression in children.   2. Depression in adolescence.   I. Goodyer, Ian M.
II. Cambridge child and adolescent psychiatry series

RJ506.D4 D44 2000
618.92'8527 – dc21   00–028925

ISBN 0 521 79426 9 paperback

Every effort has been made in preparing this book to provide accurate and up-to-date information which is in accord with accepted standards and practice at the time of publication. Nevertheless, the authors, editors and publisher can make no warranties that the information contained herein is totally free from error, not least because clinical standards are constantly changing through research and regulation. The authors, editors and publisher therefore disclaim all liability for direct or consequential damages resulting from the use of material contained in this book. Readers are strongly advised to pay careful attention to information provided by the manufacturer of any drugs or equipment that they plan to use.

This, the second edition of *The depressed child and adolescent*, is dedicated to the memory of William Parry-Jones, foundation Professor of Child and Adolescent Psychiatry in the University of Glasgow, Scotland, who was the inspiration for the series. It was his intention that every volume in this series should contain a chapter detailing the historical components of mental and behavioural disorders of young people, thereby providing the reader with an insight into some of the origins of current thought on the topic. Accordingly, I have included his original chapter from the first edition, entitled 'Historical aspects of mood and its disorders in young people', which remains perhaps the most readable and comprehensive account of how affective disorders were viewed by our predecessors.

Contents

Contributors

Adrian Angold
Department of Psychiatry
Duke University Medical Center
Box 3454
Durham, NC 27710-3454
USA

Jessica J. Auth
Center for Children and Families
Teachers' College
New York, NY 10027
USA

Jeanne Brooks-Gunn
Center for Children and Families
Teachers' College
New York, NY 10027
USA

Bruce E. Compas
Department of Psychology
John Dewey Hall
University of Vermont
Burlington, VT 05405-0134
USA

Elizabeth J. Costello
Department of Psychiatry
Duke University Medical Center
Box 3454
Durham, NC 27710-3454
USA

Erik Jan de Wilde
Faculty of Social and Behavioural Sciences
Department of Psychology
Division of Clinical and Health Psychology
University of Leiden
The Netherlands

René F. W. Diekstra
Psychosocial Department
Department of Paediatrics
University of Utrecht
Wilhelmina Children's Hospital
PO Box 18009
3501 CA Utrecht
The Netherlands

Bernadka Dubicka
University Department of Child Psychiatry
Royal Manchester Children's Hospital
Pendlebury
Manchester, M27 1HA
UK

Professor Ian M. Goodyer
Section of Developmental Psychiatry
Douglas House, 18 Trumpington Road
Cambridge, CB2 4AH
UK

Richard Harrington
University Department of Child Psychiatry
Royal Manchester Children's Hospital
Pendlebury
Manchester, M27 1HA
UK

Kim Kendall
Adolescent Health Training Program
Department of Pediatrics, WJ-10
University of Washington Medical School
Seattle, WA 98195
USA

Ineke C. W. M. Kienhorst
Psychosocial Department
Department of Paediatrics
University of Utrecht
Wilhelmina Children's Hospital
PO Box 18009
3501 CA Utrecht
The Netherlands

Israel Kolvin
Department of Child and Adolescent
Psychiatry
University of London
The Tavistock Clinic
120 Belsize Lane
London, NW3 5BA
UK

Maria Kovacs
University of Pittsburgh Medical Center
Western Psychiatric Institute and Clinic
3811 O'Hara Street
Pittsburgh, PA 15213-2593
USA

Stan Kutcher
Queen Elizabeth II Health Center
4th Floor, Suite 4018
5909 Jubilee Road
Halifax, Nova Scotia, B3H 2E2
Canada

Elizabeth McCauley
Department of Psychiatric and Behavioral
Health
CHRMC
4800 Sand Point Way NE
Seattle, WA 98105
USA

Mark Meerum Terwogt
Department of Developmental Psychology
Free University
Van der Boechorststraat 1
1081 BT Amsterdam
The Netherlands

Karen Pavlidis
Department of Psychology, NI-25
University of Washington
Seattle, WA 98195
USA

William Ll. Parry-Jones
Deceased

Anne C. Petersen
WK Kellogg Foundation
1 Michigan Avenue East
Battle Creek, MI 49017
USA

Helmut Remschmidt
Klinik für Kinder und Jugendpsychiatrie
Philipps-Universität
Hans-Sachs-Straße 6
D-35033 Marburg
Germany

Hartwin Sadowski
Department of Child and Adolescent
Psychiatry
University of London
The Tavistock Clinic
120 Belsize Lane
London, NW3 5BA
UK

Eberhard Schulz
Klinik für Kinder und Jugendpsychiatrie
Philipps-Universität
Hans-Sachs-Straße 6
D-35033 Marburg
Germany

Joel T. Sherrill
University of Pittsburgh Medical Center
Western Psychiatric Institute and Clinic
3811 O'Hara Street
Pittsburgh, PA 15213-2593
USA

Hedy Stegge
Department of Developmental Psychology
Free University
Van der Boechorststraat 1
1081 BT Amsterdam
The Netherlands

Stephen Sokolov
Mood Disorders Clinic
Sunnybrook Health Sciences Centre
2075 Bayview Avenue
North York, Ontario, M4N 3M5
Canada

Michael Strober
Adolescent Mood Disorders Program
UCLA Neuropsychiatric Institute
760 Westwood Plaza
Los Angeles, CA 90024
USA

Preface

This, the second edition of *The depressed child and adolescent*, incorporates the latest clinical and research findings.

The resurgence of interest in emotion psychology is addressed in chapters dealing with the development of affect regulation and evaluation of self and others.

A major recent advance is the discovery that comorbid disorders at presentation and over the life span are of crucial importance for delineating depressive subtypes. A precise clinical characterization results in the development of more homogeneous groupings of depressive disorders that will improve the search for genetic as well as environmental aetiologies and enhance the specificity of neuroimaging studies.

Since the first edition, a number of treatment studies have been published in psychological therapies, and psychopharmacology has also established a scientific basis for the use of selective serotonin reuptake inhibitor (SSRI) medication. These findings remain focused on adolescents, with much still needing to be determined regarding the treatment of depression in prepubertal children. There is an increased understanding that there are aetiological pathways that involve much greater interplay between brain, mind and physiological and social environments than considered hitherto.

Whilst much remains to be done, including determining the processes and mechanisms by which genes exert their effects on the environment, it seemed timely to record the progress and achievements that have been made in the last five years by scientists and clinicians alike.

Ian Goodyer

Cambridge 2001

Historical aspects of mood and its disorders in young people

William Ll. Parry-Jones

Introduction

The last 20 years have witnessed rapid expansion of clinical and theoretical interest in affective disorders in children and adolescents. Extensive historical examination of the subject has however been minimal. The primary aims of this chapter, therefore, are to assemble evidence about the wider historical background and to set some current clinical and research issues in perspective. The methodology and interpretation of historical research on affective disorder in young people need to take into consideration a number of factors.

Growth of interest in juvenile mental disorder

Prior to the mid nineteenth century, little systematic attention was given to juvenile lunatics and the existence of insanity in early life was disputed or denied. A picture of their disorders and care has to be assembled, therefore, from diverse sources, mainly reports of unusual cases (Parry-Jones, 1993). Subsequently, insanity in children and adolescents featured increasingly in asylum practice and in textbooks and journals, although it was not until the 1920s and 1930s that a recognizably separate discipline of child psychiatry emerged. The multidisciplinary speciality that took shape was the product of the confluence of expertise from paediatrics, asylum medicine, the training and custodial care of the mentally retarded, psychoanalysis, psychology, psychiatric social work, remedial education and criminology. Later, influenced by the new medical psychology and by psychoanalytic thinking, the developing speciality moved away from asylum-based psychiatry, with its concepts of organ pathology, heredity, phenomenological syndromal description and physical treatments, towards psychosocial and psychodynamic models. In the process, it distanced itself from the most severely disturbed juveniles, particularly adolescents.

Following the Second World War, there was rapid growth of hospital-based outpatient clinics, first inaugurated in the 1920s and 1930s, and the development of inpatient wards. From the mid-1960s, increasing acceptance of the need for separate services for adolescents arose out of concern about their care with adults in mental hospitals. The last 30 years have seen the emergence of British child and adolescent psychiatry as a well-established, scientific speciality, accompanied by the slow expansion, from the 1970s, of academic departments.

Changing theories of child mental development

The theories of Locke and Rousseau continued to influence concepts of child development in the first half of the nineteenth century. Darwin's theory of evolution, however, raised new problems concerning development and variation that were alien to the older psychology. By the last quarter of the century, major new interest in child study was developing rapidly in Europe and the USA, associated with biographical accounts of infant development. Such interest had clinical implications; for example, Clouston (1891) catalogued disorders associated with development up to the end of adolescence (interpreted as occurring between the ages of 18 and 25) when reproductive functions were developed and full growth attained. A recurrent theme at this time was ancestral recapitulation whereby, an individual when developing passed through stages which characterized those of his or her race. Early twentieth-century theories of child development were principally influenced by Sigmund and Anna Freud and subsequent child psychoanalytic theorists, and by Claparède, Piaget, Kohlberg, Vygotsky and Erikson.

Theories concerning the nature, development and expression of emotion

Accounts of the history of the psychology of emotion are fraught with difficulties, since 'the field is replete with theory and scantily covered with relevant experimental evidence' (Mandler, 1979). Consideration needs to be given to the influence of concepts arising from a number of different theoretical viewpoints (Gardiner et al., 1937), including: theological and philosophical perspectives; psychoanalytic and experiential theories; ethological concepts; physiological and neurobiological explanations and behavioural and cognitive interpretations. Darwin's observation (1872) that there was universal similarity of facial expression of emotions and that expressions of sadness and stress had an adaptive function was highly influential, until the advent of the James–Lange theory of emotion in the late 1880s and its subsequent critique by Cannon in the 1920s. In order to elucidate the psychology and physiology of normal emotional life, Thalbitzer (1926) drew upon the study of 'mood–psychoses', suggesting that, in children and 'very naive, primitive and uncivilised people', these states tended to be simple and uncomplicated. For many years, theories of emotional development (Bridges, 1932) indicated that emotional expressions change and become more complex and differentiated until about 2 years of age. Relatively recently, there has been an upsurge of human, and animal-based research into emotional development (Strongman, 1987; see Chapter 2).

Changing conceptions of childhood

Historical studies illustrate the changing role and status of children in the family and society (Parry-Jones, 1993). The principal issues bearing on the recognition and classification of childhood mental disorders concern the extent to which children were regarded as miniature adults, the awareness of the psychological component in children's lives and interest in the deterministic significance of early life experiences.

Terminological and conceptual confusion

A wide variety of words have been used, over the centuries, to describe and define emotional experience, expression and disturbance, generating a confusing array of theoretical concepts. 'Mania', for example, has been used for diverse excited states. In addition to the core term 'melancholia', a range of alternatives have been used to refer to depressive states, such as 'the vapours', hypochondriasis, spleen, 'hip', 'lypemania' and 'tristimania'. During the nineteenth century, the situation was complicated by inconsistent use and definition of the terms 'affect', 'mood', 'emotion' and 'feeling'. In particular, application of 'affect' and 'mood' has suffered from sustained confusion because of variation in the reliance placed, in definition, on the duration of an emotional state or the distinction between subjective and objective components.

History of affective disturbance in adults

In view of the limited consideration given to childhood disorders until the mid nineteenth century, the field is dominated by issues concerned with affective disorders in adults. Although the extensive history of this subject is receiving increasing notice (Jackson, 1986; Berrios, 1992), aspects relating to children and young people, before the mid twentieth century, have attracted minimal attention.

Diversity and variability of source material

There is only sporadic survival of heterogeneous manuscript material before 1800 and little in the way of consecutive patient-related records. With the growth of theoretical interest in childhood insanity, the availability of printed source material expanded progressively during the nineteenth century.

Primary sources, including patient records, are increasingly available from the second half of the century.

Limited historiography of child and adolescent mental disorders

Historical accounts of child and adolescent psychiatry have been mainly concerned with its development as a medical speciality and with innovative therapeutic techniques. Very limited attention has been given to the history of clinical syndromes or to the wider implications of childhood insanity (Parry-Jones, 1992).

Pre nineteenth century

Despite copious discussion of the phenomenon of melancholia from Hippocratic times onwards, the condition was very rarely alluded to among juveniles. An exception was the Greek physician, Rufus of Ephesus, in the opening years of the second century AD, who stated that melancholia 'did not occur in adolescents, but it occasionally occurred in infants and in young boys' (Jackson, 1986). Before the nineteenth century, the term 'melancholia' was used to refer to 'a rag-bag of insanity states', not necessarily including sadness and low affect, and was a subtype of mania (Berrios, 1992). Depressive states without delusions were designated by terms such as 'hypochondria', 'vapours' and 'spleen'. Although there were occasional references in the seventeenth century to 'depression' or 'defection' of spirits and 'depressed', it was only in the latter part of the eighteenth century that such terms began to feature more specifically in discussions of melancholia.

Specific references to childhood insanity and its treatment are elusive and outwardly relevant early texts covering the topics of 'melancholy', 'frensie' and 'madness', such as those by Bright in 1586 and Willis in 1683, contribute little of relevance. Burton's comprehensive work on melancholy, first published in 1621, was not primarily concerned with depressive disorders in the modern sense, but he made some observations that were pertinent to childhood. He referred to education, for example, as a source of melancholy, especially when conducted by parents. In this context, he criticized parents who were both 'too sterne, always threatning, chiding, brawling, whipping or striking; by means of which, their poor children are so disheartened and cowed, that they never after have any courage, a merry hour in their lives, or take pleasure in any thing'. At the other extreme, he criticized parents who were too indulgent. Among the other causes of melancholy in relation to children, Burton referred to melancholic parents producing offspring who inherited their characteristics. In the case of the mother, this could occur even during pregnancy and, similarly, a wet nurse could transmit melancholic tendencies to the infant. Finally, Burton emphasized that severe terror and fright could cause melancholy in the young, describing two little girls near Basle, frightened, respectively, by a body on a gibbet and a corpse in an open grave; these girls 'could not be pacified, but melancholy died' (Burton, 1827).

In the eighteenth century, neither Sauvages' seminal nosology nor Arnold's detailed account of classification and causation afforded examples of childhood melancholy, apart from a passing reference by the latter to the vulnerability of young people to 'nostalgic insanity', when away from their homes (Arnold, 1782). This condition was first described clinically in the late seventeenth century by Hofer, whose cases included a young peasant girl, pining in hospital from parental separation. Whytt (1767) described a 14-year-old boy, who become low-spirited before the onset of an eating disorder. Perfect (1791), a private madhouse owner in Kent, England, provided a comprehensive account of an 11-year-old boy treated without admission to the madhouse. He displayed 'depression and lowness', alternating with confusion and acutely disturbed 'obstreporous' states, in which he was irrational and furious, behaving like a 'raving maniac'. The disorder, which Perfect thought had no clear causation, lasted for 4–5 months and was treated with the customary polypharmacy of the period.

Nineteenth century

Melancholia and depression

Changes began to take place in the classical usage of the term 'melancholia', with its connotations of humoral physiology (black bile), leading to its emergence more specifically as a primary disorder of the emotions, which, in turn, became referred to as mental depression or simply depression (Berrios, 1988). Early nineteenth-century classificatory developments in France were particularly influential in defining new disorders. Esquirol (1845), for example, coined the term 'lypemania' for a condition characterized by 'delirium with respect to one or a small number of objects, with predominance of a sorrowful and depressing passion', although this term did not gain widespread European popularity. Esquirol considered lypemania to be 'rather the lot of adult age' whereas 'in youth, mania and monomania burst forth in all their varieties and forms'. In Germany, classifications by Griesinger, Kahlbaum and Krafft-Ebing remained influential until the publication of Kraepelin's seminal work (1921). In Britain, by the end of the nineteenth century, melancholia was clearly defined as a disorder characterized by 'a feeling of misery which is in excess of what is justified by the circumstances in which the individual is placed' (Mercier, 1892). Numerous forms were recognized, broadly grouped into those with and without delusions, including a hysterical form 'occurring principally in young girls' and a pubertal variant in which 'the patient often evinces a listless and moody apathy and perverseness of conduct' (Tuke, 1892). By the close of the century, the term 'depression' had gained greater currency, becoming a synonym for melancholia.

The growing number of case reports of juvenile lunatics in the first half of the nineteenth century rarely included melancholia and it was not until the second part of the century that there was consistent evidence of the identification, description and discussion of abnormal mood states in children and young people. Crichton-Browne (1860) made the significant observation that although melancholia 'appears incompatible with early life . . . it is so only in appearance, for the buoyancy and gladness of childhood may give place to despondency and despair and faith and confidence may be superseded by doubt and misery'. He recognized a range of disorders, principally 'pure, abstract indefinite depression' and also religious melancholy. Other forms, including hypochondriasis, were less common before puberty, 'as their existence implies subjectivity of thought'. Finally, 'simple melancholia, a mere exaggeration of that feeling of depression to which we are all at times liable, may, in youth, as in mature life, exist without at all involving the intellectual faculties'.

Maudsley (1867) included melancholia among the seven forms of childhood insanity. In his view, depression occurred in children 'with and without definite delusion or morbid impulse'. In some cases, depressive symptoms marked 'a constitutional defect of nervous element whereby an emotional or sensational reaction of a painful kind follows all impressions; the nervous or cyclical tone is radically infected with some vice of constitution so that every impression is painful'. Maudsley went on to suggest that this was often due to inherited syphilis. Deep melancholic depression was associated in older children with delusions and could lead to suicide. The concept of moral insanity, first described by Prichard (1835), was quite widely applied to young people and Maudsley referred to it as 'affective insanity' to convey 'the fundamental condition of nerve element which shows itself in affections of the mode of feeling generally, not of the special mode of moral feeling only' (Maudsley, 1879). In fact, he used the term 'affective derangement' to comprise both moral insanity and mental depression. Maudsley's principal contribution lay in the elucidation of the early onset and forms taken by childhood melancholic states and in his attempt to relate the type of melancholia to the level of development reached by the child at the time of onset. In infants, 'Feeling going before thought in the order of mental development', melancholic expression was by a 'primitive language of cries, grunts, exclamations, tones of sounds, gestures and features'. Older children aged 4 or 5 years might have 'fits of moaning, melancholy and apprehensive fears' and, later, features of typical melancholy could occur, sometimes with suicidal ideas (Maudsley, 1895). This developmental sequence differed from that of many other writers, which generally only included melancholia from the age of 10 or 12 years (Hurd, 1895). The form taken by melancholia after puberty was generally thought to resemble that in adults including, for example, the commonly occurring presentation with hypochondriacal delusions relating to bodily conditions. According to Mills (1893), delusions commonly occurring in adults, 'as of self condemnation, of the unpardonable sin, of coming to want, or of fatal organic disease' were often absent, although children brought up 'in a morbidly religious, or in distressing surroundings, sometimes exhibit a delusional state of a religious and painful character'.

In Europe, similar references to affective disorders in children began to be made. Griesinger (1867) stated that all forms of insanity occurred before puberty, albeit infrequently, including 'melancholic forms in all their varieties'. He drew specific attention to the occurrence of hypochondria, 'especially where the parents manifest excessive care of the health of the child', and to 'simple melancholic states . . . whose foundation is a general feeling of anxiety'. Later, in his influential work on 'psychic disturbance of childhood', Emminghaus (1887) demonstrated a clear understanding of the difference between child and adult disorders and identified four forms of childhood melancholia, including juvenile suicide.

Growing interest in childhood insanity in the mid nineteenth century was slow to be reflected in paediatric literature. Although West (1854), for example, referred to hypochrondriasis, malingering and moral insanity in children, no specific mention was made to mood disorder. In the early twentieth century, however, notable paediatric authors began to devote attention to functional nervous diseases of childhood, reflecting increasing awareness of the effects of emotional health, the problems of neurotic children and possible consequences in adulthood. Guthrie (1909), for example, drew attention to manifestations of fretting and home-sickness and to the effects of 'hospitalism', later studied by Spitz (1946), and Cameron (1929) recognized recurrent depression in children, including *folie circulaire*.

Mania and manic-depressive insanity

During the second half of the nineteenth century, there was increasing clarification of the concept of mania as an emotional disorder, characterized by elated affect, and its separation from general madness. By the end of the century, Maudsley (1895) divided mania, or 'insanity with excitement', into a simple form (without delusions), acute and chronic mania and 'alternating recurrent insanity'. The association between melancholic and manic states had a long history: an intimate connection between these conditions had been made as early as the second century AD by both Aretaeus and Soranus. In the medieval period, melancholia and mania were usually listed together under diseases of the head (Jackson, 1986). The position was clarified, in the mid nineteenth century, by two French alienists, Falret and Baillarger who, respectively, described and named the alternating sequence as *la folie circulaire* and *la folie à double forme*. When Kraepelin (1921) correlated the various forms, he confirmed that adolescence carried a predisposition for manic-depressive insanity, as well as dementia praecox, and observed that 0.4% of adult manic patients experienced their first episode at 10 years of age or younger.

Throughout the nineteenth century, a steady stream of published case reports recorded the occurrence of mania in children and young people, usually portrayed as early-onset examples of the 'adult-type' disorder (Morison, 1848; Mills, 1893; Fletcher, 1895). Down (1887) gave examples of infantile mania and cases 'where the various phases of insanity in the adult has been well represented'. In many of the reported cases it is difficult to distinguish primary affective disorders from states of excitement and confusion forming part of other psychotic disorders. For example, Greves (1884) gave a detailed account of 'acute mania' in a 5-year-old child, with a history of 2–3 weeks of acute disturbance but, in fact, this condition was more likely to have been a symptomatic psychotic state rather than an affective disorder.

During the last quarter of the century, many cases of *folie circulaire* in children were described. Ireland (1875), for example, reported a 13-year-old German boy, who 'had been so often punished at school . . . that he became deeply melancholy and tried to kill himself. The melancholy alternated with mania, in which he whistled and sang day and night, tore his clothes and was filthy in his habits'. Such a case was regarded as 'very rare at such an early age'. Hurd (1895) was in no doubt, however, that most cases of *folie circulaire* began at puberty, 'due to an original unstable state of the nervous system as is shown by the mental failure which follows an attempt to take on the second stage of physical and mental development'.

Pubescent and adolescent insanity

Puberty became accepted as an important physiological cause of mental disturbance and pubescent or adolescent insanity was frequently referred to during the second half of the nineteenth century. Generally, the disorders of children over the age of 12 years were thought to differ little from adult manifestations. The diverse 'insanities' of this period included abnormalities of feeling and conduct, with impaired self-control, waywardness, irritability and irresponsibility. In his entry on the 'developmental insanities' in Tuke's *Dictionary of Psychological Medicine*, Clouston (1892) detailed the special characteristics of pubescent or adolescent mania and melancholia. In summary, 'the mania of adolescence is acute, but seldom delirious; the melancholia is stuperous, and not very suicidal. Each maniacal attack is short in duration while the melancholic attacks are longer, the mania recurs from 2–20 times while the depression also recurs but not so often. The chief complications are masturbation in the males and hysterical symptoms in the females'.

Theories of causation

Melancholia and mania in juveniles have always attracted a wide range of causative explanations, generally reflecting contemporary clinical and scientific interests. Prevailing ideas of causation in the nineteenth century fall into four groups.

Physical causes

Causes thought to act primarily on the brain and nervous system included disorders such as epilepsy, febrile episodes, infections including meningitis, scarlet fever, typhoid fever and measles, intestinal parasites and trauma, particularly head injury and overexposure to the sun.

Psychological (or moral) causes

Severe shocks and frights, anxiety and distress, disappointments, bereavements, jealousy, faulty education, excessive study, religious excitement and parental brutality were the most commonly cited psychological causes. Actual or perceived loss was a recurrent theme, the consequences being particularly related to depressive states, with frequent reference to the effects of bereavement, separation and other adverse life events, such as failure in relationships and in school. Such adverse influences could be mediated by the parents. For example, Spitzka was reported to have seen 'constitutionally melancholic children in whom no other predisposing cause could be discovered than that the mother was struggling with direct or indirect results of financial crisis. In several cases the death of the father was a contributory cause of maternal depression' (Talbot, 1898). Over the last two decades of the twentieth century, earlier object loss and life stress explanations have been complemented by more specific models based on behavioural theories, the concepts of learned helplessness and cognitive distortion and, most recently, limbic-diencephalic dysfunction.

Early experience and education

The consequences of adverse early experiences, especially during child-rearing, and faulty educational practices, generated increasing comment during the nineteenth century and the role of parents and families was of special concern to many writers. Parkinson (1807), for example, drew attention to the potentially harmful effects of both 'excessive indulgence' and parental inconsistency on children. He argued that the overindulged, manipulative child could later discover his shortcomings and become depressed: 'Suffering under an accumulation of real and fancied ills, his misery becomes so great and insupportable, that sullen or furious insanity or dreadful suicide may soon be expected to succeed'. Harsh educational methods, overemphasis on scholastic attainment and the dangers of excessive 'mental exertion' in school also attracted increasing attention, especially in relation to suicide.

Hereditary transmission

The established belief in the connection between heredity and mental disease in children and adolescents was reiterated in the eighteenth century and was an enduring feature of nineteenth-century lay and medical writings and case material, with considerable preoccupation with concepts of degeneration. Distinction was made between connate disorders and hereditary susceptibilities, which could generate either disposition to disorder, for which hopes for prevention were poor, or predisposition, where the disorder was triggered by external causes and, therefore, carried the best prognosis. The role of hereditary predisposition in melancholia was recognized widely by notable alienists, including Esquirol, Heinroth, Bucknill, D. H. Tuke and Mercier.

Juveniles in asylums

Throughout the nineteenth century, severely disturbed children and adolescents were treated routinely in adult asylum wards. Mania and melancholia were common diagnoses. For example, among 592 young people admitted to Bethlem Royal Hospital, 1815–1899, who were given definite diagnoses, 345 were suffering from mania and 109 from melancholia (Wilkins, 1987). In a study of Oxfordshire asylums, Parry-Jones (1990) found evidence of a small number of young people presenting with clear evidence of depression and manic-depressive disorders.

Twentieth century

'Adultomorphic' descriptions of childhood affective disorders

A small number of essentially anecdotal case reports were published of manic and depressive states in children and adolescents (Brill, 1926; Kasanin & Kaufman, 1929), but the rarity of these early-onset adult-type disorders was acknowledged. Kasanin (1931), for example, described 10 cases under the age of 16, the youngest being 11 years, and emphasized their extreme rarity, citing the fact that only two to three children with affective psychoses presented among the 1900 new patients seen annually at the Boston Psychopathic Hospital. In the late 1930s, there was some interest in tracing aspects of the premorbid personality back to childhood (Bowman, 1934). The 1940s and 1950s, however, reflected the search for specific juvenile forms and it is noteworthy that, in 1952, a special issue of the journal, *The Nervous Child*, was devoted to manic-depressive illness in childhood. Despite such reports, however, it is significant that these disorders were not routinely included in the general textbooks of psychiatry or child psychiatry. Creak & Shorting (1944) made no reference to childhood affective disorders in their review of child psychiatry over the period of the Second World War.

Isolated descriptions of mania and hypomania, phenomenologically similar to the adult disorder, continued to appear, more frequently among adolescents than prepubertal children. Bleuler (1934), for example, reported on mania in children and Rice (1944) described manic features in a 14-year-old boy. However, the number of cases recorded was small. In 1951, Creak could only recall seeing two typically manic children – one recovering from acute encephalitis and the other, a boy of borderline intelligence, in whom 'the manic flight appeared to be a defence built around his very inadequate capacity'. In a review of world literature on juvenile manic states, Anthony & Scott (1960) found only three cases satisfying their strict inclusion criteria. More recently, however, the argument has swung in the other direction and, using a retrospective study of published cases during the period 1809–1982, Weller et al. (1986) sought to demonstrate that mania had been underdiagnosed in prepubertal children. Although the possibility of depression in adolescents was always in less doubt than in younger children, it was often argued that it posed diagnostic and treatment problems which are not present in adult patients, because of the alleged admixture of atypical, age-related features.

Deprivation reactions: effects of separation and loss

A separate theme is discernible concerned with the effects of separation and loss in infants and small children. Studies from the 1920s onwards began to draw attention to the behavioural consequences of sensory and social deprivation in institutionalized infants and the production of a syndrome, with depressive elements, resembling adult retarded depression (Levy, 1937; Freud & Burlingham, 1944; Winnicott, 1945; Scott, 1948). Spitz (1946) developed the concept of 'anaclitic depression' as a reaction, in children aged 6–12 months, to separation from their mothers, the 'love object'; features of the condition were misery, lack of expression and withdrawal. Analogies were drawn between such states and classical descriptions of mourning, pathological mourning and melancholia by Abraham (1911) and Sigmund Freud (1917), which had generated a new explanatory model of depression following the loss of a loved person. Spitz made a clear distinction between anaclitic depression and Klein's concept of the 'depressive position', which formed an integral element of the infantile psyche, arising when the infant perceives and introjects the mother as a whole person (Klein, 1991).

The description of deprivation-related depression drew comparison with the effects of separation experiences in nonhuman primates (Hinde & Spencer-Booth, 1971). It also raised questions about the role of maternal–infant bonding and led to a rapid expansion of interest in the effects of maternal deprivation, a topic pursued by many authors. Emde et al. (1965) provided a detailed account of a depressed infant in a residential nursery and, from the 1950s, influential studies were reported by the Robertsons, describing the affective response in young children detached from their mothers (Robertson & Robertson, 1971). Bowlby (1960) drew heavily on James Robertson's institutional data in his own descriptions of hospitalism and child reactions to maternal loss. In addition to these issues, the concept of anaclitic or deprivation-related depression in infants raised many other questions, especially whether or not it represented a prototype of depression in older children. Further, it was at this time that studies also commenced on the impact of early parental loss on the development of adult depression.

Doubts, challenge and denial concerning childhood depression

The developmental factors that altered a child's susceptibilities to depression, as well as the different patterns of childhood emotional responses compared

with those of adults, such as increased lability of mood, received acknowledgement during the first half of the twentieth century. Although perceptive by
modern standards, such views could also generate a very cautious approach to
the significance of mood-lowering. For example, Gillespie (1939) was in no
doubt that 'the fact that, following some disappointment, a child is found to be
depressed and to have suicidal preoccupations, does not justify us in thinking of
that child in the same terms as we would think of a similar condition in an
adult. Such depressive reactions are more akin to those of psychopathic
adolescents and young adults, i.e. emotionally immature people, than they are
to depressions (melancholia) of constitutional type'. From the late 1940s to the
1960s, doubts about affective disorder in prepubescent children increased and
its existence as a clinical entity was challenged – even denied – by many writers
(Bradley, 1945; Anthony & Scott, 1960).

   In the first edition of his influential textbook, Kanner (1947) emphasized only
the extreme rarity of 'Full-fledged thymergastic reactions' before 15 or 16 years,
although he did draw attention to mood variation occurring in normal healthy
children. Even in the second edition, depression received only passing reference in the chapter on suicide. Harms (1952), however, challenged forcefully
'the present autocratic opinion of academic psychiatry that there does not exist
manic depressive disease pattern among children', in the course of which he
claimed that Meyer's influence in discarding Kraepelinian concepts of manic-
depression had created nosological and terminological confusion. Circumspect
authors, such as Schachter (1952), sought to explain diametrically opposed
views in terms of the consequences of 'reducing' adult disorders to the infantile
scale, confusing 'periodic psychoses' in children with personality disturbances
and, above all, the absence of any long-term observation.

   The strongest views that the dynamics of adult depression, 'a superego
phenomenon', could not be applied to children, came from a number of
prominent psychoanalytic theorists. They argued that this was the case because, before the end of the latency period, children lacked well-developed
superegos (Rochlin, 1959); they were unable to tolerate the affect of hopelessness for any length of time (Rie, 1966) and lacked experience of separation till
the end of adolescence (Wolfenstein, 1966). Negative views were expressed
authoritatively. For example, Mahler (1961), contended, with great conviction,
that, 'the systematized affective disorders are unknown in childhood . . . the
immature personality structure of the infant or older child is not capable of
producing a state of depression such as that seen in the adult. It cannot survive
in an objectless state for any length of time'. An exception to this trend was
provided by the work of Sandler & Joffe (1965), who examined the

psychoanalytic records of 100 children and collated features commonly associated with depressed affect. This constituted an important step forward,
confirming that depression was seen in children and characterized by sad affect,
withdrawal, discontent, a feeling of being rejected or unloved, passivity and
insomnia.

Concept of masked depression

In order to explain the apparent difficulty in recognizing depression in children,
the concept of 'masked depression' was propounded. This proposed that an
underlying dysphoric mood could be masked by other symptoms not usually
associated with depression, e.g. somatic complaints, behavioural problems and
delinquent behaviour, school phobia and learning difficulties. In fact, such
complaints covered a large part of child and adolescent psychopathological
nosology (Toolan, 1962; Glaser, 1967; Bakwin, 1972). Depression in the mentally retarded could also be concealed in this way and Glaser emphasized that
feelings of inadequacy, helplessness, hopelessness and rejection might be expressed in acting-out behaviour rather than depression in the mentally retarded. This view was in keeping with the long-standing recognition of the
possibility of intercurrent mania and melancholia in this group. It had been
reported by Ireland (1898) and Barr (1904) suggested that insanity in the
mentally deficient could take the specific form of melancholia or 'nervous
excitability developing into acute mania'.

By recognizing that depressive affect occurred, albeit it was rarely observable, the concept of masked depression advanced understanding of affective
disturbance in children, but it remained controversial and unsatisfactory. The
diagnosis lacked operational criteria and it was impossible to tell whether or
not a common symptom was pathognomonic of depression as a 'depressive
equivalent'.

Trend towards diagnostic uniformity across age groups

Depression in childhood, in both acute and chronic forms, was included for the
first time in a major classification system by the Group for the Advancement of
Psychiatry (1966). It emphasized that it presented 'in ways somewhat different
from those manifested by adults', but childhood depression was not mentioned
in *DSM-II* in 1968. The early 1970s, however, saw a dramatic shift in thinking,
with increasing interest in phenomenology and diagnosis. There was acceptance of the existence of childhood affective disorders, especially in the prepubertal period, as distinct clinical entities, albeit rare before adolescence, and
possessing some unique features distinguishing them from adult states (From-

mer, 1968; Poznanski & Zrull, 1970; Malmquist, 1971; Anthony, 1975). This development involved growing recognition of age-related changes in language and behaviour influencing clinical expression in children, responsible for the divergence from common adult presentations (Cytryn & McKnew, 1979). Increasing reliance was now placed on the child as the best single source of information, as opposed to the conventional use of parental reports.

The recognition of the heterogeneous group of juvenile affective disorders encouraged new approaches to the specification of operational criteria for their diagnosis and classification (Cytryn & McKnew, 1972). In this context, it is interesting to note that there was a trend among American investigators to continue to claim that psychotic affective disorder was virtually nonexistent until mid-adolescence, although this was not the prevailing European view. The development of new assessment methods, using structured and semistructured interviews and rating scales, and reliable diagnostic criteria, such as Research Diagnostic Criteria, was critical in resolving confusion, particularly the differentiation between depressive affects and depressive syndromes. Epidemiological studies also began to be undertaken and the first attempts were made to clarify the pathophysiology of affective disorder. For a period, the view was sustained that child and adult depression were isomorphic, with no distinction in the diagnostic criteria for prepubertal, adolescent and adult depression, allowing the use of the same classification systems (Puig-Antich et al., 1978). The most recent studies, however, have focused again on developmental differences and age-specific features, emphasizing the necessity for their consideration during assessment and classification.

Childhood suicide and its relation to depression

Archival evidence indicates that there was a high incidence of 'self-killing' by children and adolescents in early modern England, despite the fact that, by the mid seventeenth century, legal authorities held that children under 14 years were not mentally capable of committing *felo de se*. From 1485 to 1714, for example, over 16% of recorded suicides were in juveniles under 15 years and 27% were aged 15–24 years – proportionally higher than their number in the general population (MacDonald & Murphy, 1990). According to Murphy (1986), youthful suicide at this time was an impulsive, retaliatory response to an alienating and rejecting social structure.

In the nineteenth century, the rarity of suicide in early childhood, but its increasing frequency thereafter, was well recognized. Winslow (1840), for example, referred to a small number of suicides in children of 12 or under, mentioning 'correction for a trifling fault' as a common precipitant. In 1845, Esquirol noted that, although suicide usually occurred after puberty, he had seen 'school-children terminating their existence, the victims of a vicious education, which teaches that a state of nothingness lies beyond the limits of this life, and it is lawful for a man to deprive himself of his existence, whenever it becomes disagreeable to him'. Later, a study of suicide in children by a French physician, Durand-Fardel (1855), attracted widespread interest. The adverse effects which parents and teachers could have on a child's feelings were emphasized and attention drawn to the importance of the child's emotional life, as well as to its education. Maudsley incorporated considerable discussion of childhood suicide in his principal textbooks (1867, 1879, 1895). Although regarded as a definite manifestation of melancholia, Maudsley (1895) noted that suicide 'is often done without any previous depression, on a sudden impulse springing out of the sad mood of the moment and the most trifling motive; not presumably with actual realisation of the momentous consequences, but rather perhaps as an outlet of temper or in unthinking immitation of a suicide which has been lately heard or read of'.

In the late nineteenth century, child suicide was thought to be increasing (Beach, 1898; Ireland, 1898) and, while acknowledging the difficulty of obtaining reliable statistics, serious attempts were made to monitor developments. From 1861 to 1888 in England and Wales, for example, suicides in juveniles under 15 numbered 148 boys and 113 girls (Strahan, 1893). In addition to such factors as fear of reprimand or maltreatment, excessive educational pressure was consistently thought to be a contributory factor and Westcott (1885) referred to 'several English cases of children killing themselves because unable to perform school tasks; yet it must be allowed that the most modern alteration in school life – the abolition of corporal punishment – has removed one fertile cause of suicide in childhood'.

During the first half of the twentieth century, anecdotal reports of suicide in children and young adolescents continued to appear in the psychiatric literature, but association with depression, however, tended not to be made (Bender & Schilder, 1937). Despert (1952) noted the paucity of reports of children's depressive reactions and suicide and concluded that depression was rarely associated with suicidal preoccupation, unlike the case for adults. Instead, 'suicide in children is predominantly of an impulsive character', with multiple potential motives. More recent studies have indicated much higher rates of suicidal ideation and suicide attempts in prepubertal children (Pfeffer et al., 1980), suggesting clearly that in the past such features were underrepresented (Schaffer, 1974).

Treatment

There is no evidence of specific treatment regimes for children with mania or melancholia until the 1920s and 1930s and the same range of restraints, physical methods and moral management techniques employed with adults would have been applied. Institutional care was resorted to for severe states of elation or depression, and especially to provide protection against destructiveness and suicide. In mental hospitals, it has to be assumed in the absence of positive information that children received the same range of physical treatments and opportunities for employment and recreation as adults (Kanner, 1947). Medication was always used extensively, despite its frequently nonspecific therapeutic characteristics. Antidepressants began to be given to children in the 1960s, although stimulants had been used in treating behaviourally disordered children since the 1940s. Frommer (1967), for example, reported the use of monoamine oxidase inhibitor drugs and Annell (1969) described the successful use of lithium for children and adolescents.

Conclusions

The rapid growth of clinical and research interest in mood disorders in juveniles over the last 20 years was preceded by a long period in which these conditions were discussed only cursorily, or not at all, in textbooks of psychiatry, child psychiatry or paediatrics. Nevertheless, it is evident that these disorders did not go unrecognized and the sweeping generalization that, until relatively recently, 'affective disorders in childhood were completely disregarded as a clinical entity' (Cytryn & McKnew, 1979) is not, in fact, supported by the historical evidence. On the contrary, case reports and references to affective disorders in children and adolescents had been occurring sporadically in previous centuries, with increasing frequency from the mid nineteenth century onwards. In common with all forms of juvenile insanity, however, melancholia and mania were considered to be rare before puberty and the occurrence and nature of the disorder in this age group was always more controversial than that arising in pubescence or adolescence. In general, until the last quarter of the present century, free recognition of prepubertal affective disorder was held back by doubts, misconceptions and lack of knowledge and awareness about the extent to which the child's limited cognitive and emotional development permitted the expression of sadness, hopelessness and depression. During the 1950s and 1960s, when the domination of child and adolescent psychiatry by psychoanalytic theory reached its peak, particularly in the USA, notions about superego development and its role in the definition of depression took their turn as the prime factors negating the recognition of childhood depression. With the subsequent return to near-Kraepelinian concern for descriptive diagnosis and the search for organic causes, fostered by new knowledge and pharmacological treatments, clinical and scientific interest in mood disorders and their pathophysiology began to surface. Underdiagnosis of major mood disorders in adolescents has also occurred, in part related to the alleged difficulty of their distinction from schizophrenia.

Modern reviewers of the history of child psychiatry have underestimated, or neglected, the level of awareness before the present century of child development and the aetiological implications for mental disorder of early life experiences and other factors influencing child behaviour, such as changing parent–child relationships. Serious attempts were made, in the second half of the nineteenth century, to clarify the distinctive nature of childhood disorders and classification was not simply an exercise in superimposing adult nosology. The influence of developmental levels and age of onset on the manifestation of the disorder was recognized, in addition to hereditary factors. This broad interest in the connections between the pattern of mental disorder and the underlying processes of normal physical and mental development, however, was not pursued actively in the early twentieth century and, since major affective morbidity in juveniles was managed in adult mental hospitals, an emphasis on adult-type disorders continued to prevail. The transition from the application to children of advances in the study of adult depression to the specific study of psychopathology in children was only to take place during the last two decades of the twentieth century.

The historical study of mood disorders in children and adolescents draws attention to many of the issues and questions that continue to call for clinical and research attention. The complex array of meanings attached to the term 'depression', ranging from depressive feelings and behaviours to depressive disorders, highlights the persisting need to strive for greater definitional precision. Uncertainty about continuities and discontinuities between the mood disorders of children, adolescents and adults has been an enduring theme in the literature. This raises questions about the extent to which they represent aspects of the same spectrum of disorders, whether childhood depression leads on to, or predisposes to, adult depression and whether there are juvenile antecedents to adult disorder. The necessity for a focus on the developmental variation of disorders, therefore, is overriding, without losing sight of the continuities across age groups.

REFERENCES

Abraham, K. (1911). *On Character and Libido Development*, pp. 15–34. New York: W. W. Norton.

Annell, A. L. (1969). Lithium in the treatment of children and adolescents. *Acta Psychiatrica Scandinavica* (Supplement), **207**, 19–30.

Anthony, E. J. (1975). Childhood depression. In *Depression and Human Existence*, ed. E. J. Anthony & T. Benedek. Little, Brown, Boston.

Anthony, J. & Scott, P. D. (1960). Manic-depressive psychosis in childhood. *Journal of Child Psychology and Psychiatry*, **1**, 53–70.

Arnold, T. (1782). *Observations on the Nature, Kinds, Causes, and Prevention of Insanity, Lunacy or Madness*, vol. 1, pp. 265–72. Leicester: G. Robinson.

Bakwin, H. (1972). Depression – a mood disorder in children and adolescents. *Maryland State Medical Journal*, **21**, 55–61.

Barr, M. W. (1904). *Mental Defectives: Their History, Treatment and Training*. Philadelphia: P. Blakiston's Son.

Beach, F. (1898). Insanity in children. *Journal of Mental Science*, **44**, 459–74.

Bender, L. & Schilder, P. (1937). Suicidal preoccupations and attempts in children. *American Journal of Orthopsychiatry*, **7**, 225–34.

Berrios, G. E. (1988). Melancholia and depression during the nineteenth century: a conceptual history. *British Journal of Psychiatry*, **153**, 298–304.

Berrios, G. E. (1992). History of the affective disorders. In *Handbook of Affective Disorders*, 2nd edn, ed. E. S. Paykel, pp. 43–56. Edinburgh: Churchill Livingstone.

Bleuler, E. (1934). *Textbook of Psychiatry*. New York: Macmillan.

Bowlby, J. (1960). Grief and mourning in infancy and early childhood. *Psychoanalytic Study of the Child*, **15**, 9–52.

Bowman, K. M. (1934). A study of the pre-psychotic personality in certain psychoses. *American Journal of Orthopsychiatry*, **4**, 473–98.

Bradley, C. (1945). In *Modern Trends in Child Psychiatry*, ed. N. Lewis & B. Pacella. New York: International Universities Press.

Bridges, K. M. B. (1932). Emotional development in early infancy. *Child Development*, **3**, 324–41.

Bright, T. (1586). *A Treatise of Melancholie*. London: T. Vautrollier.

Brill, A. A. (1926). Psychotic children: treatment and prophylaxis. *American Journal of Psychiatry*, **5**, 357–64.

Burton, R. (1827). *The Anatomy of Melancholy*, vol. I. London: Longman, Rees, Orme.

Cameron, H. C. (1929). *The Nervous Child*, 4th edn, pp. 77–8. London: Oxford University Press.

Clouston, T. S. (1891). *The Neurosis of Development, Being the Morison Lectures for 1890*. Edinburgh: Oliver & Boyd.

Clouston, T. S. (1892). Developmental insanities and psychoses. In *A Dictionary of Psychological Medicine*, vol. 1, ed. D. H. Tuke, pp. 357–71. London: Churchill.

Creak, M. (1951). Psychoses in childhood. *Journal of Mental Science*, **97**, 545–54.

Creak, E. M. & Shorting, B. J. (1944). Child psychiatry. *Journal of Mental Science*, **90**, 365–81.

Crichton-Browne, J. (1860). Psychical diseases of early life. *Journal of Mental Science*, **6**, 284–320.

Cytryn, L. & McKnew, D. H. (1972). Proposed classification of childhood depression. *American Journal of Psychiatry*, **129**, 149–55.

Cytryn, L. & McKnew, D. H. (1979). Affective disorders. In *Basic Handbook of Child Psychiatry*, vol. 2, ed. J. D. Noshpitz. New York: Basic Books.

Darwin, C. (1872). *The Expression of the Emotions in Man and Animals*. London: Murray.

Despert, J. L. (1952). Suicide and depression in children. *Nervous Child*, **9**, 378–89.

Down, J. L. (1887). *On Some of the Mental Affections of Childhood and Youth*. London: J. & A. Churchill.

Durand-Fardel, M. (1855). Etude sur le suicide chez les enfants. *Annales Médico-Psychologiques*, **1**, 61–79.

Emde, R. N., Polak, P. R. & Spitz, R. A. (1965). Anaclitic depression in an infant raised in an institution. *Journal of the American Academy of Child Psychiatry*, **4**, 545–53.

Emminghaus, H. (1887). *Die Psychischen Storungen der Kindesalters*. Tubingen.

Esquirol, E. (1845). *Mental Maladies. A Treatise on Insanity* (trans. E. K. Hunt), pp. 33–4. Philadelphia: Lea & Blanchard.

Fletcher, W. B. (1895). Mental development and insanity of children. *International Clinics*, **1**, 138–47.

Freud, S. (1917). *Mourning and Melancholia. Collected Papers, IV*. London: Hogarth Press.

Freud, A. & Burlingham, D. (1944). *Infants Without Families*. New York: International Universities Press.

Frommer, E. A. (1968). Treatment of childhood depression with antidepressant drugs. *British Medical Journal*, **1**, 729–32.

Gardiner, H. M., Metcalf, R. C. & Beebe-Center, J. G. (1937). *Feelings and Emotion: A History of Theories*. New York: American Book Company.

Gillespie, R. D. (1939). *A Survey of Child Psychiatry*. London: Oxford University Press.

Glaser, K. (1967). Masked depression in children and adolescents. *American Journal of Psychotherapy*, **21**, 565–74.

Greves, E. H. (1884). Acute mania in a child of five years. *Lancet*, **ii**, 824–6.

Griesinger, W. (1867). *Mental Pathology and Therapeutics*, p. 143. London: New Sydenham Society.

Group for the Advancement of Psychiatry (1966). *Psychopathological Disorders in Childhood: Theoretical Considerations and a Proposed Classification*. Report no. 62, pp. 236–7, 287. New York: Group for the Advancement of Psychiatry.

Guthrie, L. G. (1909). *Functional Nervous Disorders in Childhood*. London: H. Frowde/Hodder & Stoughton.

Harms, E. (1952). Differential pattern of manic-depressive disease in childhood. *Nervous Child*, **9**, 326–56.

Hinde, R. A. & Spencer-Booth, Y. (1971). Effects of brief separation from mother on rhesus monkeys. *Science*, **173**, 111–18.

Hurd, H. M. (1895). *Some Mental Disorders of Childhood and Youth*. Baltimore: Friedenwald.

Ireland, W. W. (1875). German retrospect. *Journal of Mental Science*, **20**, 615–31.

Ireland, W. W. (1898). *The Mental Affections of Children, Idiocy, Imbecility and Insanity*. London: J. & A. Churchill.

Jackson, S. W. (1986). *Melancholia and Depression. From Hippocratic Times to Modern Times.* New Haven: Yale University Press.

Kanner, L. (1947). *Child Psychiatry,* 5th edn, p. 506. Springfield, IL: C. Thomas.

Kasanin, J. (1931). The affective psychoses in children. *American Journal of Psychiatry,* **10**, 897–926.

Kasanin, J. & Kaufman, M. R. (1929). A study of the functional psychoses in childhood. *American Journal of Psychiatry,* **9**, 307–84.

Klein, M. (1991). The emotional life and ego development of the infant with special reference to the depressive position (paper read 1944). In *The Freud–Klein Controversies 1941–45,* ed. P. King & R. Steiner, pp. 752–97. London: Tavistock/Routledge.

Kraepelin, E. (1921). *Manic Depressive Insanity and Paranoia.* Edinburgh: E. & S. Livingstone.

Levy, D. M. (1937). Primary affect hunger. *American Journal of Psychiatry,* **94**, 643–52.

MacDonald, M. & Murphy, T. R. (1990). *Sleepless Souls. Suicide in Early Modern England,* pp. 250–6. Oxford: Clarendon Press.

Mahler, M. S. (1961). On sadness and grief in infancy and childhood. *Psychoanalytic Study of the Child,* **16**, 332–54.

Malmquist, C. P. (1971). Depressions in childhood and adolescence. I. II. *New England Journal of Medicine,* **284**, 887–93, 955–61.

Mandler, G. (1979). Emotion. In *The First Century of Experimental Psychology,* ed. E. Hearst, pp. 275–391. Hillsdale, NJ: Lawrence Erlbaum Associates.

Maudsley, H. (1867). *The Physiology and Pathology of the Mind,* pp. 259–93. London: Macmillan.

Maudsley, H. (1879). *The Pathology of Mind,* p. 280. London: Macmillan.

Maudsley, H. (1895). *The Pathology of Mind,* pp. 163–233. London: Macmillan.

Mercier, C. (1892). Melancholia. In *A Dictionary of Psychological Medicine,* vol. II, ed. D. H. Tuke, pp. 787–96. London: J. & A. Churchill.

Mills, C. K. (1893). Some forms of insanity and quasi-insanity in children. *Transactions of the Medical Society of Pennsylvania,* **24**, 204–13.

Morison, T. C. (1848). Case of mania occurring in a child six years old. *Journal of Psychological Medicine and Mental Pathology,* **1**, 317–18.

Murphy, T. R. (1986) 'Woful childe of parents rage': suicide of children and adolescents in early modern England, 1507–1710. *Sixteenth Century Journal,* **XVII**, 259–70.

Parkinson, J. (1807). *Observations on the Excessive Indulgence of Children, Particularly Intended to Show its Injurious Effects on their Health, and the Difficulties it Occasions in their Treatment during Sickness.* London: H. D. Symonds.

Parry-Jones, W. Ll. (1990). Juveniles in nineteenth-century Oxfordshire asylums. *British Journal of Clinical and Social Psychiatry,* **7**, 51–8.

Parry-Jones, W. Ll. (1992). Historical research in child and adolescent psychiatry: scope, methods and application. *Journal of Child Psychology and Psychiatry,* **33**, 3–12.

Parry-Jones, W. Ll. (1993). History of child and adolescent psychiatry. In *Child and Adolescent Psychiatry, Modern Approaches,* 3rd edn, ed. M. Rutter, L. Hersov & E. Taylor, pp. 794–812. Oxford: Blackwell Scientific.

Perfect, W. (1791). *A Remarkable Case of Madness, with the Diet and Medicines used in the Cure.* Rochester: for the author.

Pfeffer, C. R., Conte, H. R., Plutchik, R. & Jerrett, I. (1980). Suicidal behavior in latency-age children: an out-patient population. *Journal of the American Academy of Child Psychiatry*, **19**, 703–10.

Poznanski, E. & Zrull, J. P. (1970). Childhood depression: clinical characteristics of overtly depressed children. *Archives of General Psychiatry*, **23**, 8–15.

Prichard, J. C. (1835). *A Treatise on Insanity and Other Disorders Affecting the Mind*. London: Sherwood, Gilbert & Piper.

Puig-Antich, J., Blau, S., Marx, N., Greenhill, L. & Chambers, W. (1978). Prepubertal major depressive disorder: pilot study. *Journal of the American Academy of Child Psychiatry*, **17**, 695–707.

Rice, K. K. (1944). Regular 40 to 50 day cycle of psychotic behavior in a 14 year old boy. *Archives of Neurology and Psychiatry*, **51**, 478–80.

Rie, H. E. (1966). Depression in childhood. A survey of some pertinent contributions. *Journal of the American Academy of Child Psychiatry*, **5**, 653–85.

Robertson, J. & Robertson, J. (1971). Young children in brief separation: a fresh look. *Psychoanalytic Study of the Child*, **26**, 264–315.

Rochlin, G. (1959). The loss complex. *Journal of the American Psychoanalytic Association*, **7**, 229–316.

Sandler, J. & Joffe, W. G. (1965). Notes on childhood depression. *International Journal of Psychoanalysis*, **46**, 88–96.

Schachter, M. (1952). The cyclothymic states in the pre-pubescent child. *Nervous Child*, **9**, 357–62.

Schaffer, D. (1974). Suicide in childhood and early adolescence. *Journal of Child Psychology and Psychiatry*, **15**, 275–91.

Scott, W. C. M. (1948). The psychoanalytic concept of the origin of depression. *British Medical Journal*, **i**, 538.

Spitz, R. A. (1946). Anaclitic depression. *Psychoanalytic Study of the Child*, **2**, 313–42.

Strahan, S. A. K. (1893). *Suicide and Insanity. A Physiological and Sociological Study*. London: Swan Sonnenschein.

Strongman, K. T. (1987). *The Psychology of Emotion*, 3rd edn, pp. 141–66. Chichester: Wiley.

Talbot, E. S. (1898). *Degeneracy its Causes, Signs and Results*, p. 60. Chichester: W. Scott.

Thalbitzer, S. (1926). *Emotion and Insanity*, pp. 70–1. London: Kegan Paul, Trench, Trubner.

Toolan, J. H. (1962). Depression in children and adolescents. *American Journal of Orthopsychiatry*, **32**, 404–15.

Tuke, D. H. (ed.) (1892). *A Dictionary of Psychological Medicine*, p. 797. London: J. & A. Churchill.

Weller, R. A., Weller, E. B., Tucker, S. G. & Fristad, M. A. (1986). Mania in prepubertal children: has it been underdiagnosed? *Journal of Affective Disorders*, **11**, 151–4.

West, C. (1854). *Lectures on the Diseases of Infancy and Childhood*, 3rd edn, pp. 185–206. London: Longman, Brown, Green & Longmans.

Westcott, W. W. (1885). *Suicide; its History, Literature, Jurisprudence, etc.* London.

Whytt, R. (1767). *Observations on the Nature, Causes and Cures of Those Disorders which have been Commonly Called Nervous, Hypochondriac or Hysteric*. Edinburgh: Royal College of Physicians.

Wilkins, R. (1987). Hallucinations in children and teenagers admitted to Bethlem Royal Hospital in the nineteenth century and their possible relevance to the incidence of schizophrenia. *Journal of Child Psychology and Psychiatry*, **28**, 569–80.

Willis, T. (1683). *Two Discourses Concerning the Soul of Brutes Which is that of the Vital and Sensitive of Man* (trans. S. Pordage). London: Thomas Dring, Ch. Harper & John Leigh.

Winslow, F. (1840). *The Anatomy of Suicide*. London: Henry Renshaw.

Winnicott, D. W. (1945). Primitive emotional development. *International Journal of Psychoanalysis*, **26**, 137–43.

Wolfenstein, M. (1966). How is mourning possible? *Psychoanalytic Study of the Child*, **21**, 93–123.

This chapter was written by the Late Professor William Parry-Jones for the first edition of this book. It has been reprinted unaltered in this, the second edition, as a tribute to his memory and scholarship. It still remains as possibly the most outstanding review of the recent history of affective disorders in young people available in the literature.

2

The development of emotional intelligence

Mark Meerum Terwogt and Hedy Stegge

Introduction

All animals, including humans, are equipped with a number of more or less autonomic emotion programmes: perceived danger immediately elicits a tendency to flee (the basic fear programme), obstructive entities elicit an automatic tendency to attack (the basic anger programme), and so on. Such basic emotional reactions are mainly controlled by subcorticolimbic brain structures (MacLean, 1993; Schore, 1994). From a Darwinistic point of view, these prewired response syndromes are clearly functional, in the sense that they promote survival. This functionalist perspective seems to be in sharp contrast with the everyday life conception of emotions as disorganizing forces that interfere with one's ability to reason, which is presumably caused by the intrusive quality of emotions: our regular thought processes are often overruled by the emotion programme.

In daily life, we need these automatic emotion programmes on many occasions. Since cognition is much too slow to deal with immediate danger (Arnold, 1960), the primitive fear programme will sometimes literally function as a life-saving mechanism. Now what about less urgent circumstances? Even then, emotions are still functional in that they warn us that some interest is at stake (Frijda, 1986). However, under these circumstances, the accompanying primitive action impulse does not always serve our best interests in the complex society in which we live. We cannot attack everything that stands in our way or run away from everything that makes us nervous. Basic routines have to be adjusted to social requirements.

The first question that arises is how do we break up an automatic routine? Human emotions have three interacting components. Next to the behavioural-expressive component, there is a physiological-biochemical one: the organism has to prepare itself for action. But the development of the human brain, not only by adding new brain structures but also, more importantly, by further integration among components emerging through more elaborated and differentiated pathways in the brain (Tucker, 1992) created a third component: the cognitive-experiential one. Human beings are able to reflect on their own emotional functioning, and it is this latter element that allows for the necessary flexibility.

Making an automatism the object of attention is enough to disrupt the normal execution of the routine. There are numerous examples from other domains that illustrate this phenomenon. Suppose we ask someone who is keeping his balance on a balancing beam to tell us how he manages to do so. The person who tries to answer this question falls off; the highly organized and automatic act of balancing is disturbed. The same phenomenon can be observed if we ask an experienced driver how she changes gears. By making the act the object of attention, she is likely to make a mistake that she would otherwise never have made. In both examples, reflection interrupts a highly successful automatic program. Of course, in these cases, such an action is counterproductive; there is no need to alter the program. In fact, if routines like driving skills in the second example become automatized during development, we have given up cognitive control exactly because they are always successful. Where basic emotion programs are concerned, the exact opposite holds true. In the course of development there are fewer and fewer situations in which the acting-out of the original programmes is advantageous or even permitted. And although cognition may not always be able to modify intense emotional impulses (I was so angry, I hit him before I knew what I was doing), there are many situations in which we might attend to our emotional impulse in time to break up the primitive program.

The temporary blockage of an emotional impulse provides us with the opportunity to substitute the original program with a more adaptive alternative. From the moment of interruption, the emotion process is strongly influenced by our cognitive abilities. Since the primary intuitive appraisal that elicited the initial emotional reaction is not open for introspection (Zajonc, 1980), this process starts with a reappraisal of the situation in emotional terms (Lazarus et al., 1982). Our experience or emotional awareness stems from this second analysis, elaborated by the steps that follow. Like any other problem-solving task, we then have to set our goals, generate strategic options to deal with the problem and evaluate these in terms of our goals and the situational constraints (Garber et al., 1991).

These mental activities may well change our emotional state. If we discover, for instance, that there is no acceptable way to deal with a situation that initially aroused our anger, that anger may easily turn into something like frustration or sadness. Once we have gained insight into how cognition and emotion interact, we may start to use this knowledge more strategically in order actively to change an emotional state. For example, we may search for information that tells us whether or not our adversary has hurt us on purpose. This cognitive analysis does not change the outcome as such, but it does influence the emotional impact of the situation. In the case of a negative outcome caused by another person, we may actively look for mitigating circumstances in order to improve our angry mood (H. Stegge, unpublished dissertation).

Knowing that children's cognitive abilities become increasingly powerful, we may describe emotional development as follows. Initially, the young child's emotional behaviour is determined by relatively rigid, wired-in programs. The child has no cognitive access to these programs and no knowledge of them. Emotional behaviour is entirely determined by environmental input. We will describe how, after this initial biological stage, the child gradually gains an insight into the determinants of emotional behaviour. As a result, the child's emotional behaviour will no longer be completely 'data-driven'. That is, behaviour will no longer be based entirely on elements directly derived from the actual situation, but on the child's own subjective cognitive representation of events within the context of his or her theory of emotion. In the course of development, we can observe an accumulating body of emotional knowledge, and we will see that situational characteristics will increasingly trigger these knowledge structures. Or, stated otherwise: data-driven emotional behaviour will gradually be replaced by knowledge-driven behaviour.

In principle, all knowledge about emotion is derived from three sources. Harris & Olthof (1982) named them the solipsistic, the behaviouristic and the sociocentric source. The first source refers to introspection: people may gain knowledge by trying to retrace their own private processes. The behaviouristic source concerns the observable elements of human functioning. Emotional knowledge can also be obtained by observing one's own and other people's reactions to different situations. Finally, the sociocentric source depicts people as the passive recipients of information provided by the (verbal) community. It is impossible to say which of these sources is the most important one, and in the remainder of the chapter we will see that it is often a combination of information from different sources that helps build a new form of understanding. Children are known to be active information processors, but knowledgable others can be very helpful, not only by directing the child's attention to relevant internal and external phenomena, but also by providing whole chunks of information that may help the child to link the two environments together.

There is a large set of cognitive abilities involved in the understanding and regulation of emotions, known collectively as emotional intelligence: 'the ability to perceive emotions, to access and generate emotions so as to assist thought, to understand emotions and emotional knowledge, and to reflectively regulate emotions so as to promote emotional and intellectual growth' (Mayer & Salovey, 1997). This chapter aims to address some of the major developments in this domain.

First, we will discuss early concept formation, including children's understanding of the link between situation and emotion. We will then discuss the development of emotional knowledge within the more general context of the development of a theory of mind. We will show how children's increasing abilities to analyse cognitively emotional situations results in the understanding of more complex emotions such as guilt, shame and pride. We will turn to the important issue of emotion regulation, as most of the emotional knowledge that children acquire during the course of development ultimately serves to adapt their emotional reactions adequately in the service of personal or social goals. While we will mainly discuss the influence of cognition on the emotion process in the earlier sections, we will also address the reciprocal relation between cognition and emotion. We will do so by discussing examples of a so-called emotional bias, when cognition and emotion are tightly knit together in a rigid affective organization. We will illustrate the relevance of the abilities discussed by giving examples of a problematic development. In our concluding remarks we suggest that these problems may be countered by early interventions along the lines of cognitive behaviour therapy.

Early emotion concepts

Children start to use emotion terms quite early – around the beginning of their second year (Bretherton et al., 1986; Smiley & Huttenlocher, 1989). Words like 'laugh' and 'cry' are understood earlier than words like 'happy' and 'sad' (Honkavaara, 1961), indicating that the overt elements of the emotional process are easier to grasp than the internal states. By 2–3 years of age, children realize that there can be a variety of personal reasons for an emotional reaction and they start asking spontaneously for these reasons (Cairns & Hsu, 1977; Bretherton & Beeghly, 1982). Connections between emotional states and situational determinants are sorted out. Around the age of 4, there is a fair consensus among children about the kinds of situations that will provoke the basic emotions of happiness, fear, sadness and anger (Barden et al., 1980).

Knowledge of the meaning of other emotions will develop in a fairly stable order that seems to be determined by a number of factors. The early understanding of basic emotions is probably related to the fact that these emotions are characterized by a unique facial expression that makes them easy to identify (Reichenbach & Masters, 1983). The order of acquisition is also determined by the simple opportunity to learn. For example, disgust is often considered one of the basic emotions (Ekman & Friesen, 1974) but, unlike the labels of the other basic emotions, the word is not frequently used in children's immediate environment. Therefore, its understanding comes relatively late. On the other hand, the concept of shyness is understood not much later than happiness, fear, sadness and anger (Harris et al., 1987). Shyness is not accompanied by a unique expression (at least, not a unique facial expression), but the concept is used quite frequently in the presence of children. The third and probably most influential factor that determines the order of acquisition is the complexity of the emotions involved (Harris et al., 1987). For example, understanding of social emotions like shame, guilt or pride requires an appreciation of social standards or rules, the ability to recognize violations of those standards or rules, and the ability to anticipate other people's reactions to such violations. It is often argued that, even at the age of 10, we cannot be sure that children have acquired an adult concept of these emotions (Colby et al., 1983).

Children's knowledge of the antecedents of different emotions is an important step in their learning process. At first, they seem to assume a one-to-one correspondence between situation and emotion. This makes it hard for them to understand the complexity of daily emotional life, in which situations often have a multiple emotional impact. As we will see shortly, the explicit recognition of emotional ambivalence seems to pose difficulties for young children.

At a behavioural level, ambivalence can be observed in early childhood (Meerum Terwogt, 1987). Older siblings often vacillate between tenderness and hostility in their approach to a younger sibling (Dunn, 1984). Yet, if we ask them to tell us how they feel in these situations, they are likely to acknowledge only one of these feelings (Harter, 1983; Harter & Buddin, 1987). Around the age of 6, children acknowledge that one can experience two different emotions immediately after one another, although they still find it hard to accept that those emotions can be completely opposite ones, like happiness and sadness (Olthof et al., 1987). It is only much later, at about the age of 10, that children accept the co-occurrence of conflicting emotions (Meerum Terwogt et al., 1986a; Harter & Buddin, 1987).

What makes it so difficult to acknowledge the existence of mixed feelings? One explanation might be that young children still find it difficult to change perspectives in one and the same situation: 'I'm sad because Blacky is ill, but happy since he seems to be recovering quite well'. Harris (1989) suggests that they may have adopted the logical notion that happy and sad are mutually exclusive opposites, which may interfere with a conscious awareness of their own ambivalent feelings. Their cognitive appraisal of the situation might stop at the first emotional source detected. The link between emotion and situation is then stored accordingly. It is only when both conflicting elements are very salient that the child may become aware of the presence of mixed feelings. Such experiences will gradually weaken the initial model of a one-to-one relationship between situations and emotions and replace it with a more complex one.

Children's understanding of mixed emotions seems to be an important step in the development of emotional competence. This becomes especially clear when we look at children with emotional problems. One of the basic difficulties of emotionally disturbed children seems to be an inability to acknowledge conflicting feelings, which may have an impact on different domains of their lives (Meerum Terwogt, 1990). For example, when we ask them for self-evaluative statements, they are inclined to look at themselves as 'all smart' or 'all dumb', respectively, 'all good' or 'all bad'. In this case, the inability to combine positive and negative elements makes it hard for them to acquire a realistic self-image (Harter, 1977).

The development of a theory of emotion

We have seen how theoretical notions may delay and boost development. Now we will address the question of how children acquire a more general framework theory, known as the theory of mind (Wellman, 1990; Mitchell, 1996), and the place of the emotion concept within this theory.

Although an understanding of the common causal relations between particular situations and particular emotions is very important, it is not sufficient for a full understanding of emotion. Children must also be able to go beyond the objective characteristics of a situation. In fact, the emotional impact of an event is determined by a person's subjective appraisal of the situation, an appraisal which is (de)formed by personal beliefs, expectations and desires (Harris, 1989). A gift will not elicit happiness if the recipient does not want it or suspects the motive of the donor.

Even very young children acknowledge the fact that other people may have desires or beliefs which are different from their own. This can easily be observed in pretend play (Piaget, 1962; Leslie, 1987). In most children, the first signs of pretend play emerge somewhere in their second year of life. A young girl acts as if her doll is a genuine person (Wolf et al., 1984). At first, the young 'mother' treats her 'child' as a passive recipient of her own actions, but later on she makes the doll talk and act independently and eventually supplies it with desires, sensations and emotions. Around $3\frac{1}{2}$–4 years of age, we can even hear the child use a different voice if she talks for the doll.

In the more advanced forms of pretend play, the child clearly acknowledges that her make-believe companion is not simply an extension of herself. The other person has distinct qualities, and can do things that the child pretends not to know about. When playing hide-and-seek, we can see how the child first puts her doll in the cupboard, while shouting directly afterwards: 'Where are you?' Similarly, the preferences and feelings of the doll may be different from those of her creator. She likes spinach, while the child herself does not.

Three-year-olds still show a limited appreciation of the subjective character of desires; they are often influenced by an egocentric perspective. They understand that someone can hold a preference that is slightly different from their own (for instance, 'going to the zoo' versus 'going to the park') as long as both activities are clearly agreeable from their perspective (Wellman, 1990). However, they find it hard to accept that other people may hold a less obvious desire (Moore et al., 1995; Rieffe et al., 2000), for example, preferring potatoes over chocolate.

The appreciation of deviant beliefs is even more difficult. This is often demonstrated by the so-called false belief paradigm (Wimmer & Perner, 1983). In the original set-up, the children see the doll Maxi put away his bar of chocolate in the cupboard. After Maxi has left the room, his mother comes in and moves the chocolate. When he returns to the scene, the participants are asked where Maxi will look for his chocolate. It is not until the age of 4 that children acknowledge that Maxi's actions are governed by a false belief. Around that time, children make the conceptual shift from a simple desire theory, in which actions are directly motivated by desires, to the adult-like belief desire theory which states that someone's actions have to be understood in terms of the combined impact of beliefs and desires (Wellman, 1990).

Belief desire reasoning is not only of vital importance for understanding other people's overt behaviour, it also allows us to make assumptions about their internal state – their emotions. Even very young children appreciate that there is a fundamental connection between desires and emotions: William feels happy when he gets the ice cream he wants and he starts crying when his mother denies him one. Whether someone experiences a positive or a negative emotion depends on the fulfilment of desires. Or, to be more accurate, on your beliefs about the fulfilment of desires: you are happy as long as you believe that your desires will be met. In order to study children's understanding of the connection between beliefs and emotions, Harris et al. (1989) used a puppet play, quite similar to the original Wimmer & Perner false belief experiment. They presented children with a situation in which Elly the elephant is going for a walk. She leaves her beloved can of Coke on the kitchen table for her return. Meanwhile, the children observe how Mickey the monkey tricks his elephant friend: he secretly replaces the Coke with milk. Elly returns and the children are asked two questions: How would she feel now? (that is, just before she discovers the deceit) and How would she feel after having taken a sip from the can? (that is, when she has discovered the true state of affairs). It was shown that even 3-year-old children understand that Elly will be disappointed at the moment she discovers the trick. But it is not before the age of 5 that most children predict that, until that discovery is made, Elly will still be happy in the anticipation of her favourite drink.

Children's newly acquired theory of mind clearly slowly starts to affect their general conception of emotion. When asked, for instance, 'How do you know that you are happy?' 6-year-olds typically answer with statements like 'Because it's my birthday' or 'Because I'm laughing'; they refer to the observable antecedents and consequences of the emotional state. Only one out of 10 children at this age gives an answer that refers to the inner state. By the age of 10, the mental component has a much more central position in the child's concept of emotion. Although observable components are still mentioned, about 90% of 10-year-olds typically answer the question by saying something like: 'I'm happy since I feel happy (inside)', thereby showing that they consider the internal mental state an important identifying element (Harris et al., 1981). By then, children have learned that not everybody appreciates a situation in the same way and that emotional expressions can be deceptive (Saarni, 1997). Therefore, what really counts in the identification of emotions is the subjective feeling state. The 6-year-old behaviourists have changed into 10-year-old mentalists (Harris & Olthof, 1982).

Social emotions: norms and values

We have seen how young children begin to understand simple emotions like anger, happiness or sadness in terms of private mental states. We will now extend this analysis to some of the more complex emotions: guilt, shame and pride. Although the terms 'guilt' and 'shame' are often used interchangeably, it is now generally acknowledged that the two terms refer to phenomenologically different experiences (Tangney, 1990; Ferguson & Stegge, 1995, 1998). Guilt is a self-critical reaction to a specific act of wrong-doing that is perceived to be immoral in nature. The person feels responsible for the resulting consequences, ruminates about what he or she has done, wants to confess and to make reparation. Shame, in contrast, involves a negative evaluation of the entire self which conveys a sense of fundamental defectiveness. The person feels weak and isolated. Since there is a fear of being ridiculed and rejected, the person who feels ashamed reveals a strong desire to hide from other people.

Guilt, shame and pride are so-called social emotions, due to the fact that social norms and values play a critical role in their experience. Young children do not yet acknowledge the importance of this kind of social information. They simply pursue their goals and analyse a situation in terms of the outcome (Thompson, 1989). Getting what you want leads to happiness, while not getting it results in feelings of sadness or frustration. A very young boy who completes a jigsaw puzzle for the 20th time is as happy as he was after completing it for the first time. Being successful is all that counts. But soon, his appreciation that some tasks are easy and some tasks are difficult (in relation to his own norms and skills) will start to make a difference. When accomplishing something for the first time he will experience pride, whereas this emotion will no longer be felt if the job is considered easy on later occasions.

In the course of development, children come to realize that, whereas some behaviours are approved of by other people, others are reacted to with disapproval. Gaining other people's approval now becomes an important goal that guides children's behaviour. Normative standards for behaviour become more and more important. And as children start causally to analyse their own behaviour and the behaviour of others in greater depth, personal responsibility becomes an important determinant of affective experience. In the achievement domain, children realize, for example, that there is a difference between failure that is due to controllable causes (such as the amount of effort put in), and failure caused by uncontrollable factors (such as lack of ability). The former attribution results in feelings of guilt, while the latter causes feelings of shame (Stipek & DeCotis, 1988). Likewise, in the moral domain, blaming others for harm becomes increasingly dependent on the other's intentions and the avoidability of the event. Intentional and avoidable harm results in more anger and aggression towards the perpetrator than accidental and unavoidable harm (Ferguson & Rule, 1983; Olthof et al., 1989).

Between the age of 5 and 10, the relevance of personal responsibility and normative standards is increasingly acknowledged and taken into account (Graham et al., 1984; Ferguson et al., 1991). Again, we observe a developmental time lag between children's actual knowledge in a certain domain and their judgement of the relevance of this knowledge on an emotional and a behavioural level. Although 5- and 6-year-old children know the difference between accidental success and success that is the result of hard work, they do not include that information in their emotional evaluation of the situation (Graham, 1988). The same goes for knowledge in the moral domain. Young children do have a fair sense of right and wrong. Even 3-year-olds provide differentiated judgements about 'very bad things' like 'stealing' and 'killing', and things that are only 'a little bad', like 'not saying your prayers before you go to sleep' and 'not tidying your room in time' (Smetana, 1981). However, this knowledge does not have an impact on their course of action (Harris, 1989).

Why is it that young children do not acknowledge the relevance of this information? First, they may lack the cognitive capacities that are needed to combine effectively all the different perspectives in their emotional evaluation. Second, the fact that young children know the difference between good and bad does not tell us anything about the question of whether or not they have internalized the rules they express. Clearly, there is a big difference between knowing the rule, and really subscribing to it and behaving accordingly. For instance, we all know that we have to pay taxes. However, many of us see no harm in trying to dodge them if we can. We know the rule, but it is not an effective guideline for behaviour. No feelings of guilt are elicited to stop us from breaking the rule. Children initially need an actual audience to make them realize that norms and values are important. The child with the jigsaw puzzle, in our earlier example, can probably count on his mother's approval when he finishes the puzzle for the first few times. Later on, his accomplishment gets less and less admiration. If the child were a bit older, the mother would probably even openly react in an annoyed way if the child tried to attract her attention for the 20th time. Reissland (1988) argues that the onset of pride is marked by the fact that it is exactly this approval rather than the experience of success itself that elicits the pleasure in the child. In fact, this is what Cooley refers to as the 'looking glass self' (Cooley, 1902; see also Harris, 1989). At first, feeling pride or shame is dependent on the close proximity of another person and his or her approval or disapproval. Later on, the child will experience these emotions with greater autonomy. The internalization of norms and values is completed and the proximity of the audience is no longer critical. Children are able to judge their own actions with respect to their own normative standards of conduct. This is also reflected in the child's language. Whereas young children refer to other people when talking about pride and shame, 8-year-olds speak about feeling proud or ashamed of themselves (Harter & Whitesell, 1989).

Social emotions become mechanisms of spontaneous self-control provided that several prerequisites are fulfilled, including an awareness of standards of conduct, a felt obligation to regulate behaviour with respect to these standards and an ability to recognize discrepancies between one's own behaviour and these internalized values (Ausubel, 1955). As such, these emotions serve an important function as they stimulate children to behave in accordance with social norms and values. However, development can also take a more maladaptive course. As they grow older, children become more vulnerable to the experience of discrepancies, since they are increasingly able to detect them. Moreover, these experienced discrepancies have longer-lasting implications for the child's self-esteem and his or her future expectations and motivations, since children begin to describe themselves as well as other people's ideas about them in more stable terms (Ruble & Rholes, 1981; Moretti & Higgins, 1990). They start to do so in behavioural terms (4–6 years), but later on (9–11 years) they are inclined to use more generalized trait-like descriptions. As a consequence, it becomes more and more difficult for the child to reduce a certain discrepancy, since not only must the behaviour itself be changed, but also certain features of the self. Hence, children may be increasingly vulnerable to the feelings of helplessness and hopelessness that are so characteristic of depression (Moretti & Higgins, 1990).

Regulation of emotions

In the previous sections, we have discussed the development of children's understanding of different components of the emotion process. It was shown that, with increasing age, children come to understand the broad variety of emotions (including the more complex ones) that people have available to help them function adequately in a complex world. Moreover, we have shown how children gain insight into the basic components of human behaviour (they develop a 'theory of mind') and start to apply this knowledge to the domain of emotions. An increasing understanding of the subjective nature of emotions helps children to understand better not only their own emotional reactions, but also those of others.

As has already been argued, emotionally competent or intelligent behaviour calls for emotion regulation: the adjustment of basic emotion programs in the service of personal or social goals (Meerum Terwogt & Olthof, 1989). We will now discuss the development of emotion regulation in more detail, with a focus on the central role that emotional understanding plays in this process.

A lot of emotional behaviour does not meet social standards. Laughing at a funeral and hitting your boss when you are angry are just a few of the endless list of emotional reactions that will elicit severely negative reactions from the environment. From a social point of view, it is often merely the expressive component that needs adaptation. However, we need to realize that successful masking (of improper emotions) or simulation (of proper ones) may prevent stressful situations from getting worse, but does not necessarily serve more personal goals which are aimed at altering the problematic situation or the inner feeling state. Therefore, it is important to make a distinction between the regulation of emotional expressions and the regulation of subjective feelings in order to improve one's mood.

The deliberate regulation of emotional expressions can be observed quite early in life (Meerum Terwogt et al., 1986b). Girls aged 3–4 years, for instance, tended to produce a kind of half-smile upon receiving a disappointing gift from the experimenter: an expression that was quite different from the frank disappointment they showed when the experimenter was not around (Cole, 1986). Probably, these early accomplishments have relatively little to do with social and emotional competence. Harris (1989) suggests that these behaviours could very well be the result of indoctrination practices. Over and over again, we instruct our children to smile and to say 'thank you' in reaction to a present. Children who are able to meet these instructions have proved not much more than that they have learned a simple rule of politeness. We can hardly expect children as young as 3 to be aware of the fact that they are showing an emotion that does not correspond to what they feel, let alone appreciate the potentially misleading impact of this action on other people. In fact, all participants in Cole's experiment, whether they were able to conceal their disappointment or not, claimed that the experimenter would know how they really felt.

In contrast, 6-year-olds know that facial expressions can be misleading. They appreciate the difference between real and apparent emotions (Saarni, 1979, 1984; Gross & Harris, 1988); the difference between the private world of experience known only to the self, and the public world, in which behaviours and facial expressions are visible to others. Once the child acknowledges the possible advantages of hiding an emotion, we might expect deliberate attempts to disguise vulnerability by misleading actions. P. L. Harris & G. R. Guz (unpublished paper) illustrated this in a nice field study. They interviewed a group of 8-year-old boys soon after their arrival at preparatory boarding school, which was a stressful situation for most of them. At the same time, the children knew that showing fear and worry was not appropriate and would have social repercussions. Deceptive behaviour was the only way out: 'Well, you'd have to act cheerfully (irrespective of how you feel) and try and make friends with everybody'.

Again, the importance of the regulation of emotional expressions for our social life becomes very clear when we look more closely at a group of emotionally disturbed children. These children also appreciate that you can hide your feelings from others, i.e. manipulate the expression (Meerum Terwogt et al., 1990). However, their strategic use of this knowledge shows an important limitation. Between 7 and 11 years of age, normal children use the option of hiding or pretending emotions for two reasons: as a means of protecting the self and out of consideration for others ('I didn't want my sister to know that I felt sad on her birthday'). Emotionally disturbed children from the same age group tended to adopt display rules just for selfish reasons (Taylor & Harris, 1984; S. Adlam-Hill & P. L. Harris, unpublished paper). This can be interpreted in terms of a general developmental delay. The notion of deception to protect the feelings of others takes an extra cognitive step: a change of perspective. Alternatively, one can argue that emotionally disturbed children have grown up in a family environment that gave them little opportunity to learn the rules governing the emotional dialogue that normally takes place between people (Jones et al., 1998). How can you learn the subtle rules of mutual influence when the reactions of your care-takers bear almost no relation to your own behaviour, as seems to be the case with both neglecting and overprotective parents? Whatever the origins of these children's problems, the fact that they do not seem to consider others' feelings when showing their own emotional reactions will most likely harm the quality of their social interactions.

As has already been argued, children who limit their regulation efforts to the display of emotions may still have to endure their private feeling state. Mood improvement often calls for a different course of action. Actually, there are two ways of diminishing the emotional impact of stressful situations: problem-focused and emotion-focused strategies (Lazarus & Folkman, 1984). Problem-focused coping aims at removing or diminishing the problems presented by the actual situation, whereas emotion-focused strategies seek to improve the resulting emotional state. As the use of problem-focused coping changes the emotional state as well, albeit indirectly, both types of strategies can be seen as equally effective from an emotion perspective. Effectively, the same bipartition is made by Rothbaum et al. (1982), who prefer to talk about primary versus secondary coping. These labels follow from the assumption that people always attempt first to change the situation to their advantage and consider alternative strategies only after these primary attempts seem to be blocked. Secondary (or emotion-focused) strategies are particularly useful in situations that are beyond a person's control. If we are, for instance, confronted with the death of a close friend, we can only learn to live with it, or, as Rothbaum et al. (1982) phrase it, try 'to maximize our goodness of fit with the conditions as they are'. Secondary control options are also effective in situations in which primary solutions are expected to have social repercussions. While it may be unwise to leave a boring meeting, nothing prevents us from shortening the time by thinking of more interesting things.

Generally, it can be argued that most secondary or emotion-focused strategies appear later in life. Whereas 6-year-old children are able to produce a wide variety of primary strategies when asked how to deal with negative emotions, they rarely claim to use secondary strategies. Reactions like avoidance, direct behavioural intervention and asking the help of powerful others are considered earlier in life than mental distraction or a cognitive reappraisal of the situation (Band & Weisz, 1988; Altshuler & Ruble, 1989). Earlier on (Meerum Terwogt & Stegge, 1995), we showed that this developmental sequence can at least partly be explained by the child's growing understanding of emotion as a mental phenomenon. Problem-focused strategies acquire some kind of behavioural action. If your little brother has broken one of your toys, there are a number of actions that may help. You can try to mend it yourself. You can ask the help of others to repair it. Or you can go to the shop and buy a new one. Each of these actions may help you to feel better. But what if the toy is beyond repair and you have no money? In this case, you cannot change the outcome and you have to look for other options. An important category of alternative strategies shows up when children start to appreciate that people do not react to the situation as such, but to their subjective representation of the situation – that is, when children have acquired a basic 'theory of mind' – they come to understand that the emotional impact of a situation depends on how you look at it. Mood improvement can thus also be accomplished by mental manipulation. You will be less angry once you are able to convince yourself that your little brother did not act on purpose (changing beliefs), and less sad when you remind yourself that it was not you favourite toy anyway (changing desires). Once children are aware of these mental phenomena, they may start to look for an acceptable reappraisal that enables them to adapt to the situation as it is (H. Stegge & M. Meerum Terwogt, unpublished paper).

The use of mental strategies is stimulated by socialization. Just like older children learn that they are no longer allowed to display their emotions in any situation without repercussions, they also discover that at their age some of the behavioural patterns they used earlier in life are no longer acceptable. Whereas a younger child may be allowed to run away from a distressing situation, older children are expected to use alternative ways to deal with their emotions. On the one hand, this may result in the use of more adaptive problem-focused behaviours – which explains why the use of problem-focused approaches stays relatively constant throughout childhood (Compas et al., 1988) – while on the other hand, it may stimulate the use of mental strategies. No one can control your thoughts, so you are always free to use this type of strategy!

Emotionally biased thinking

So far, we have discussed how cognition may modify the emotion process. However, the relation between cognition and emotion goes both ways: emotions also influence cognitions. Research with both adults and children has shown, for example, that happy people perceive and evaluate ambiguous situations differently from sad people (Stegge, 1995; Stegge et al., 1995). Cole et al. (1994) have aptly expressed this reciprocal relation between cognition and emotion by referring to emotions as both regulated and regulatory phenomena.

Previously, we have seen some examples of a problematic emotional development. We will now discuss more generally the issue of maladaptiveness, using the concept of emotion dispositions of emotional biases introduced by Magai & McFadden (1995; see also Malatesta & Wilson, 1988). From this perspective, pathological functioning can be described as a situation in which affect and the associated cognitions and behaviours are tightly knit together and consolidated into an emotional bias. In the clinical literature, ample evidence can be found for the existence of systematic affective biases. Here, we will discuss some of the more obvious examples (Stegge, 1996; Stegge et al., 1998).

Dodge and his colleagues (Quiggle et al., 1992; Crick & Dodge, 1994) have extensively documented a pattern of emotions, cognitions and behaviours in agressive children that can be interpreted in terms of an anger bias: anger is reported in a wider range of situations, situations are more frequently perceived as harmful for the self and other people are relatively often seen as enemies with bad intentions. On a behavioural level, these children also act in accordance with their angry feelings: they tend to generate aggressive 'solutions' to problem situations and often opt for one.

Similarly, anxious children seem to organize their experiences in terms of fear. They are inclined to perceive ambiguous situations as threatening or dangerous, and do not engage in a more detailed analysis of the situation in order to test the reality of their initial perception (Chorpita et al., 1996). Instead, they try to reduce their anxiety immediately by seeking avoidance or distraction (Daleiden & Vasey, 1997).

In depression, sadness can be seen as the emotion that shapes experiences. The cognitions of depressed children are strongly dominated by the themes of personal loss or failure so characteristic of this emotion. Depressed children seem to intensify further their negative cognitions by a ruminative cognitive process in which they tend to attribute failure or loss experiences to their own inadeqaucy or inability, which finally results in a very low self-esteem (Harter, 1990). In this respect, Hammen (1990) talks about a cognitive triad: low self-esteem complemented by feelings of helplessness and hopelessness. As these biased cognitions promote total passivity, it is not very surprising that research has shown that depressed children deal with problematic situations mainly by withdrawal and, when possible, avoidance (Garber et al., 1991; Quiggle et al., 1992; see Chapter 3 for a full discussion of the negative cognitive biases associated with the onset of depressive states).

The maladaptive constellations of feelings, cognitions and behaviours of psychiatrically disturbed children are generally more complex than the ones we have just described. Anxiety and depression are often comorbid (Crowley & Emerson, 1996), just as anxiety and anger are (Wenar, 1994). Moreover, the content of these abnormal states may be complicated by the influence of guilt and shame dispositions. These latter emotions are frequently underdeveloped in behaviourally disturbed children, whereas anxious and depressed children seem to suffer from a surfeit of guilt and shame (Ferguson & Stegge, 1995, 1998).

Naturally, the biasing influence of dominant emotions is not restricted to the clinical domain. Some children are easily frightened, whereas others are known to be rebellious or stubborn. However, it is only in extreme cases that these biases prevent children from adaptive behaviour (Magai & McFadden, 1995). Problems may arise when children either gradually lose the awareness of an emotion that is always present and neglect its implications, or simply feel unable to change it. In the former case, they will no longer consider the need to correct for an emotional bias (I evaluated him badly only because I was so angry; he's probably nicer than I thought). In the latter case, they only have the option of giving in to the emotional impulse (I was so angry, I simply had to hit him).

Concluding remarks

In this chapter, we have discussed how children come to understand the basic connections between emotions and their causes and consequences. We have shown the importance of the skills that need to be acquired to become an emotionally competent or intelligent person. There are several problems that may hamper this learning process. Children may be reared in an environment that provides emotional information that is more confusing than helpful. Moreover, they may have learned to ignore emotional signals. 'Wrong' information, as well as not heeding one's emotions at the proper moment, can result in distorted ideas about emotions. Children may have failed to learn some of the important connections, or may not have learned how to use this information in order to exercise emotional control. A proper insight may also have been hampered by imbalance in the emotional system. In this case, children's experiences around one or a few dominant emotions tend to consolidate into an emotional bias. Here, it is not so much the failure of making certain connections but the prevalence of systematically biased connections that causes the problem. Whatever the problem, it is important to emphasize the dynamic principles behind the emotion process in order to put development on the right track again: control can only be obtained if children realize that emotions are subjective experiences (that can be influenced by cognition). This is exactly the focus of cognitive behavioural therapy, which aims to re-establish control by providing people with an insight into the basic relations between cognition, emotion and behaviour.

We have pointed out that children acquire an understanding of the basic principles of human emotional behaviour at a rather young age. The development of the core elements of a theory of mind takes place somewhere between the age of 3 and 6. And although children still have a lot to learn about emotions after the age of 6, their acknowledgement of the fundamental principles of a theory of mind allows for the possibility of some form of cognitive behavioural therapy even at this young age. Of course, when attempting such an approach we have to keep in mind the child's limitations. Research on the development of emotional understanding (as discussed in this chapter) may provide a useful starting point for devising specific treatment programmes adapted to the child's age.

REFERENCES

Altshuler, J. L. & Ruble, D. N. (1989). Developmental changes in children's awareness of strategies for coping with uncontrollable stress. *Child Development*, **60**, 1337–49.

Arnold, M. B. (1960). *Emotion and Personality*, vol. 1. New York: Columbia University Press.

Ausubel, D. P. (1955). Relationships between shame and guilt in the socialization process. *Psychological Review*, **62**, 378–90.

Band, E. B. & Weisz, J. R. (1988). How to feel better when it feels bad: children's perspectives on coping with everyday stress. *Developmental Psychology*, **24**, 247–53.

Barden, R. C., Zelko, F. A., Duncan, S. W. & Masters, J. C. (1980). Children's consensual knowledge about the experiential determinants of emotion. *Journal of Personality and Social Psychology*, **39**, 368–76.

Bretherton, I. & Beeghly, M. (1982). Talking about internal states of mind: the acquisition of an explicit theory of mind. *Developmental Psychology*, **18**, 906–21.

Bretherton, I., Fritz, J., Zahn-Waxler, C. & Ridgeway, D. (1986). Learning to talk about emotions: a functionalist perspective. *Child Development*, **57**, 529–48.

Cairns, H. & Hsu, J. (1977). Who, why, when, and how: a developmental study. *Journal of Child Language*, **5**, 477–88.

Chorpita, B. F., Albano, A. M. & Barlow, D. H. (1996). Cognitive processing in children: relationship to anxiety and family influences. *Journal of Clinical Child Psychology*, **25**, 170–6.

Colby, A., Kohlberg, L., Gibbs, J. & Lieberman, M. (1983). *A Longitudinal Study of Moral Judgement. Monographs of the Society for Research in Child Development*, vol. 200. Chicago, IL: University of Chicago Press.

Cole, P. M. (1986). Children's spontaneous control of facial expression. *Child Development*, **57**, 1309–21.

Cole, P. M., Michel, M. K. & O'Donnell Teti, L. (1994). The development of emotion regulation and dysregulation: a clinical perspective. In *The Development of Emotion Regulation*, vol. 9, ed. N. A. Fox. *Monographs of the Society of Research in Child Development*. Chicago, IL: University of Chicago Press.

Compas, B. E., Malcarne, V. L. & Fondacaro, K. M. (1988). Coping with stressful events in older children and young adolescents. *Journal of Consulting and Clinical Psychology*, **56**, 405–11.

Cooley, C. H. (1902). Human nature and the social order. New York: Charles Scribner's Sons.

Crick, N. R. & Dodge, K. A. (1994). A review and reformulation of social information-processing mechanisms in children's social adjustment. *Psychological Bulletin*, **115**, 74–101.

Crowley, S. L. & Emerson, E. N. (1996). Discriminant validity of self-reported anxiety and depression in children: negative affectivity or independent constructs? *Journal of Clinical Child Psychology*, **25**, 139–46.

Daleiden E. L. & Vasey, M. W. (1997). An information-processing perspective on childhood anxiety. *Clinical Psychology Review*, **17**, 407–29.

Dunn, J. (1984). *Sisters and Brothers*. London: Fontana.

Ekman, P. & Friesen, W. V. (1974). Detecting deception from body and face. *Journal of Personality and Social Psychology*, **29**, 288–98.

Ferguson, T. J. & Rule, B. G. (1983). An attributional perspective on anger and aggression. In *Aggression: Theoretical and Empirical Reviews*, vol. I, ed. R. G. Green & E. I. Donnerstein. New York: Academic Press.

Ferguson, T. J. & Stegge, H. (1995). Emotional states and traits in children: the case of guilt and shame. In *Self-conscious Emotions*, ed. J. P. Tangney & K. W. Fischer, pp. 174–97. New York: Guilford Press.

Ferguson, T. J. & Stegge, H. (1998). Assessing guilt in children: a rose by any other name still has thorns. In *Guilt and Children*, ed. J. A. Bybee, pp. 19–74. New York: Academic Press.

Ferguson, T. J., Stegge, H. & Damhuis, I. (1991). Children's understanding of guilt and shame. *Child Development*, **62**, 827–39.

Frijda, N. H. (1986). *The Emotions*. Cambridge: Cambridge University Press.

Garber, J., Braafladt, N. & Zeman, J. (1991). The regulation of sad affect: an information processing perspective. In *The Development of Emotion Regulation and Dysregulation*, ed. J. Garber & K. A. Dodge, pp. 208–40. Cambridge: Cambridge University Press.

Graham, S. (1988). Children's developing understanding of the motivational role of affect: an attributional analysis. *Cognitive Development*, **3**, 71–88.

Graham, S., Doubleday, C. & Guarino, P. A. (1984). The development of relations between perceived controllability and the emotions of pity, anger, and guilt. *Child Development*, **55**, 561–5.

Gross, D. & Harris, P. L. (1988). Understanding false beliefs about emotions. *International Journal of Behavioural Development*, **11**, 475–88.

Hammen, C. (1990). Cognitive approaches to depression. In *Advances in Clinical Child Psychology*, vol. 13, ed. B. B. Lahey & A. E. Kazdin, pp. 139–73. New York: Plenum.

Harris, P. L. (1989). *Children and Emotion. The Development of Psychological Understanding*. Oxford: Blackwell.

Harris, P. L. & Olthof, T. (1982). The child's concept of emotion. In *Social Cognition; Studies of the Development of Understanding*, ed. G. Butterworth & P. Light, pp. 188–209. Brighton: Harvester Press.

Harris, P. L., Olthof, T. & Meerum Terwogt, M. (1981). Children's knowledge of emotion. *Journal of Child Psychology and Psychiatry*, **22**, 247–61.

Harris, P. L., Olthof, T., Meerum Terwogt, M. & Hardman, C. E. (1987). Children's knowledge of situations that provoke emotion. *International Journal of Behavioral Development*, **10**, 319–43.

Harris, P. L., Johnson, C. N., Hutton, D., Andrews, G. & Cooke, T. (1989). Young children's theory of mind and emotion. *Cognition and Emotion*, **3**, 379–400.

Harter, S. (1977). A cognitive-developmental approach to children's expression of conflicting feelings and a technique to facilitate such expression in play therapy. *Journal of Consulting and Clinical Psychology*, **45**, 417–32.

Harter, S. (1983). Children's understanding of multiple emotions: a cognitive-developmental approach. In *The Relationship between Social and Cognitive Development*, ed. W. F. Overton, pp. 147–94. Hillsdale, NJ: Erlbaum.

Harter, S. (1990). Causes, correlates, and the functional role of global self-worth: a life-span perspective. In *Competence Considered*, ed. R. J. Sternberg & J. Kolligan, pp. 67–97. New Haven: Yale University Press.

Harter, S., & Buddin, B. (1987). Children's understanding of the simultaneity of two emotions: a five-stage acquisition sequence. *Developmental Psychology*, **23**, 388–99.

Harter, S. & Whitesell, N. (1989). Developmental changes in children's emotion concepts. In *Children's Understanding of Emotions*, ed. C. Saarni & P. L. Harris, pp. 81–116. New York: Cambridge University Press.

Honkavaara, S. (1961). *The Psychology of Expression. British Journal of Psychology Monograph*

Supplements, vol. 32. London: British Journal of Psychology.

Jones, D. C., Abbey, B. B. & Cumberland, A. (1998). The development of display rule knowledge: linkages with family expressiveness and social competence. *Child Development*, **69**, 1209–22.

Lazarus, R. S. & Folkman, S. (1984). *Stress, Appraisal, and Coping*. New York: Springer.

Lazarus, R. S., Coyne, J. C. & Folkman, S. (1982). Cognition, emotion and motivation: the doctoring of Humpty-Dumpty. In *Psychological Stress and Psychopathology*, ed. R. W. Neufield, pp. 218–39. New York: McGraw-Hill.

Leslie, A. M. (1987). Pretence and representation: the origins of 'theory of mind'. *Psychological Review*, **94**, 412–26.

MacLean, P. D. (1993). Cerebral evolution of emotion. In *Handbook of Emotions*, ed. M. Lewis & J. M. Haviland, pp. 67–86. New York: Guilford Press.

Magai, C. & McFadden, S. H. (1995). *The Role of Emotions in Social and Personality Development*. New York: Plenum.

Malatesta, C. Z. & Wilson, A. (1988). Emotion–cognition interaction in personality development: a discrete emotions, functionalist analysis. *British Journal of Social Psychology*, **27**, 91–112.

Mayer, J. D. & Salovey, P. (1997). What is emotional intelligence? In *Emotional Development and Emotional Intelligence*, ed. P. Salovey & D. J. Sluyter, pp. 3–34. New York: Basic Books.

Meerum Terwogt, M. (1987). Children's behavioral reactions in situations with a dual emotional impact. *Psychological Reports*, **61**, 100–2.

Meerum Terwogt, M. (1990). Disordered children's acknowledgement of multiple emotions. *Journal of General Psychology*, **117**, 59–69.

Meerum Terwogt, M. & Olthof, T. (1989). Awareness and self-regulation of emotion in young children. In *Children's Understanding of Emotion*, pp. 209–37. New York: Cambridge University Press.

Meerum Terwogt, M. & Stegge, H. (1995). Children's understanding of the strategic control of negative emotions. In *Everyday Concepts of Emotion: an introduction to the psychology, anthropology and linguistics of emotion*, ed. J. A. Russell, J. Fernandez-Dols, A. S. R. Manstead & J. C. Wellenkamp, vol. 81, pp. 373–90. NATO ASI series. Dordrecht: Kluwer Academic.

Meerum Terwogt, M., Koops, W., Oosterhoff, T. & Olthof, T. (1986a). Development in processing of multiple emotional situations. *Journal of General Psychology*, **113**, 109–19.

Meerum Terwogt, M., Schene, J. & Harris, P. L. (1986b). Self-control of emotional reactions by young children. *Journal of Child Psychology and Psychiatry*, **27**, 357–66.

Meerum Terwogt, M., Schene, J. & Koops, W. (1990) Concepts of emotion in institutionalized children. *Journal of Child Psychology and Psychiatry*, **31**, 1131–43.

Mitchell, P. (1996). *Acquiring a Concept of Mind*: a review of psychological research and theory. Hove: Psychological Press.

Moore, C., Jarrold, C., Russell, J. & Lumb, A. (1995). Conflicting desire and the child's theory of mind. *Cognitive Development*, **10**, 467–82.

Moretti, M. M. & Higgins, E. T. (1990). The development of self-esteem vulnerabilities: social and cognitive factors in developmental psychopathology. In *Competence Considered*, ed. R. J. Sternberg & J. Kolligan, Jr., pp. 286–314. New Haven: Yale University Press.

Olthof, T., Meerum Terwogt, M., van Panthaleon van Eck, O. & Koops, W. (1987). Children's knowledge of the integration of successive emotions. *Perceptual and Motor Skills*, **65**, 407–14.

Olthof, T., Ferguson, T. J. & Luiten, A. (1989). Personal responsibility antecedents of anger and blame reactions in children. *Child Development*, **60**, 1328–66.

Piaget, J. (1962). *Play Dreams and Imitation*. New York: Norton.

Quiggle, N., Garber, J., Panak, W. & Dodge, K. A. (1992). Social-information processing in aggressive and depressed children. *Child Development*, **63**, 1305–20.

Reichenbach, L. & Masters, J. (1983). Children's use of expressive and contextual cues in judgments of emotion. *Child Development*, **54**, 993–1004.

Reissland, N. (1988). Neonatal imitation in the first hour of life: observations in rural Nepal. *Developmental Psychology*, **24**, 464–9.

Rieffe, C., Meerum Terwogt, M., Koops, W., Stegge, H. & Oomen, A. (2000). Preschoolers' appreciation of uncommon desires and subsequent emotions. *British Journal of Developmental Psychology* (in press).

Rothbaum, F., Weisz, J. R. & Snyder, S. S. (1982). Changing the world and changing the self: a two-process model of perceived control. *Journal of Personality and Social Psychology*, **42**, 5–37.

Ruble, D. & Rholes, W. (1981). The development of children's perceptions and attributions about their social world. In *New Directions in Attribution Research*, vol. 3, ed. J. Harvey, W. Ickes & R. Kidd, pp. 3–36. Hillsdale, NJ: Lawrence Erlbaum.

Saarni, C. (1979). Children's understanding of display rules for expressive behaviour. *Developmental Psychology*, **15**, 424–9.

Saarni, C. (1984). Observing children's use of display rules: age and sex differences. *Child Development*, **55**, 1504–13.

Saarni, C. (1997). Emotional competence and selfregulation in childhood. In *Emotional Development and Emotional Intelligence*, ed. P. Salovey & D. J. Sluyter, pp. 35–66. New York: Basic Books.

Schore, A. N. (1994). *Affect Regulation and the Origin of the Self: the neurobiology of emotional development*. Hillsdale, NJ: Erlbaum.

Smetana, J. G. (1981). Preschool children's conception of moral and social rules. *Child Development*, **52**, 1333–6.

Smiley, P. & Huttenlocher, J. (1989). Young children's acquisition of emotion concepts. In *Children's Understanding of Emotion*, ed. C. Saarni & P. L. Harris, pp. 27–49. New York: Cambridge University Press.

Stegge, H. (1996). De invloed van emoties op cognities en gedrag (Influences of emotions on cognitions and behaviour). In *Jaarboek Ontwikkelingspsychologie, Orthopedagogiek en Kinderpsychiatry 2* [*Annual Review of Developmental Psychology, Special Education and Child Psychiatry*] vol. 2, ed. J. D. Bosch et al., pp. 235–61. Houten: Bohn, Stafleu, Van Loghum.

Stegge, H., Meerum Terwogt, M. & Koops, W. (1995). Mood congruity in children: effects of age, imagery capability and demand characteristics. *International Journal of Behavioral Development*, **18**, 177–91.

Stegge, H., Meerum Terwogt, M. & Bijstra, J. (1998). Emoties als aangrijpingspunt voor de diagnostiek van psychische stoornissen (Emotions as a criterium for diagnosing developmental psychopathology). In *Van Lastig tot Misdadig (From Problematic to Criminal)*, ed. W. Koops & W. Slot, pp. 67–80. Houten: Bohn, Stafleu, Van Loghum.

Stipek, D.J. & DeCotis, K. M. (1988). Children's understanding of the implications of causal attributions for emotional experiences. *Child Development*, **59**, 1601–16.

Tangney, J. P. (1990). Assessing individual differences in proneness to shame and guilt: development of the self-conscious affect and attribution inventory. *Journal of Personality and Social Psychology*, **59**, 102–11.

Taylor, D. A. & Harris, P. L. (1984). Knowledge of strategies for the expression of emotion among normal and maladjusted boys: a research note. *Journal of Child Psychology and Psychiatry*, **24**, 223–9.

Tompson, R. A. (1989). Causal attribution and children's emotional understanding. In *Children's Understanding of Emotion*, ed. C. Saarni & P. L. Harris, pp. 117–50. New York: Cambridge University Press.

Tucker, D. M. (1992). Developing emotions and cortical networks. In *Minnesota Symposia on Child Psychology*, vol. 24, *Developmental Behavioral Neuroscience*, ed. M. R. Gunnar & C. A. Nelson, pp. 75–128. Hillsdale, NJ: Erlbaum.

Wellman, H. M. (1990). *The Child's Theory of Mind*. Cambridge, MA: MIT Press/Bradford.

Wenar, C. (1994). *Developmental Psychopathology: from infancy through adolescence*. New York: McGraw-Hill.

Wimmer, H. & Perner, J. (1983). Beliefs about beliefs: representations and constraining function of wrong beliefs in young children's understanding of deception. *Cognition*, **13**, 103–28.

Wolf, D. P., Rygh, J. & Altshuler, J. (1984). Agency and experience: actions and states in play narratives. In *Symbolic Play*, ed. I. Bretherton. Orlando, FL: Academic Press.

Zajonc, R. B. (1980). Feeling and thinking: preferences need no inferences. *American Psychologist*, **35**, 151–73.

3

Developmental precursors of depression: the child and the social environment

Elizabeth McCauley, Karen Pavlidis and Kim Kendall

Introduction

An episode of clinical depression during childhood or adolescence has a negative impact on social, academic and family functioning, as well as being associated with an increased risk for recurrence (McCauley & Myers, 1992) and impairment in social-emotional functioning that extends into adult life (Harrington et al., 1990). Efforts to identify effective prevention and treatment strategies for depression in children are ongoing (Myers & McCauley, 1997). Prevention and treatment approaches need to be informed by a developmentally sensitive understanding of the mechanisms that underlie the onset of depression in young people.

Understanding the underpinnings of clinical depression is a complex task, which must include consideration of a multitude of factors. Depression is not simply a disorder of mood regulation but involves alterations in physiological and cognitive functioning. Moreover, the study of depression requires careful attention to developmental issues, especially the challenges of adolescence. While the general incidence of psychopathology increases only moderately during the adolescent years, the frequency of depression increases significantly, particularly in females (Rutter et al., 1976; Lewinsohn et al., 1993; Hankin et al., 1998). Furthermore, recent research suggests a discontinuity between prepubertal and postpubertal depression. Depression which first presents during the prepubertal period appears to be more strongly linked to environmental factors while postpubertal depression is best explained by a model of interaction between genetic and environmental factors (Thapar & McGuffin, 1996). More importantly, prepubertal depression represents a strong, but nonspecific risk for adult adjustment problems whereas adolescent depression is strongly linked to recurrent depressive episodes during adult life (Harrington et al., 1996). The striking age and gender patterns in depression rates indicate that a developmental theoretical framework is needed to understand factors that may increase vulnerability to depression, with close attention to risk factors for adolescent depression.

This chapter will explore developmental variables, including family, individual and environmental, that might contribute to, or constitute, a predisposition to onset of depression during adolescence. Developmental processes that are central to the adolescent's formation of emotion regulation skills and sense of self will be reviewed with the goal of presenting a working model of how developmental factors could contribute to lowering the threshold for depression.

Family studies and intergenerational transmission

An increased prevalence of depressive disorder has been observed in relatives of depressed youth in comparison to relatives of youth with no psychiatric disturbance (Puig-Antich et al., 1989). Furthermore, offspring of depressed parents have a sixfold increase in risk for depression, with additional risk conferred if both parents are affected (Weissman et al., 1987; Mitchell et al., 1989; Downey & Coyne, 1990). Elevated rates of affective disorders in children of depressed parents have been documented in clinical (Downey & Coyne, 1990) and nonreferred samples (Beardslee et al., 1993). Although children of parents with affective disorders are at risk for a host of behavioural and emotional problems, childhood depression seems to be specifically associated with parental depression (Downey & Coyne, 1990; Beardslee & Wheelock, 1994).

A variety of mechanisms have been proposed to explain why offspring of depressed parents may be vulnerable to developing affective disturbances. Although genetic factors may increase risk for depression (Beardslee & Wheelock, 1994; see Chapter 7 of this volume for review), there is evidence that it is the interaction of genetic and environmental factors which is critical in the development of more severe forms of depression (Rende et al., 1993). For example, depressed parents' styles of interacting with their children may increase their child's vulnerability to developing depression. Depressed mothers are more likely to use withdrawal, conflict avoidance or overcontrolling strategies rather than negotiation to cope with child noncompliance compared to nondepressed mothers (Downey & Coyne, 1990; Gelfand & Teti, 1990; Beardslee & Wheelock, 1994; Cummings & Davies, 1994). Depressed mothers also tend to be more hostile and irritable compared to controls (Beardslee & Wheelock, 1994). Hammen (1992) has described a pattern of increased and persistent stressors in families with a depressed mother, given the impact depression has on the mother's ability to cope constructively, problem-solve and use social support. Thus, a depressed parent may serve as a model for depressive thinking and coping or may contribute to an overall home environment which increases risk for depression. There is also evidence that, in homes of adolescents with a history of depression, family environment is more impaired if the youth's mother also has a history of depression (Shiner & Marmorstein, 1998).

An insecure attachment history has also been proposed as a mechanism for the intergenerational transmission of depression. During the attachment process two extremely important aspects of development begin to take shape; the establishment of an internal working model of the world based on the mental representation of the attachment relationship (Cassidy, 1988; Kobak & Sceery, 1988) and the initial development of emotion regulation skills. The development of effective emotional regulation and coping skills, as well as a positive sense of the self, will depend on the care-giver's role in assisting the infant in controlling his or her emotional state through social interaction and routines established during the early years of life (Als, 1978; Kopp, 1982). Increased risk of both insecure attachment and disruptions in emotional regulation have been associated with maternal depression (Cummings & Davies, 1994). Dawson and colleagues have shown that disruptions in emotion regulation systems exist in insecurely attached infants of depressed mothers (Dawson et al., 1992).

Longitudinal studies are clearly needed to confirm a link between early attachment history and the development of depression. Kobak & Sceery (1988) looked at the correlates of type of attachment in first-year college students who completed the Adult Attachment Interview. They found that secure attachment was related to constructive affect regulation, low anxiety, low distress, low hostility, higher social competence and higher evidence of ongoing family support in late adolescence. Dismissive attachment was related to more loneliness, hostility with peers, peer ratings of low self-esteem and high anxiety, self-ratings of relationships with others as distant and less ongoing support from families. Preoccupied attachment led to peer ratings of high anxiety, self-ratings of low competence and high symptoms.

Family interaction with depressed youths

Attachment during the school age and adolescent years can be conceptualized using the central features of attachment during infancy through early childhood. As in earlier development, parents continue to provide a secure base from which the adolescent can explore (Bowlby, 1988; Allen et al., 1994). During adolescence, attachment themes generally take the form of parental support of the adolescent's autonomy and independence while maintaining a warm and supportive parent–adolescent relationship (Bowlby, 1980). Healthy adolescent development is thought to be facilitated by a family environment characterized by close family relationships that, at the same time, foster the development of autonomy.

Studies of depressed youths and their families: family warmth, support and cohesion

Studies of children and adolescents have consistently shown that low levels of parental warmth and support are associated with both depressive symptoms and clinical depression. In community samples, adolescents who perceive themselves as receiving low parental support report higher levels of depressive symptoms (Conrad Schwarz & Zuroff, 1979; Armsden & Greenberg, 1987; Burbach et al., 1989; Slavin & Rainer, 1990; Kobak et al., 1991; Papini et al., 1991; Papini & Roggmann, 1992; Gonzales, 1993; Lamborn & Steinberg, 1993; Lewinsohn et al., 1994; McFarlane et al., 1995). A clinic sample of depressed youth and their mothers reported poorer communication and less warmth compared to a nonclinic sample of adolescent–mother dyads (Puig-Antich et al., 1993). Adolescent depressive symptoms have also been shown to relate to adolescent reports of low family cohesion (Burt et al., 1988; Feldman et al., 1988; Reinherz et al., 1989; Garrison et al., 1992; Prange et al., 1992; Rudd et al., 1993; Cumsille & Epstein, 1994). Longitudinal studies have provided evidence that adolescents with positive family relationships are less likely to become depressed several years later (Petersen et al., 1991; Reinherz et al., 1993; Lewinsohn et al., 1994). The link between a perception of a less positive family environment and depressive symptoms has also been documented in younger children (Kaslow et al., 1984; Kaslow et al., 1990) and in adult depressives' retrospective accounts of their family relationships (Burbach & Borduin, 1986; Lopez et al., 1989).

Research that has examined the specificity of family relatedness problems to depression in youths suggests that perceptions of low parental warmth, support and family cohesion may be more strongly associated with depressive than nondepressive disorders (Armsden et al., 1990; Stark et al., 1990; Barrera & Garrison-Jones, 1992). However, in a study of inpatient children with a variety of psychiatric disorders, including depression, all reported lower family cohesion (Asarnow et al., 1987).

Parental rejection, hostility and family conflict

Depressive symptoms in youths have also been associated with parental rejection (Poznanski & Zrull, 1970; Lefkowitz & Tesiny, 1984; Robertson &

Simons, 1989; Whitbeck et al., 1992). More extreme forms of negative parent behaviour, such as severe punishment and maltreatment, have also been associated with childhood depression (Downey & Walker, 1992). Puig-Antich et al. (1993) found that mothers and their clinically depressed adolescents reported more corporal punishment relative to healthy controls. However, Lefkowitz & Tesiny (1984) found that parental rejection of their 8-year-olds was a better predictor of depressive symptoms 10 years later than was parental use of punishment.

Although family conflict may be predictive of depressive symptoms both currently (Burt et al., 1988; Forehand et al., 1988; Stark et al., 1990) and prospectively (Forehand et al., 1988; Reinherz et al., 1993), family conflict and hostility appear to be characteristic of families of adolescents with a variety of emotional and behavioural problems (Asarnow et al., 1987; Kashani et al., 1988). Parental hostility, rejection, family conflict and coercive discipline strategies are most consistently reported by studies on families of externalizing children (Olweus, 1980; Patterson et al., 1984; Campbell, 1987; DiLalla et al., 1988; Haddad et al., 1991).

Interestingly, observational studies indicate that depressed youths may not express overtly negative affect (especially anger) and may, in fact, show higher levels of positive affect relative to controls (Dadds et al., 1992; Sanders et al., 1992). There is evidence that especially high levels of positive validation towards mothers are more likely to occur with depressed girls than boys (K. Pavlidis & E. McCauley, unpublished paper). Such findings suggest that families of youths with depressive symptoms may try to deflect overt conflict. It may be that depressed youths, especially girls, are more invested in maintaining positive connections with family members, which may require avoiding an assertive stance.

Development of autonomy

Less work has investigated the link between family support for autonomy and depression in youths. There is some evidence that a perception of mothers as intrusive, controlling or overinvolved is associated with depressive symptoms in college students (Lopez et al., 1989; Zemore & Rinholm, 1989). In addition, the parenting literature on community samples of adolescents has provided evidence for a link between a lack of parent support of adolescent autonomy and adolescent internalizing problems. Baumrind (1991a) found that parents who value conformity, closely monitor their adolescents and are intrusive have adolescents with elevated rates of internalizing behaviour relative to those with parents who display assertive control but are still responsive to their adolescent's needs. Interestingly, Baumrind's work has suggested that the association between parent overcontrolling behaviour and internalizing problems may be stronger for girls (Baumrind, 1991b). Other investigators have also found that high levels of parental control in the context of low responsiveness are associated with adolescent internalizing symptoms (Steinberg et al., 1994). There is also evidence that parent psychological control, such as withdrawal of love, guilt and pressure to change, is associated with internalizing symptoms in offspring (Fauber et al., 1990; Barber et al., 1994). Gonzales (1993) investigated differential parent–adolescent interaction predictors of adolescent internalizing and externalizing symptoms in a sample of African-American female teens. Adolescent perceptions of maternal behavioural control and less secure attachment were associated with internalizing symptoms, while high conflict and low maternal behavioural control were the best predictors of externalizing symptoms.

A few studies have investigated parental overcontrol and overprotection as it relates specifically to depression in youths. Burt et al. (1988) found an association between adolescent perceptions of more parent control and depressive symptoms, and Stark et al. (1990) found that a less democratic parenting style and an enmeshed family environment were associated with depression, but not anxiety, in youths. While one study of depressed adolescents did not reveal differences in adolescent perceptions of parental overprotection relative to either normal or nondepressed psychiatric controls (Burbach et al., 1989), another found parent reports of overprotection associated with greater depression reported by the child (Magnussen, 1991). Findings from these self-report studies are corroborated by observational studies, which have shown that adolescent depressive symptoms are associated with family interactions characterized by high levels of maternal dominance and low levels of adolescent communicative assertiveness (Kobak et al.,1993; Kobak & Ferenz-Gillies,1995). Among a sample of psychiatric and community controls, higher scores on adolescent behaviours that interfered with autonomy and lower scores on behaviours that interfered with positive relating were associated with depressed affect. In contrast, externalizing symptoms were predicted by higher levels of negative behaviours such as hostility (Allen et al., 1994). There is also evidence that sadness in boys is associated with observed maternal encouragement of dependence and other maternal controlling behaviours (Inoff-Germain et al., 1988).

In summary, depressive symptoms and depression in youths appear to be associated with maternal dominance, deficits in autonomy and problems in attachment. While these families may appear fairly cohesive to outsiders, it appears that they have difficulty encouraging autonomy and providing emotional support. Although parents may appear to be highly involved, depressed youths perceive their parents as lacking in warmth and support and possibly as intrusive. It also appears that depression in males and females may have somewhat different family interaction correlates, with males more likely to express anger overtly and females more likely to try to deflect conflict. In contrast to families of depressed youths, parent–adolescent interactions of externalizing youths are more consistently associated with overt hostility, conflict and parental rejection, as well as a deficit in parental limit-setting and monitoring of the adolescent's activities. These findings suggest that both sets of youths experience an impoverished sense of interpersonal connectedness. However, while depressed adolescents receive little support for developing autonomy, it seems that externalizing adolescents receive little guidance in determining boundaries for their autonomy.

Finally, investigators have attempted to identify specific family demographic characteristics, such as socioeconomic status and family structure, that are risk factors for depression. Evidence does not suggest that low socioeconomic status is a risk factor for the development of major depression (Velez et al., 1989; Lewinsohn et al., 1994).

Findings regarding family structure are somewhat mixed and it appears that family interaction may be more important in predicting adolescent depression than socioeconomic status or family structure (Feldman et al., 1988; Garrison et al., 1992; Puig-Antich et al., 1993; Cumsille & Epstein, 1994; McKeown et al., 1997).

Individual characteristics

Problems in the family environment appear to be clearly associated with depression in young people. However, there is evidence that child characteristics are associated with depression independently of family characteristics (Downey & Walker, 1992). All children develop a number of individual characteristics or response patterns as a result of their interactions within their family and broader environment. These response styles build on basic temperamental characteristics, the quality of attachment formation and ongoing learning at home, school and in the community. These patterns gradually come together to form a more cohesive whole which is frequently referred to as personality. Personality is used as a unifying construct or organizing system which includes the emotional, behavioural and cognitive components of an individual's characteristic style of interacting with the world as it has been shaped by experience. In the following sections we will consider how key elements of the child's and adolescent's developing personality contribute to increased risk for depression.

Temperament

Biologically determined factors such as health status, cognitive and physical attributes, maturational rate (e.g. timing of developmental milestones, puberty) and temperament may play a role in the development of emotional disturbances such as depression. Temperament refers to the infant's characteristic way of interacting with the world which is moulded by both genetically transmitted traits and interactions with the environment that begin at birth or before (see review by Prior, 1992). The characteristics thought to be temperamentally based in young children include negative emotionality, difficultness, adaptability to novelty, reactivity, attention regulation, sociability and positive reactivity (Bates, 1989). These styles have been categorized into broad patterns that differ in terms of how 'easy' or 'difficult' a child is, with 'difficult' temperament constituting a risk factor for poorer outcome over the course of development.

The importance of temperament in the developmental process depends on the continuity and stability of these traits over time. Prior's (1992) comprehensive review of the temperament literature identified considerable variability in the data on continuity and stability, depending on the specific trait studied, the details of the study design and the sex of the child followed. Kagan and colleagues (1989) tracked the course of socially inhibited children from 3 to 7 years of age, and found considerable stability in these traits. Moreover, these youngsters were more fearful than socially outgoing controls at age 7, and exhibited greater physiological reactivity. These findings led to speculation that children who are extremely socially inhibited may have a 'lower threshold for limbic-hypothalamic arousal to unexpected changes in the environment'. Temperamental differences in sensitivity to the environment and in reaction to arousal, such as those identified by Kagan and colleagues (1989), may play a central role in shaping a child's coping responses well beyond infancy. Risk factors for depression such as social inhibition and increased negative affect, may be part of the child's initial, biologically programmed make-up.

Children with difficult temperament are overrepresented in clinical samples (Maziade et al., 1990) and support exists for a relation between difficult temperament and later externalizing disorders (Maziade et al., 1990; Prior, 1992). Data supporting a link between temperamental factors and depression are less prevalent. Shyness has been associated with later depression (Lazarus, 1982), as well as with anxiety disorders in Kagan's sample of behaviourally inhibited children (Hirschfeld et al., 1992). However, in Chess and colleagues'

(1983) classic longitudinal study, no infant or toddler temperamental characteristics differentiated the children who became clinically depressed in childhood or adolescence. Rende (1993) assessed the ability of the early temperamental dimensions of sociability, emotionality, and activity to predict delinquency, depression and hyperactivity at age 7. Temperamental traits were significantly associated with later behavioural profiles, as measured by maternal ratings on the Child Behavior Checklist, but the patterns of relations differed for boys and girls. Higher ratings of anxiety/depression were related to early temperament ratings of greater emotionality and less sociability in girls. For boys, greater emotionality was related to later anxiety/depression, and higher activity ratings predicted later attention problems but sociability was not predictive of later behavioural profiles. Kashani and colleagues (Kashani et al., 1991a, b) found 'difficult' temperament to be associated with higher levels of psychopathology in a community sample of children and with higher levels of hopelessness in a sample of children hospitalized because of psychiatric or behavioural problems. However, these studies included only concurrent assessments of both temperament and psychopathology.

Follow-up studies that extend into adolescence are now becoming available. Recently, Kagan and colleagues (Schwartz et al., 1996) assessed the behavioural adjustment at age 13 of the original sample of inhibited and noninhibited children. Based on both self (Youth Self Report) and parent report (Child Behavior Checklist), the youth who had been uninhibited were rated as significantly higher than the inhibited group on externalizing behaviours. Group differences were not as clearcut in terms of internalizing problems. There were no significant differences based on youth self-report but parents of inhibited youth rated these young adolescents as demonstrating more withdrawn behaviour, although this trend was not statistically significant. It should be noted, however, that although there were group differences, most scores were not elevated into the clinical range and no group differences in terms of school or social competence emerged. Smith & Prior (1995) examined the role of temperament in determining stress resilience among a group of 'high-risk' adolescents. Teachers' ratings of positive temperament, characterized as low emotional reactivity and high social engagement, was the strongest predictor of resilience both in the school and home setting. This provides another example of how temperament could contribute to, or modulate, risk for depression.

Few studies have directly explored temperamental characteristics of depressed children. In an epidemiological study of children in an English secondary school, Goodyer and colleagues (1993) observed a significant association between the temperamental quality of increased emotionality and depression.

However, as noted by the researchers, the number of children in this sample who met criteria for clinical depression was quite small (16 girls and 3 boys in a sample of 193). Furthermore, reports of temperamental style might have been confounded by prodromal depressive symptomatology or by depression itself.

In summary, having a difficult or inhibited temperament appears to increase risk for later behavioural problems, although the mechanism of transmission is not clearly articulated. Perhaps temperament contributes to risk for depression by impacting the child's relationships with others. Parental qualities and goodness of fit between mother and child play a critical role in how difficult temperament is expressed over time (Prior, 1992). This is particularly important if temperamental factors impact the resolution of early developmental tasks, which in turn might contribute to the development of depression.

Coping and emotion regulation

The ability to regulate negative emotions and develop adaptive coping skills are important in protecting against the onset of depression. Adaptive coping skills refer to the child's ability to respond in a manner that diminishes the intensity of negative emotion such that the child can effectively function in his or her environment (with respect to interpersonal, school-related and other demands). A distinction is made between problem-focused coping and emotion-focused coping (Lazarus & Folkman, 1984). Problem-focused coping refers to how a person responds to the demands of a stressful situation in terms of active problem-solving efforts. Emotion-focused coping, in contrast, refers to the individual's attempts to mediate the emotion experienced and encompasses passive and avoidant coping responses.

Rumination, which is considered a form of emotion-focused coping, has been linked to depression in adults as well as in children (Nolen-Hoeksema, 1998). Ruminative coping responses refer to a tendency to focus passively and repetitively on one's symptoms of depression and the possible reasons for those symptoms without taking actions to relieve them. Nolen-Hoeksema (1998) conducted a series of studies that have indicated that rumination and lack of distraction strategies predict current and future depression in adults.

There is also evidence that females are more likely than males to engage in ruminative coping responses, and that this gender difference may account in part for the preponderance of female depression that emerges during the teen years (Nolen-Hoeksema, 1998). Sethi & Nolen-Hoeksema (1997), in a study of eighth-graders (13–14 years old), found that girls were more likely to engage in internally focused thoughts (e.g. thinking about themselves) than boys. In contrast, boys reported engaging in more externalized focusing and positive thoughts (sports, music, etc.). The tendency for girls to ruminate was found for events that were positive and neutral, as well as for negative situations. Similarly, Gomez (1998) found that girls were more likely to engage in avoidant coping responses than boys were. The depression literature has supported the notion that passive and avoidant coping is associated with elevated levels of depressive symptoms. Children with elevated levels of depressive symptoms are more likely to offer avoidant coping responses in response to hypothetical stressful situations (Garber et al., 1991; Gomez, 1998). Elevated levels of depression are also associated with a lower likelihood of engaging in support-seeking and cognitive restructuring (Garber et al., 1995; Spirito et al., 1996). Spirito et al. (1996) found that social withdrawal as a coping response may be associated with psychiatric difficulties in general as opposed to a specific characteristic of depression, while deficits in cognitive restructuring may be specific to depression.

In line with the gender differences in rates of adolescent depression, some research has found that a link between coping style and depressive symptoms may hold only for females (Compas et al., 1988). Gomez (1998) found that, for girls in their later teen years, high levels of competitiveness served as a buffer against depression for those who presented with a tendency to engage in avoidant coping.

Aggression as a coping response has also been implicated as a risk for depression. Several studies have found that children who offer aggressive responses to hypothetical stresses were more likely to have elevated levels of depression (Garber et al., 1991). While some research has found this connection to hold only for females (Compas et al., 1988), other research has found that aggression and depression are linked for boys only (Garber et al., 1995).

Garber and colleagues (1991) also investigated whether depressed children differed from nondepressed children in their evaluation of the effectiveness of different coping strategies. Depressed children tended to have a lower expectation of the effectiveness of various coping responses than did nondepressed children. These results suggest that, in addition to a tendency to use maladaptive coping strategies, depressed children may be less likely to utilize active coping due to the expectation that it may not make them feel better. This outcome is consistent with the expectations of self and others predicted by poor attachment quality. Indeed, Garber and colleagues (1991) suggest that the lower effectiveness ratings of coping strategies made by depressed children may be a reflection of their actual experiences with their parents, with whom their efforts at regulating their emotions were ineffective.

In summary, elevated levels of depression in youths are associated with a tendency to engage in passive and avoidant coping responses and a deficit in active problem-solving, support-seeking and cognitive restructuring. Although such a coping style serves as a risk factor for both genders, females are more likely to exhibit this pattern and ineffective coping may explain, in part, the gender difference in depression that emerges in early adolescence.

Cognitive styles

How a child copes with negative emotion and stressful life events is influenced in part by his or her cognitive style. Particular cognitive styles are associated with, and predict depression in both children and adults. According to Beck's (1967) cognitive model of depression, the depressed individual has a negative view about the world, the self and the future, as well as a negative organizing self-schema or filter. This, in turn, colours how both old experiences are perceived and new experiences are interpreted, leading to cognitive distortions such that new information is processed within a negative frame while more positive cues are ignored or misread. Abramson et al. (1989) propose a model of depression which stresses the importance of attributional style. Depressed individuals are described as attributing the occurrence of negative events in their lives to stable, integral characteristics of themselves, while positive events are seen as chance occurrences outside the depressed person's control. This pattern of thinking contributes to feelings of hopelessness and helplessness. A depressogenic cognitive style refers to the tendency to see the self and the environment in a negative light, as reflected in low self-esteem, hopelessness about the future and a negative attributional style or the tendency always to see the cup as half-empty rather than half-full.

Several studies have found associations between cognitive styles and depression in children that are consistent with these models (Seligman et al., 1984; Haley et al., 1985; Bodiford et al., 1988; McCauley et al., 1988). Research on the ability to reframe negative events cognitively has shown that children who demonstrate a pessimistic explanatory style (one in which the causes of bad events are seen as internal, stable and global, and causes of good events are seen as external, unstable and specific) are at increased risk for future depression, and children who become depressed develop a more pessimistic explanatory style which persists even after remission of depression (Nolen-Hoeksema & Girgus, 1995). Garber & Flynn (1998) found, in three studies of the short-term, prospective effects of stressful events such as disappointing grades and peer rejection, that cognitive set measured before the experience of a stressful event 'moderated the effect of the event on the expression of depressive symptoms'.

Cognitive distortions are not always a component of depression in adolescence but have been shown to differentiate depressed from nondepressed youth, and to be more strongly associated with severe depression (Marton & Kutcher, 1995). Furthermore, in these studies the depressive cognitive style persisted, although in a less severe form after remission of the depressive episode (Gotlib et al., 1993; Marton et al., 1993). However, it remains unclear if a negative cognitive style constitutes a vulnerability which increases risk for depression in the face of significant life stressors, or if this style develops as a result of discouraging events and/or a depressive episode itself.

To clarify this issue, Teasdale and colleagues (Teasdale, 1988, 1999; Teasdale & Barnard, 1993; Teasdale et al., 1998) have developed and tested the 'differential activation hypothesis'. According to this hypothesis, there are individual differences in the cognitive response patterns which become activated during periods of even mild depression. Those individuals who respond with negative cognitions are more vulnerable to significant depression. A more negative cognitive response to dysphoric mood induction has been associated with history of past depression and higher ratings of subsequent depressive symptoms in adult and college-age samples (Teasdale & Dent, 1987). Similar findings have recently been reported in a study of a community sample of adolescents with no history of psychiatric disorder (Kelvin et al., 1999). In this study adolescents who were rated by parents as high in emotionality on a temperament scale responded to dysphoric mood induction with significantly more negative self-descriptors than they did to neutral mood induction. Thus, the cognitive vulnerability which increases risk for depression may be a latent variable not sensitive to self-report assessment unless activated by dysphoric mood or stressful live events.

Although there has been a significant amount of research investigating the association between particular cognitive styles and depression, there has been less research examining the origins of these cognitive styles. Bowlby (1980) theorized that these negative cognitive styles emerge as a result of the individual's internal representations of his or her relationship with an attachment figure. If the attachment process has left the child insecure, the internal representation of the self is that he or she is a failure or unlovable, therefore there is the expectation of negative events, hostility or rejection by others. This position finds initial support in studies of one group of children at increased risk for depression – children of depressed mothers. These children have been found to endorse lower self-esteem, and to have a more negative attributional style than children being raised by mothers with no mental health problems (Goodman et al., 1994; Garber & Flynn, 1998).

Garber & Flynn (1998) have engaged in a longitudinal study to understand better the origins of a depressive cognitive style. Children in sixth grade (11–12 years old) were initially recruited and a sample was selected to include children with and without a maternal history of mood disorder. The study explored the role of the mother's own cognitive style, parenting style and stressful life events in relation to child self-report of self-worth, attributional style and hopelessness. Findings on cognitive style revealed a significant association between mother and child ratings on global self-worth but not on the measures of attributional style, hopelessness or perceived competence except in the domain of scholastic competence. However, when mothers completed the attributional question-naire, having been asked to respond as their child would, mother and child ratings were significantly correlated. On parenting practices, the mothers' report of greater use of psychological control and less acceptance at time one, was associated with youths' report of lower self-worth and a more depressive attributional style 1 year later. Finally, negative life events over the year, after controlling for cognitive variables at time one, predicted depressive attribu-tional style and hopelessness, but not ratings of self-worth at subsequent follow-up points. Thus, a somewhat different constellation of factors was associated with each of the three cognitive variables considered. Moreover, the interactions among variables was also critical; for instance, negative life events were more strongly linked to increased hopelessness in youth with low self-worth. These findings underscore the complexity of the issues at hand.

Self-schema and self-worth

Also consistent with the idea of the child's internal representations of the self and others contributing to depressogenic cognitions is the work of Hammen and colleagues (Hammen et al., 1985; Zupen et al., 1987; Hammen & Good-man-Brown, 1990), who have shown associations between particular self-schemas and vulnerability to depression. Self-schema is the child's cognitions or beliefs about the self; how one views one's own traits such as worthiness and competence. Hammen & Goodman-Brown (1990) investigated children's self-schemas via their patterns of recalled associations to a set of questions. They were able to classify the subjects into two groups based on the predominant patterns of recalled events. If the child recalled mostly events pertaining to interpersonal relationships they were classified as interpersonally vulnerable; if recall focused on performance or achievement, they were classified as achieve-ment-vulnerable. Next, Hammen & Goodman-Brown (1990) demonstrated that children who rated interpersonal events as particularly important to their sense of self were more likely to experience depression when faced with an interpersonal threat than were children with a self-efficacy or achievement type of self-schema classification.

Harter and colleagues (Renouf & Harter, 1990; Harter et al., 1992) also provide support for an integral relation between self-schema as reflected in sense of self-worth and depressed affect in early adolescence. Sense of self-worth was highly correlated with depressed mood among their sample of middle-school children, with almost one-to-one correspondence of depressed mood and low self-worth among the 'depressed' group (Renouf & Harter, 1990). Mood and self-worth ratings also changed in unison over a 1-year follow-up period. Moreover, two clusters of self-concept features were found to be related to depression and hopelessness as well as suicidal ideation in young adolescents. One cluster included a sense of competency in terms of physical appearance, peer likability and athletics, while the other cluster included scholastic competence and behavioural conduct. In addition to competence in the domain of importance to the individual, Harter identifies social support from parents and peers as the second key source of self-worth (Harter & Whitesell, 1996). The importance of sense of self-worth or self-esteem in depression is underscored by a recent study in which Lewinsohn and colleagues (1997) investigated 44 psychosocial variables to determine which ones were specifically associated with depression as opposed to nonaffective disorders. Self-consciousness, self-esteem and inactivity secondary to an illness or injury were the only variables which demonstrated a specific association with depression.

In summary, a depressive cognitive style, as reflected in low sense of self-worth, negative attributional style, hopelessness and a negative self-schema does appear to be associated with greater risk for depression in children and adolescents. Moreover, there is growing evidence that these cognitive features may be shaped by the nature of the parent–child interaction as well as the child's exposure to stressful life events. It remains unclear if a depressive cognitive set is a trait which increases an individual's risk for depression or if stressful life events or the experience of depression triggers it. In general, cognitive style is considered a risk factor for depression, not a sufficient causal factor in itself. Chapter 8 provides a comprehensive review of the role life stress plays in the onset and maintenance of depression in young people.

Personality

As the child matures, the various components of response style begin to form a more cohesive whole, which is frequently referred to as personality. In the study of depression in adults, considerable attention has been paid to personality characteristics as risk factors for subsequent depression. This literature initially grew out of the psychoanalytic tradition (Chodoff, 1972; Blatt et al.,

1982) but has come to include cognitive behavioural perspectives as well (Beck, 1983). The underlying assumption is that certain individuals, because of unsuccessful resolution of earlier developmental tasks (e.g. attachment), form personality styles that put them at risk for depression.

Within the personality literature, two clusters of characteristics are most consistently linked with depression. The characteristics are remarkably consistent across theoretical frameworks (Blatt et al., 1982; Akiskal et al., 1983; Beck, 1983). The first cluster includes helplessness, fears of abandonment, and a neediness for love or caring – the dependent personality. The second cluster focuses more on achievement themes with core characteristics including heightened guilt, sense of worthlessness and a feeling of not living up to standards. Individuals within these two groups might evidence the same depressive symptoms but have different internal models (or experiences of depression) which stem from their individual early experiences and resulting self-system. The two personality types parallel the self-concept clusters described by Harter and her co-workers (1992). Blatt and colleagues (1982) propose that the issues of dependence and self-criticism are activated in the experience of normal, transitory depressed mood. Furthermore, individuals with dependent or self-critical personality styles are at increased risk for significant clinical bouts of depression in times of stress. A number of theorists have suggested that it is the particular type of stress – loss in terms of either a personal relationship or personal status – that combines with these personality vulnerabilities to culminate in depression (Blatt et al., 1982; Hammen, 1992).

Unfortunately, empirical support delineating the role of preexisting personality features is scant. Although there has been long-standing interest in the question of predisposing personality factors, research in this area has faced a number of complex methodological barriers. The most central limitation is that few studies have looked prospectively at personality factors as precursors of clinical depression. The bulk of the research has been conducted on nonclinical samples or samples of individuals in the midst of, or recovering from, an episode of clinical depression. Both acute and resolving depressions have been found to impact responses to personality assessments (Akiskal et al., 1983; Hirschfeld et al., 1989), making clear interpretation of what came first impossible. However, two prospective studies have become available. Hirschfeld and colleagues (1989) assessed the personality characteristics of 438 first-degree relatives and spouses of clinically depressed individuals as part of the National Institute of Mental Health collaborative study. The original personality assessments of those who became depressed ($n = 29$) reflected significantly less 'emotional strength', more introspection, increased emotional arousal and greater need for attention than the nondepressed group. The analyses also revealed some interesting age effects. Subjects were divided into two groups based on age at first evaluation; the younger group included those aged 17–30, while the older group included subjects aged 31–41. Within the younger group, the personality assessments of those who became depressed ($n = 15$) could not be differentiated from the never depressed subjects, in part because of the marked variability on the personality measures demonstrated across the entire group of younger subjects. In the older subjects, measures of personality variables among those who did not become depressed, reflected considerable emotional stability, which was not apparent in the subgroup of older subjects who became depressed. The failure to find predictive value of personality measures among younger subjects may reflect an overall immaturity in personality formation, with more stable emotional characteristics coming with age. However, cohort effects or the possibility that depression in the younger sample had a more dominant biological diathesis could not be ruled out.

The second study that looked at personality factors in a prospective way was done with a sample of older adolescents. As part of Block and Block's longitudinal study of development (Gjerde et al., 1988; Block et al., 1991), a group of 87 young people, followed since age 3, completed a self-report depression scale at the time of their evaluation age 18 years. All subjects had participated in detailed assessments of personality and cognitive development at ages 3–4, 7, 11, 14 and 18. Boys and girls differed significantly in the pattern of early characteristics related to later depressive symptoms (Block & Gjerde, 1990; Block et al., 1991; Gjerde & Block, 1996). Girls who later endorsed greater depressive tendencies were described as 'oversocialized, intropunitive', and overcontrolled, whereas later depression was associated with a more externalized pattern of behaviour in boys. For instance, items assessed at the 7-year-old evaluation and associated with later depression in girls included shyness, liking to be alone, as well as greater ability to develop close and lasting relationships. By the 14-year-old evaluation, concern over self-adequacy, increased vulnerability, anxiety and tendency to ruminate emerged as characteristics predictive of greater depression at 18 in girls.

For the boys, a different pattern emerged. Depressive symptoms at 18 were associated with more transient relationships with peers and a willingness to stretch limits, observed even in early childhood years. By early adolescence boys who later endorsed depressive symptoms were described as negativistic, sensitive to criticism and distrustful. Another important sex difference emerged: higher IQ scores at preschool assessment were related to greater chance of later depression in girls, while lower IQ was associated with later depression in boys.

Block and colleagues (Block & Gjerde, 1990; Block et al., 1991) view problems with accomplishment and hostility as central to the early presentation of boys who later endorse depressive features, while for girls self-esteem issues appear more critical. They place these gender differences in early trajectories within the larger context of differential socialization of boys and girls within our society (Block et al., 1991). This research group also reported extensive data from personality assessments of the subjects obtained at the same time as the assessment of depressive tendencies (Gjerde et al., 1988). The findings were quite consistent with earlier developmental patterns. The males with greater self-reported depression continued to have a more externalized pattern of behaviour with greater interpersonal antagonism, unrestraint, discontent with self and unconventionality than less depressed 18-year-old males. Depression in girls was associated with increased rumination or introspection and sense of inadequacy.

In sum, there is considerable support for a developmental model of vulnerability to depression. Mediating between early, biologically based temperamental characteristics and the emergence of a cohesive personality structure are a host of critical interactions with the environment and developing features such as coping skills and cognitive style. We have suggested that these experiences or, more importantly, how the child interprets these experiences, depends in great part on the attachment process which provides children with their internalized models of both self and the world around them. Much more careful research is needed to determine the viability of this developmental model. There are some very compelling common threads which emerge from quite divergent research areas. It is, however, difficult to know if, for instance, shyness as identified in the temperament literature refers to the same behaviour profile as the shyness described in the studies by Block and colleagues of early personality characteristics of girls who become depressed. Careful definition of variables, plus attention to validity of measurements, especially those taken at very different periods in development, is needed.

Peer relationships and social competence

A final area of consideration is how the child, with his or her emerging sense of self and personality, interacts with the world beyond the family unit. There is evidence that depressed youths perceive their peer relationships to be lower in supportiveness (Armsden & Greenberg, 1987; Rudolph et al., 1997; Shirk et al., 1997) and view themselves as less socially competent (Rudolph et al., 1997) relative to their nondepressed counterparts. Parents of depressed children rate their children as having a more difficult time maintaining friendships relative to parents of nondepressed psychiatric controls (Puig-Antich et al., 1985a). Although some studies have found that children with depressive symptoms tend to be categorized as rejected on sociometric ratings (Kennedy et al., 1989; Boivin et al., 1994), other research has not found sociometric ratings to relate to depressive symptoms (Blechman et al., 1986). Blechman et al. (1986), however, did find that peers may accurately perceive their depressed peers as depressed. Little & Garber (1995) in a longitudinal project found that depression only predicted peer rejection at a 3-month follow-up for those youths who experienced low levels of life stress. They interpreted their findings to suggest that life stress mediates the impact of depressive symptoms on peer relationships, and that peers may be more accepting of other children's depressive symptoms if they occur in the face of a significant life stressor (Little & Garber, 1995).

Studies that are limited to the depressive episode have indicated that, although perceptions of low social support are associated with current depression, they may not be predictive of onset of depression (Reinherz et al., 1989; Lewinsohn et al., 1994). There is also evidence that social relationships improve substantially with recovery of a depressive episode but may not reach levels of success reported in normal controls (Puig-Antich et al., 1985b).

There have been efforts to clarify the association between perceived social interaction deficits and actual social behaviour. Analysis of free-play interactions between youths with low scores on depressive symptoms and high scores indicated that children who reported high levels of depressive symptoms spent more time alone, were more aggressive and experienced fewer initiations by peers relative to their nondepressed counterparts (Altmann & Gotlib, 1988). In another study, peer confederates rated clinically depressed adolescents, particularly females, lower in social interest and social skills following a 10-minute interaction compared to normal controls (Connolly et al., 1992). Another study compared interactions between dyads with a dysphoric and nondysphoric adolescent and dyads with two nondysphoric adolescents. Dysphoric adolescents were more likely to perceive their partners as more critical and less friendly, and their nondysphoric partners viewed them as more critical and negative and expressed feelings of rejection toward the dysphoric adolescent (Baker et al., 1996).

There is evidence that the relation between social difficulties and depressive symptoms may be mediated by depressive cognitions (Cole & Turner, 1993).

Boivin et al. (1995) found that negative peer experiences were more likely to predict depressed mood at a later time when peer interactions led children to feel badly about their social situations. In contrast to the above findings, a longitudinal study found that youths with depressive symptoms may actually underestimate their social acceptance, and that this perception is a consequence as opposed to a predictor of depression (Cole et al., 1998).

In summary, difficulties with social relationships appear to accompany depression in young people. Interestingly, it seems that social problems reflect in part the depressed youth perception of others as critical and rejecting; which in turn may spark critical and defensive behaviour on their part, which puts peers off, and this leads to isolation.

Adolescent challenges

The material presented so far has focused on factors which might constitute increased vulnerability to depression. The second part of the risk equation suggests that depression occurs when the vulnerable individual is faced with significant life stress (see Chapter 8 for a complete review). Since the prevalence of depression increases significantly during the adolescent years, there may be something unique about adolescence, and the stresses encountered during this developmental period, which triggers the expression of depression. Adolescents begin to function as part of the larger world and the ongoing process of separation and individuation from family becomes more significant as the young person strives to establish his or her own independent identity. Resolution of these challenges builds on skills acquired throughout the developmental process. Thus, the child with poorly resolved issues of attachment, poor affect regulation skills and a negative coping and cognitive style is highly vulnerable in the face of the multitude of adolescent challenges.

Most young adolescents are faced with significant changes in every aspect of their lives; pubertal development, cognitive maturation, school transition and increased performance pressures in all arenas – academics, sports, social and family. Some have hypothesized that the increase in depression during the adolescent period, which is particularly noteworthy in girls, is secondary to the hormonal changes and brain maturation which accompany pubertal development (Susman et al., 1987; Brooks-Gunn & Warren, 1989; Petersen et al., 1991; Angold & Rutter, 1992). Drawing on data from a longitudinal study of children moving through puberty, Angold and colleagues (1998) found differential risk patterns for boys and girls. For boys, pubertal development, as marked by transition to Tanner stage III or higher, had at least a short-term effect of reducing prevalence of depression. In girls, however, mid-puberty marked an emergence of increased risk for depression (Angold et al., 1998). It was initially unclear whether this increased risk for girls was related to the direct influence of the changing neuroendocrine environment or whether it was an indirect effect of the social and emotional implications of the girls' change in physical presentation.

Angold and colleagues (1999) explored this further by investigating the role of physical development as reflected in Tanner stage and changes in hormone levels. These analyses indicated that hormone levels – specifically increasing levels of oestrogen and testosterone levels above the 60th percentile – were significantly associated with depression. Moreover, the association between pubertal status and depression was accounted for in the regression models by the hormonal data. The researchers conclude that while hormonal changes are not sufficient to cause depression, they do place developing girls into a hormonal risk pool more similar to that of adult women. Hormonal changes, while related to change in mood, may not be as important in explaining depressed mood as other environmental stressors (Brooks-Gunn & Warren, 1989). However, the physical, environmental and developmental changes, and the stressors associated with these changes, appear to play an important role in the onset of depression in adolescence.

The greater increase in prevalence of depression among girls than boys during the adolescent years suggests there may be other factors in addition to the differential impact of pubertal changes that distinguish how girls – especially vulnerable girls – experience the stresses of adolescence.

As suggested in the work reviewed above by Block and colleagues (Block & Gjerde, 1990; Block et al., 1991), there is growing evidence that boys and girls follow different developmental pathways before presenting with depressive symptomatology. Petersen and colleagues (1991) also found problems through-out development in boys who became depressed during middle-school years, whereas the depressed girls in their sample were less likely to have histories of previous adjustment difficulties. Thus, it may be that the stressors of adolescence have more of an impact on girls than boys. Pubertal development is one adolescent change that appears to impact boys and girls differently. Early puberty has been associated with increased self-esteem in boys while girls who develop early have lower self-esteem and more negative body image than those with later adolescent development. Pubertal changes *per se* do not appear to be critical in the onset of depression but may play a critical role in setting the stage for depression by influencing how the young adolescent girl feels about her body and her subsequent self-esteem (Petersen et al., 1991; Harter et al., 1992).

Furthermore, it appears that the number of stressors faced at once is important (N. Garmezy, unpublished paper). Simmons et al. (1987) found lowest self-esteem among young adolescent girls who experienced a change in school while going through their pubertal growth, whereas both boys and girls whose growth spurt occurred after transitioning into a new school setting reported more positive self-concept. Petersen et al. (1991) also found this synchronicity of change to be an important factor which had a greater impact on girls because they were more likely, given the earlier time of their growth spurt, to experience pubertal and school changes simultaneously. Petersen and colleagues (1991) concluded from their study of 335 young adolescents that girls were at greater risk for developing depressed affect by 12th grade (age 17–18) because they experienced more challenges in early adolescence than did boys.

Gender socialization is another crucial factor to consider when investigating factors associated with depression. Several aspects of gender socialization have been implicated in the preponderance of female depression, one of which has been described as a conflict between connectedness and autonomy. Adolescent girls may place greater value on maintaining a sense of connectedness, especially to their mothers, than has traditionally been acknowledged in studies looking at the individuation process in groups of boys and girls together (Rich, 1990). It has been observed that depressed females often view their own autonomous behaviour as a threat to relationships, and therefore they will inhibit their own independence (Kaplan, 1986). The task of achieving autonomy-relatedness during adolescence appears particularly challenging for females, and may relate in part to the preponderance of female depression beginning in adolescence.

Developmental model

This chapter has attempted to pull together multiple research areas to explore the factors that currently appear to be the developmental underpinnings of depression in adolescence and perhaps adulthood as well. We found remarkable consistency between various research areas, a consistency that continually reinforced the notion that attachment begins the developmental processes that later affect one's ability to cope effectively with both a stressful internal process, such as individuation, and external stressors, such as adverse life events. Each area of research built upon the other, exposing various aspects of the complex developmental process that underlies good coping and vulnerability to depression. We have attempted to illustrate how various aspects of development affect the onset of depression in Figure 3.1.

Our model is similar to one suggested by Hammen (1992) in its emphasis on

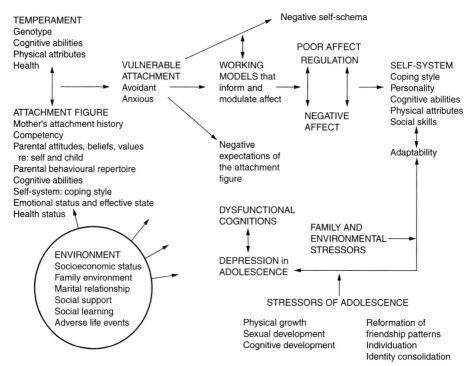

Figure 3.1. Factors affecting vulnerability to depression in adolescence.

viewing unsuccessful resolution of the attachment process as the precursor to the development of a negative self-schema and a subsequent compromised ability to regulate negative affect. The model presented in this chapter further elaborates on factors that may lead to compromised attachment, incorporates the role of emotion regulation and focuses on a more holistic view of the development of depression. Hammen's model places more emphasis on cognitive components in isolation from other factors. In addition, our model allows for the specification of stressors unique to any developmental state across the life cycle, as well as the delineation of broader environmental factors that interact with these stressors. In this case, the stressors unique to adolescence have been highlighted in terms of their likely contribution to the onset of depression in adolescence.

REFERENCES

Abramson, L. Y., Metalsky, G. I. & Alloy, L. B. (1989). The hopelessness theory of depression: does the research test the theory? In *Social Cognition and Clinical Psychology*: a synthesis, ed. L.

Y. Abramson, pp. 33–65. New York: Guilford Press.

Akiskal, H. S., Hirschfeld, R. M. A. & Yerevanian, B. I. (1983). The relationship of personality to affective disorders. *Archives of General Psychiatry*, **40**, 801–10.

Allen, J. P., Hauser, S. T., Bell, K. L. & O'Connor, T. G. (1994). Longitudinal assessment of autonomy and relatedness in adolescent–family interactions as predictors of adolescent ego development and self-esteem. *Child Development*, **65**, 179–94.

Als, H. (1978). Assessing an assessment: conceptual considerations, methodological issues, and a perspective on the future of the Neonatal Behavioral Assessment Scale. In *Organization and Stability: A Commentary on the Brazelton Neonatal Behavioral Assessment Scale*, ed. A. J. Sameroff. Monographs of the Society for Research in Child Development, vol. 43, pp. 14–28. Chicago, IL: University of Chicago Press.

Altmann, E. O. & Gotlib, I. H. (1988). The social behavior of depressed children: an observational study. *Journal of Abnormal Child Psychology*, **16**, 29–44.

Angold, A. & Rutter, M. (1992). Effects of age and pubertal status on depression in a large clinical sample. *Development and Psychopathology*, **4**, 5–28.

Angold, A., Costello, E. J. & Worthman, C. M. (1998). Puberty and depression: the roles of age, pubertal status, and pubertal timing. *Psychological Medicine*, **28**, 51–61.

Angold, A., Costello, E. J., Erkanli, A. & Worthman, C. M. (1999). Pubertal changes in hormone levels and depression in girls. *Psychological Medicine*, **29**, 1043–53.

Armsden, G. C. & Greenberg, M. T. (1987). The inventory of parent and peer attachment: individual differences and their relationship to psychological well-being in adolescence. *Journal of Youth and Adolescence*, **16**, 427–54.

Armsden, G. C., McCauley, E., Greenberg, M., Burke, P. M. & Mitchell, J. R. (1990). Parent and peer attachment in early adolescent depression. *Journal of Abnormal Child Psychology*, **18**, 683–97.

Asarnow, J. R., Carlson, G. A. & Guthrie, D. (1987). Coping strategies, self-perceptions, hopelessness, and perceived family environments in depressed and suicidal children. *Journal of Consulting and Clinical Psychology*, **55**, 361–6.

Baker, M., Milich, R. & Manolis, M. B. (1996). Peer interactions of dysphoric adolescents. *Journal of Abnormal Child Psychology*, **24**, 241–55.

Barber, B. K., Olsen, J. E. & Shagle, S. C. (1994). Associations between parental psychological and behavioral control and youth internalized and externalized behaviors. *Child Development*, **65**, 1120–36.

Barrera, M. & Garrison-Jones, C. (1992). Family and peer social support as specific correlates of adolescent depressive symptoms. *Journal of Abnormal Child Psychology*, **20**, 1–16.

Bates, J. E. (1989). Concepts and measures of temperament. In *Temperament in Childhood*, ed. G. A. Kohnstamm, J. E. Bates & M. K. Rothbart, pp. 3–26. New York: Wiley.

Baumrind, D. (1991a). The influence of parenting style on adolescent competence and substance use. *Journal of Early Adolescence*, **11**, 56–95.

Baumrind, D. (1991b). Effective parenting during the early adolescent transition. In *Family Transitions*, ed. P. A. Cowen & M. Hetherington, pp. 111–64. New Jersey: Lawrence Erlbaum.

Beardslee, W. R. & Wheelock, I. (1994). Children of parents with affective disorders: empirical findings and clinical implications. In *Handbook of Children and Adolescents*, ed. W. M. Reynolds & H. F. Johnson, pp. 463–79. New York: Plenum Press.

Beardslee, W. R., Keller, M. B., Lavori, P. W., Staley, J. & Sacks, N. (1993). The impact of parental affective disorder on depression in offspring: a longitudinal follow-up in a nonreferred sample. *Journal of the American Academy of Child and Adolescent Psychiatry*, **32**, 723–30.

Beck, A. T. (1967). *Depression: Causes and Treatment*. Philadelphia: University of Pennsylvania.

Beck, A. T. (1983). Cognitive therapy of depression: new perspectives. In *Treatment of Depression: old controversies and new approaches*, P. I. Clayton & J. Barrett, pp. 265–90. New York: Raven Press.

Blatt, S. J., Quinlan, D. M., Chevron, E. S. & McDonald, C. (1982). Dependency and self-criticism: psychological dimensions of depression. *Journal of Consulting and Clinical Psychology*, **50**, 113–24.

Blechman, E. A., McEnroe, M. J., Carella, E. T. & Audette, D. P. (1986). Childhood competence and depression. *Journal of Abnormal Psychology*, **95**, 223–7.

Block, J. & Gjerde, P. F. (1990). Depressive symptoms in late adolescence: a longitudinal perspective on personality antecedents. In *Risk and Protective Factors in the Development of Psychopathology*, ed. J. Rolf, A. S. Masten, D. Cicchetti, K. H. Nuechterlein & S. Weintraub, pp. 334–60. Cambridge: Cambridge University Press.

Block, J., Gjerde, P. F. & Block, J. H. (1991). Personality antecedents of depressive tendencies in 18-year-olds: a prospective study. *Journal of Personality and Social Psychology*, **60**, 726–38.

Bodiford, C. A., Eisenstadt, T. H., Johnson, J. H. & Bradlyn, A. S. (1988). Comparisons of learned helpless cognitions and behavior in children with high and low scores on the Children's Depression Inventory. *Journal of Clinical Child Psychology*, **6**, 483–98.

Boivin, M., Poulin, F. & Vitaro, F. (1994). Depressed mood and peer rejection in childhood. *Development and Psychopathology*, **6**, 483–98.

Boivin, M., Mymel, S. & Burkowski, W. M. (1995). The roles of social withdrawal, peer rejection, and victimization by peers in predicting loneliness and depressed mood in childhood. Special issue: developmental processes in peer relations and psychopathology. *Development and Psychopathology*, **7**, 765–86.

Bowlby, J. (1980). *Attachment and Loss*, vol. III: *Loss*. New York, Basic Books, Inc.

Bowlby, J. (1988). *A Secure Base: parent–child attachment and healthy human development*. New York, Basic Books.

Brooks-Gunn, J. & Warren, M. P. (1989). Biological and social contributions to negative affect in young adolescent girls. *Child Development*, **60**, 40–55.

Burbach, D. J. & Borduin, C. M. (1986). Parent–child relations and the etiology of depression: a review of methods and findings. *Clinical Psychology Review*, **6**, 133–53.

Burbach, D. J., Kashani, J. H. & Rosenberg, R. K. (1989). Parental bonding and depressive disorders in adolescents. *Journal of Child Psychology and Psychiatry*, **3**, 417–29.

Burt, C. E., Cohen, L. H. & Bjorck, J. P. (1988). Perceived family environment as a moderator of young adolescent life stress adjustment. *American Journal of Community Psychology*, **16**, 101–22.

Campbell, A. (1987). Self-reported delinquency and home life: evidence from a sample of British girls. *Journal of Youth and Adolescence*, **16**, 167–77.

Cassidy, J. F. (1988). Child–other attachment and the self in 6-year-olds. *Child Development*, **59**, 121–34.

Chess, S., Thomas, A. & Hassibi, M. (1983). Depression in childhood and adolescence: a prospective study of six cases. *Journal of Nervous and Mental Disease*, **171**, 411–20.

Chodoff, P. (1972). The depressive personality: a critical review. *Archives of General Psychiatry*, **27**, 666–73.

Cole, D. A. & Turner, J. E. (1993). Models of cognitive mediation and moderation in child depression. *Journal of Abnormal Psychology*, **102**, 271–81.

Cole, D. S., Martin, J. M., Peeke, L. G., Seroczynski, A. D. & Hoffman, K. (1998). Are cognitive errors of underestimation predictive or reflective of depressive symptoms in children: a longitudinal study. *Journal of Abnormal Psychology*, **107**, 481–98.

Compas, B. E., Malcarne, V. L. & Fondacaro, K. M. (1988). Coping with stressful events in older children and young adolescents. *Journal of Consulting and Clinical Psychology*, **56**, 405–11.

Connolly, J., Geller, S., Marton, P. & Kutcher, S. (1992). Peer responses to social interaction with depressed adolescents. *Journal of Clinical Child Psychology*, **21**, 365–70.

Conrad Schwarz, J. & Zuroff, D. C. (1979). Family structure and depression in female college students: effects of parental conflict, decision-making power, and inconsistency of love. *Journal of Abnormal Psychology*, **88**, 398–406.

Cummings, E. M. & Davies, P. T. (1994). Maternal depression and child development. *Journal of Child Psychology and Psychiatry*, **35**, 73–112.

Cumsille, P. E. & Epstein, N. (1994). Family cohesion, family adaptability, social support, and adolescent depressive symptoms in outpatient clinic families. *Journal of Family Psychology*, **8**, 202–14.

Dadds, M. R., Sanders, M. R., Morrison, M. & Rebgetz, M. (1992). Childhood depression and conduct disorder: II. An analysis of family interaction patterns in the home. *Journal of Abnormal Psychology*, **101**, 505–13.

Dawson, G., Grofer Klinger, L., Panagiotides, H., Spieker, S. & Frey, K. (1992). Infants of mothers with depressive symptoms: electroencephalograph and behavioral findings related to attachment status. *Development and Psychopathology*, **4**, 67–80.

DiLalla, L. F., Mitchell, C. M., Arthur, M. W. & Paglioca, P. M. (1988). Aggression and delinquency: family and environmental factors. *Journal of Youth and Adolescence*, **17**, 233–46.

Downey, G. & Coyne, J. C. (1990). Children of depressed parents: an integrative review. *Psychological Bulletin*, **108**, 50–76.

Downey, G. & Walker, E. (1992). Distinguishing family-level and child-level influences on the development of depression and aggression in children at risk. *Development and Psychopathology*, **4**, 81–95.

Fauber, R., Forehand, R., Thomas, A. M. & Wierson, M. (1990). A mediational model of the impact of marital conflict on adolescent adjustment in intact and divorced families: the role of disrupted parenting. *Child Development*, **62**, 1112–23.

Feldman, S. S., Rubenstein, J. L. & Rubin, C. (1988). Depressive affect and restraint in early adolescents: relationships with family structure, family process, and friendship support. *Journal of Early Adolescence*, **8**, 279–96.

Forehand, R., Brody, G., Slotkin, J. et al. (1988). Young adolescent and maternal depression: assessment, interrelations, and family predictors. *Journal of Consulting and Clinical Psychology*, **56**, 422–6.

Garber, J. & Flynn, C. (1998). Origins of the depressive cognitive style. In *The Science of Clinical Psychology: Accomplishments and Future Directions*, ed. D. K. Routh & R. J. DeRubeis, pp. 53–93. Washington, DC: American Psychological Association.

Garber, J., Braafladt, N. & Zeman, J. (1991). The regulation of sad affect: an information-processing perspective. In *The Development of Emotion Regulation and Dysregulation*, ed. J. Garber & K. A. Dodge, pp. 208–42. New York: Cambridge University Press.

Garber, J., Braafladt, N. & Weiss, B. (1995). Affect regulation in depressed and nondepressed children and young adolescents. Special issue: emotions in developmental psychopathology. *Development and Psychopathology*, **7**, 93–115.

Garrison, C. Z., Addy, C. L., Jackson, K. L., McKeown, R. & Waller, J. L. (1992). Major depressive disorder and dysthymia in young adolescents. *American Journal of Epidemiology*, **135**, 792–802.

Gelfand, D. M. & Teti, D. M (1990). The effects of maternal depression on children. *Clinical Psychology Review*, **10**, 329–53.

Gjerde, P. F. & Block, J. (1996). A developmental perspective on depressive symptoms in adolescence gender differences in autocentric–allocentric modes of impulse regulation. In *Adolescence: Opportunities and Challenges*, ed. D. Cicchetti & S. Toth. Rochester Symposia on Developmental Psychopathology, vol. 7, pp. 167–96. Rochester, NY: University of Rochester Press.

Gjerde, P. F., Block, J. & Block, J. H. (1988). Depressive symptoms and personality during late adolescence: generic differences in the externalization–internalization of symptom expression. *Journal of Abnormal Psychology*, **97**, 475–86.

Gomez, R. (1998). Impatience–aggression, competitiveness and avoidant coping: direct and moderating effects on maladjustment among adolescents. *Personality and Individual Differences*, **25**, 649–61.

Gonzales, N. A. (1993). Parent–adolescent relations and adolescent adjustments in African-American families. *Dissertation Abstracts International*, **53**, 4975.

Goodman, S. H., Adamson, L. B., Riniti, J. & Cole, S. (1994). Mothers' expressed attitudes: associations with maternal depression and children's self-esteem and psychopathology. *Journal of the American Academy of Child and Adolescent Psychiatry*, **33**, 1265–74.

Goodyer, I. M., Ashby, L., Altham, P. M. E., Vize, C. & Cooper, P. J. (1993). Temperament and major depression in 11 to 16 year olds. *Journal of Child Psychology and Psychiatry*, **34**, 1409–23.

Gotlib, I. H., Lewinsohn, P. M., Seeley, J. R., Rohde, P. & Redner, J. E. (1993). Negative cognitions and attributional style in depressed adolescents: an examination of stability and specificity. *Journal of Abnormal Psychology*, **102**, 607–15.

Haddad, J. D., Barocas, R. & Hollenbeck, A. R. (1991). Family organization and parent attitudes of children with conduct disorder. *Journal of Clinical Child Psychology*, **20**, 152–61.

Haley, G. M., Fine, S., Marriage, K., Moretti, M. M. & Freeman, R. J. (1985). Cognitive behavior and depression in psychiatrically disturbed children and adolescents. *Journal of Consulting and Clinical Psychology*, **53**, 535–7.

Hammen, C. (1992). Cognitive, life stress, and interpersonal approaches to a developmental psychopathology model of depression. *Development and Psychopathology*, **4**, 189–206.

Hammen, C. & Goodman-Brown, T. (1990). Self-schemas and vulnerability to specific life stress in children at risk for depression. *Cognitive Therapy and Research*, **14**, 215–27.

Hammen, C., Marks, T., Mayol, A. & deMayo, R. (1985). Depressive self-schemas, life stress, and vulnerability to depression. *Journal of Abnormal Psychology*, **94**, 308–19.

Hankin, B. L., Abramson, L. Y., Moffitt, T. E. et al. (1998). Development of depression from preadolescence to young adulthood: emerging gender differences in a 10-year longitudinal study. *Journal of Abnormal Psychology*, **107**, 128–40.

Harrington, R., Fudge, H., Rutter, M., Pickles, A. & Hill, J. (1990). Adult outcomes of childhood and adolescent depression: I. Psychiatric status. *Archives of General Psychiatry*, **47**, 465–73.

Harrington, R., Rutter, M. & Fombonne, E. (1996). Developmental pathways in depression: multiple meanings, antecedents, and endpoints. *Development and Psychopathology*, **8**, 601–16.

Harter, S. & Whitesell, N. (1996). Multiple pathways to self-reported depression and psychological adjustment among adolescents. *Development and Psychopathology*, **8**, 761–77.

Harter, S., Marold, D. B. & Whitesell, N. R. (1992). Model of psychosocial risk factors leading to suicidal ideation in young adolescents. *Development and Psychopathology*, **4**, 167–88.

Hirschfeld, R. M. A., Klerman, G. L., Lavori, P. et al. (1989). Premorbid personality assessments of first onset of major depression. *Archives of General Psychiatry*, **46**, 345–50.

Hirschfeld, D. R., Rosenbaum, J. F., Biederman, J. et al. (1992). Stable behavioral inhibition and its association with anxiety disorder. *Journal of the American Academy of Child and Adolescent Psychiatry*, **31**, 103–11.

Inoff-Germain, G., Nottelmann, E. D., Arnold, G. S. & Susman, E. J. (1988). Adolescent aggression and parent–adolescent conflict: relations between observed family interactions and measures of the adolescents' general functioning. *Journal of Early Adolescence*, **8**, 17–36.

Kagan, J., Reznick, S. & Snidman, N. (1989). Biological bases of childhood shyness. *Science*, **240**, 167–71.

Kaplan, A. (1986). The 'self-in-relation': implications for depression in women. *Psychotherapy*, **23**, 234–42.

Kashani, J. H., Burbach, D. J. & Rosenberg, T. K. (1988). Perception of family conflict resolution and depressive symptomatology in adolescents. *Journal of the American Academy of Child and Adolescent Psychiatry*, **27**, 42–8.

Kashani, J. H., Ezpeleta, L., Dandoy, A. C., Doi, S. & Reid, J. C. (1991a). Psychiatric disorders in children and adolescents: the contribution of the child's temperament and the parents' psychopathology and attitudes. *Canadian Journal of Psychiatry*, **36**, 569–73.

Kashani, J. H., Soltys, S. M., Dandoy, A. C., Vaidya, A. F. & Reid, J. C. (1991b). Correlates of hopelessness in psychiatrically hospitalized children. *Comprehensive Psychiatry*, **32**, 330–7.

Kaslow, N. J., Rehm, L. P. & Siegel, A. W. (1984). Social–cognitive and cognitive correlates of depression in children. *Journal of Abnormal Child Psychology*, **12**, 605–20.

Kaslow, N. J., Rehm, L. P., Pollack, S. L. & Siegel, A. W. (1990). Depression and perception of family functioning in children and their parents. *American Journal of Family Therapy*, **18**, 227–35.

Kelvin, R. G., Goodyer, I. M., Teasdale, J. D. & Brechin, D. (1999). Latent negative self-schema and high emotionality in well adolescents at risk for psychopathology. *Journal of Child Psychology and Psychiatry*, **40**, 959–68.

Kennedy, E., Spence, S. H. & Hensley, R. (1989). An examination of the relationship between childhood depression and social competence amongst primary school children. *Journal of Child Psychology and Psychiatry*, **30**, 561–73.

Kobak, R. R. & Ferenz-Gillies, R. (1995). Emotion regulation and depressive symptoms during adolescence: a functionalist perspective. *Development and Psychopathology*, **7**, 183–92.

Kobak, R. R. & Sceery, A. (1988). Attachment in late adolescence: working models, affect regulation, and representations of self and others. *Child Development*, **59**, 135–46.

Kobak, R. R., Sudler, N. & Gamble, W. (1991). Attachment and depressive symptoms during adolescence: a developmental pathway analysis. *Development and Psychopathology*, **3**, 461–74.

Kobak, R. R., Cole, H. E., Ferenz-Gillies, R., Fleming, W. & Gamble, W. (1993). Attachment and emotion regulation during mother–teen problem solving: a control theory analysis. *Child Development*, **64**, 231–45.

Kopp, C. B. (1982). Antecedents of self-regulation: a developmental perspective. *Developmental Psychology*, **18**, 199–214.

Lamborn, S. D. & Steinberg, L. (1993). Emotional autonomy redux: revisiting Ryan and Lynch. *Child Development*, **64**, 483–99.

Lazarus, P. J. (1982). Incidence of shyness in elementary school age children. *Psychological Reports*, **51**, 904–6.

Lazarus, R. & Folkman, S. (1984). *Stress, Appraisal, and Coping*. New York: Springer.

Lefkowitz, M. M. & Tesiny, E. P. (1984). Rejection and depression: prospective and contemporaneous analyses. *Developmental Psychology*, **20**, 776–85.

Lewinsohn, P. M., Hops, H., Roberts, R. E., Seeley, J. R. & Andrews, J. A. (1993). Adolescent psychopathology: I. Prevalence and incidence of depression and other DSM-III-R disorders in high school students. *Journal of Abnormal Psychology*, **102**, 133–44.

Lewinsohn, P. M., Roberts, R. E., Seeley, J. R. et al. (1994). Adolescent psychopathology: II. Psychosocial risk factors for depression. *Journal of Abnormal Psychology*, **103**, 302–15.

Lewinsohn, P. M. Gotlib, I. H. & Seeley, J. R. (1997). Depression-related psychosocial variables: are they specific to depression in adolescents? *Journal of Abnormal Psychology*, **3**, 365–75.

Little, S. A. & Garber, J. (1995). Aggression, depression, and stressful life events predicting peer rejection in children. Special issue: developmental processes in peer relations and psychopathology. *Development and Psychopathology*, **7**, 845–56.

Lopez, F. G., Campbell, V. L. & Watkins, C. E. (1989). Constructions of current family functioning among depressed and nondepressed college students. *Journal of College Student Development*, **30**, 221–8.

Magnussen, M. G. (1991). Characteristics of depressed and non-depressed children and their parents. *Child Psychiatry and Human Development*, **21**, 185–91.

Marton, P. & Kutcher, S. (1995). The prevalence of cognitive distortion in depressed adolescents. *Journal of Psychiatry and Neuroscience*, **20**, 33–8.

Marton, P., Churchard, M. & Kutcher, S. (1993). Cognitive distortion in depressed adolescents. *Journal of Psychiatry and Neuroscience*, **18**, 103–7.

Maziade, M., Caron, C., Cote, R., Boutin, M. P. & Thivierge, J. (1990). Extreme temperament and diagnosis. *Archives of General Psychiatry*, **47**, 477–84.

McCauley, E. & Myers, K. (1992). The longitudinal clinical course of depression in children and adolescents. *Child and Adolescent Psychiatric Clinics of North America*, **1**, 183–96.

McCauley, E., Mitchell, J. R., Burke, P. & Moss, S. (1988). Cognitive attributes of depression in children and adolescents. *Journal of Consulting and Clinical Psychology*, **56**, 903–8.

McFarlane, A. H., Bellissimo, A. & Norman, G. R. (1995). The role of family and peers in social self-efficacy: links to depression in adolescence. *American Journal of Orthopsychiatry*, **65**, 402–10.

McKeown, R. E., Garrison, C. Z., Jackson, K. L. et al. (1997). Family structure and cohesion, and depressive symptoms in adolescents. *Journal of Research on Adolescence*, **7**, 267–81.

Mitchell, J., McCauley, E., Burke, P., Calderon, R. & Schloredt, K. (1989). Psychopathology in parents of depressed children and adolescents. *Journal of the American Academy of Child and Adolescent Psychiatry*, **28**, 352–7.

Myers, K. & McCauley, E. (1997). Treatment of depressive disorders in adolescence. In *Current Psychiatric Therapy*, ed. D. Dunner, pp. 458–67. Philadelphia: W. B. Saunders.

Nolen-Hoeksema, S. (1998). Ruminative coping with depression. In Motivation and Self-regulation across the Life Span, ed. J. Heckhausen, & C. S. Dweck, pp. 237–56. Cambridge: Cambridge University Press.

Nolen-Hoeksema, S. & Girgus, J. S. (1995). Explanatory style and achievement, depression, and gender differences in childhood and early adolescence. In Explanatory Style, ed. G. M. Buchanan & E. P. Seligman, pp. 57–70. Mahwan: Lawrence Erlbaum.

Olweus, D. (1980). Familial and temperamental determinants of aggressive behavior in adolescent boys: a causal analysis. *Developmental Psychology*, **16**, 644–60.

Papini, D. R. & Roggman, L. A. (1992). Adolescent perceived attachment to parents in relation to competence, depression, and anxiety: a longitudinal study. *Journal of Early Adolescence*, **12**, 420–40.

Papini, D. R., Roggman, O. A. & Anderson, J. (1991). Early-adolescent perceptions of attachment to mother and father: a test of the emotional-distancing and buffering hypotheses. *Journal of Early Adolescence*, **11**, 258–75.

Patterson, G. R., Dishion, T. J. & Bank, L. (1984). Family interaction: a process model of deviancy training. *Aggressive Behavior*, **10**, 253–67.

Petersen, A. C., Sarigiani, P. A. & Kennedy, R. E. (1991). Adolescent depression: why more girls? *Journal of Youth and Adolescence*, **20**, 247–71.

Poznanski, E. & Zrull, J. P. (1970). Childhood depression: clinical characteristics of overtly depressed children. *Archives of General Psychiatry*, **23**, 8–15.

Prange, M. E., Greenbaum, P. E., Silver, S. E. et al. (1992). Family functioning and psychopathology among adolescents with severe emotional disturbances. *Journal of Abnormal Child Psychology*, **20**, 83–102.

Prior, M. (1992). Childhood temperament. *Journal of Child Psychology and Psychiatry*, **33**, 249–79.

Puig-Antich, J., Lukens, E., Davies, M. et al. (1985a). Psychosocial functioning in prepubertal major depressive disorders: I. Interpersonal relationships during the depressive episode. *Archives of General Psychiatry*, **42**, 500–7.

Puig-Antich, J., Lukens, E., Davies, M. et al. (1985b). Psychosocial functioning in prepubertal major depressive disorders: II. Interpersonal relationships after sustained recovery from affective episode. *Archives of General Psychiatry*, **42**, 511–17.

Puig-Antich, J., Goetz, D., Davies, M. et al. (1989). A controlled family history study of prepubertal major depressive disorder. *Archives of General Psychiatry*, **46**, 406–18.

Puig-Antich, J., Kaufman, J., Ryan, N. D. et al. (1993). The psychosocial functioning and family environment of depressed adolescents. *Journal of the American Academy of Child and Adolescent Psychiatry*, **32**, 244–53.

Reinherz, H. Z., Stewart-Berghauer, G., Pakiz, B. et al. (1989). The relationship of early risk and current mediators to depressive symptomatology in adolescence. *Journal of the American Academy of Child and Adolescent Psychiatry*, **28**, 942–7.

Reinherz, H. Z., Giaconia, R. M., Pakiz, B. et al. (1993). Psychosocial risks for major depression in late adolescence: a longitudinal community study. *Journal of the American Academy of Child and Adolescent Psychiatry*, **32**, 1155–63.

Rende, R. (1993). Longitudinal relations between temperament traits and behavioral syndromes in middle childhood. *Journal of the American Academy of Child and Adolescent Psychiatry*, **32**, 287–90.

Rende, R. D., Plomin, R., Reiss, D. & Hetherington, E. M. (1993). Genetic and environmental influences on depressive symptomatology in adolescence: individual differences and extreme scores. *Journal of Child Psychology and Psychiatry and Allied Disciplines*, **34**, 1387–98.

Renouf, A. G. & Harter, S. (1990). Low self-worth and anger as components of the depressive experience in young adolescents. *Development and Psychopathology*, **2**, 293–310.

Rich, S. (1990). Daughters' view of their relationships with their mothers. In *Making Connections: the relational worlds of adolescent girls at the Emma Willard School*, ed. C. Gilligan, N. P. Lyons & T. J. Hanmer, pp. 258–73. Cambridge: Harvard University Press.

Robertson, J. F. & Simons, R. L. (1989). Family factors, self-esteem, and adolescent depression. *Journal of Marriage and the Family*, **51**, 125–38.

Rudd, N. M., Stewart, E. R. & McKenry, P. C. (1993). Depressive symptomatology among rural youth: a test of the circumplex model. *Psychological Reports*, **72**, 56–8.

Rudolph, K. D., Hammen, C. & Burge, D. (1997). A cognitive–interpersonal approach to depressive symptoms in preadolescent children. *Journal of Abnormal Child Psychology*, **25**, 33–45.

Rutter, M., Grahm, P., Chadwick, O. F. D. & Yule, W. (1976). Adolescent turmoil: fact or fiction? *Journal of Child Psychology and Psychiatry*, **17**, 35–56.

Sanders, M. R., Dadds, M. R., Johnston, B. M. & Cash, R. (1992). Childhood depression and conduct disorder: I. Behavioral, affective, and cognitive aspects of family problem-solving interactions. *Journal of Abnormal Psychology*, **101**, 495–504.

Schwartz, C. E., Snidman, N. & Kagan, J. (1996). Early childhood temperament as a determinant of externalizing behavior in adolescence. *Development and Psychopathology*, **8**, 527–37.

Seligman, M. E. P., Peterson, C., Kaslow, N. et al. (1984). Attributional style and depressive symptoms among children. *Journal of Abnormal Psychology*, **93**, 235–8.

Sethi, S. & Nolen-Hoeksema, S. (1997). Gender differences in internal and external focusing among adolescents. *Sex Roles*, **37**, 687–700.

Shiner, R. L. & Marmorstein, N. R. (1998). Family environments of adolescents with lifetime depression: associations with maternal depression history. *Journal of the American Academy of Child and Adolescent Psychiatry*, **37**, 1152–60.

Shirk, S. R., Van Horn, M. & Leber, D. (1997). Dysphoria and children's processing of supportive interactions. *Journal of Abnormal Child Psychology*, **25**, 239–49.

Simmons, R. G., Burgeson, R., Carlton-Ford, S. & Blyth, D. A. (1987). The impact of cumulative change in early adolescence. *Child Development*, **58**, 1220–34.

Slavin, L. A. & Rainer, K. L. (1990). Gender differences in emotional support and depressive symptoms among adolescents: a prospective analysis. *American Journal of Community Psychology*, **18**, 407–21.

Smith, J. & Prior, M. (1995). Temperament and stress resilience in school-age children: a within-families study. *Journal of the American Academy of Child and Adolescent Psychiatry*, **34**, 168–79.

Spirito, A., Francis, G., Overholser, J. & Frank, N. (1996). Coping, depression, and adolescent suicide attempts. *Journal of Clinical Child Psychology*, **25**, 147–55.

Stark, K. D., Humphrey, L. L, Crook, K. & Lewis, K. (1990). Perceived family environments of depressed and anxious children: child's and maternal figure's perspectives. *Journal of Abnormal Child Psychology*, **18**, 527–47.

Steinberg, L., Lamborn, S. D., Darling, N., Mounts, N. S. & Dornbusch, S. M. (1994). Over-time changes in adjustment and competence among adolescents from authoritative, authoritarian, indulgent, and neglectful families. *Child Development*, **65**, 754–70.

Susman, E. J., Inoff-Germain, G., Nottelmann, E. D. et al. (1987). Hormones, emotional dispositions, and aggressive attributes in young adolescents. *Child Development*, **48**, 1114–34.

Teasdale, J. D. (1988) Cognitive vulnerability to persistent depression. *Cognition and Emotion*, **2**, 247–74.

Teasdale, J. D. (1999). Emotional processing, three modes of mind and the prevention of relapse in depression. *Behavioral Research and Therapy*, **37** (Suppl. 1), S53–77.

Teasdale, J. D. & Barnard, P. J. (1993). *Affect, Cognition and Change: remodelling depressive thought*. Hillsdale, NJ: Lawrence Erlbaum.

Teasdale, J. D. & Dent, J. (1987). Cognitive vulnerability to depression: an investigation of two hypotheses. *British Journal of Clinical Psychology*, **26**, 113–26.

Teasdale, J. D., Lloyd, C. A. & Hutton, J. M. (1998). Depressive thinking and dysfunctional schematic mental models. *British Journal of Clinical Psychology*, **37**, 247–57.

Thapar, A. & McGuffin, P. (1996). The genetic etiology of depressive symptoms: a developmental perspective. *Development and Psychopathology*, **8**, 751–60.

Velez, C. N., Johnson, J. & Cohen, P. (1989). A longitudinal analysis of selected risk factors for childhood psychopathology. *Journal of the American Academy of Child and Adolescent Psychiatry*, **28**, 861–4.

Weissman, M. M., Gammon, G. D., John, K. et al. (1987). Children of depressed parents: increased psychopathology and early onset of depression. *Archives of General Psychiatry*, **44**, 847–53.

Whitbeck, L. B., Hoyt, D. R., Simons, R. L. et al. (1992). Intergenerational continuity of parental rejection and depressed affect. *Journal of Personality and Social Psychology*, **63**, 1036–45.

Zemore, R. & Rinholm, J. (1989). Vulnerability to depression as a function of parental rejection and control. *Canadian Journal of Behavioral Science*, **21**, 364–76.

Zupen, B., Hammen, C. & Jaenicke, C. (1987). The effects of current mood and prior depressive history of self-schematic processing in children. *Journal of Experimental Child Psychology*, **43**, 149–58.

4

Physiological processes and the development of childhood and adolescent depression

Jeanne Brooks-Gunn, Jessica J. Auth, Anne C. Petersen and Bruce E. Compas

Recent conceptualizations of developmental psychopathology provide a useful framework for studying depression in childhood and adolescence (Sroufe & Rutter, 1984; Cicchetti & Schneider-Rosen, 1986; Rutter, 1986). These conceptualizations offer a framework for how depressed mood and clinical depression develop within sociocultural, biogenetic, personality and family domains, and how both types of depression change over time as a function of these domains. A developmental perspective focuses on the continuities and discontinuities between normal growth and psychopathology, age-related and gender-related alterations in coping and in symptom expression, and behavioural reorganizations that occur around salient developmental transitions. These include internal and external sources of competence and vulnerability, and the effects of development on pathology and of pathology on development (Attie & Brooks-Gunn, 1992). More work using such a framework has been conducted on depression than on other forms of psychopathology (Cicchetti & Schneider-Rosen, 1986; Rutter et al., 1986; Goodyer, 1990; Brooks-Gunn & Petersen, 1991; Cicchetti & Toth, 1991; Cicchetti et al., 1992).

In this chapter, we examine five issues of childhood and adolescent depression that consider the interplay between continuity and risk. The first focuses on the rate of various forms of depression in the childhood and adolescence years, to see whether, and at what ages, discontinuities in the prevalence of depression exist. Since children and adolescents differ in their rates of depressed mood and clinical depression, we go on to ask about the factors that might account for these discontinuities. The second issue, then, tracks the physiological concomitants and possible predictors of depression among the physiological changes that characterize early adolescence. However, adolescence not only involves physical growth, but also social, emotional, cognitive and academic changes (Brooks-Gunn & Petersen, 1983, 1991; Lerner & Foch, 1987; Gunnar & Collins,

1988; McAnarney & Levine, 1988; Feldman & Elliott, 1990). It has been hypothesized that rises in emotional problems generally, and depression specifically, are due to the confluence of events with which the adolescent must cope. Physiological change becomes only one set of a series of challenges (Brooks-Gunn & Petersen, 1984; Brooks-Gunn & Reiter, 1990). In the third section, the timing and sequencing of biopsychosocial changes in the first half of adolescence are discussed as they shed light on increases in depression seen at this time. The fourth section considers perhaps the greatest risk factor in the development of depression – family history and rearing environment. Familial history combines both possible physiological and environmental pathways to clinical depression. Finally, we take an admittedly brief look at what is known about continuity between clinical depression and less severe forms of depressed affect, especially as the study of physiological processes might shed light on this most important aspect of continuity.

Continuity of rates of depression across age and gender

Continuity in signs and symptoms

Following others such as Kazdin (1990), we distinguish between depressed affect and symptomatology, on the one hand, and clinical depression, on the other (ignoring for the moment various forms of clinical depression, as defined by *DSM-IV* (American Psychiatric Association, 1994) and other diagnostic systems). Depressive affect refers to periods of sadness, unhappiness or dysphoric mood that most individuals experience at some point in their lives. Depressed affect may co-occur with other negative emotions, such as fear, guilt, anger and disgust (Watson & Kendall, 1989). It also represents, in part, one of two broad affective dimensions identified by Watson & Tellegen (1985) – the two being negative and positive affect. Depressed affect is distinguishable from anxiety, in part because depressed mood is inversely correlated with positive affect while anxiety is not associated with positive mood (Watson & Kendall, 1989). Depressed affect occurs in about one-third of all youth at any point in time (range across studies is 15–45%: Roberts et al., 1991; Petersen et al., 1993). Little research charts age trends over the adolescent years, although a few studies suggest that it peaks in the middle adolescent years (Brooks-Gunn, 1991; Petersen et al., 1992; Ge et al., 1994). Girls are more likely to report depressed mood than boys. Fewer children report experiencing depressed mood, and reliable gender differences do not exist until adolescence (Rutter et al., 1976).[1]

A diagnosis of clinical depression is based on *DSM-IV* criteria (American

Psychiatric Association, 1994) and, unlike mood and symptomatology, must be derived from clinical interviews, not just self-report scales. Clinical depression is much more severe and lengthy; it has a major impact on activities of daily living. Epidemiological studies suggest that the point prevalence is around 4–5% for adults, with estimates ranging from 1% to 8.3% for adolescents (Rutter et al., 1976; Blazer et al., 1985; Weissman et al., 1987; Fendrich et al., 1990; Petersen et al., 1993).[2] It should be noted that lifetime prevalence rates of depression in studies of adolescence report rates of 20% (Lewinsohn et al., 1991). The lifetime prevalence for adolescence is similar to that of adults, which has been reported as 15–20% (Lewinsohn et al., 1993; Kessler et al., 1994). This similarity suggests that the history of depression observed in adults began during adolescence (Lewinsohn et al., 1993; Birmaher et al., 1996). Rates are lower for children (Rutter et al., 1976). Additionally, gender differences in rates of depression are seen following the transition to adolescence. Whereas many studies report gender differences, with girls having higher rates of depressive mood and disorder (usually 2 : 1 for girls to boys) emerging during the ages of 12–14 (Nolen-Hoeksema & Girgus, 1994), examination of effect sizes suggests that differences may be smaller in magnitude (see Compas et al., 1998, for a discussion of the influence of sampling and design on gender differences in rates of depression). Compas and colleagues (1997) demonstrated that gender differences in adolescents' depressed mood were nonsignificant or very small in a sample of adolescents with no history of referral for mental health services. (These important issues regarding prevalence and gender differences are discussed in more detail in Chapter 6.)

In summary, depressed mood and clinical depression increase during the adolescent years, as compared to the childhood years, with adolescent girls, especially those with a history of referral for mental health services, being at more risk for both aspects of depression than adolescent boys.

Comorbidity with other mental disorders

Research suggests that a high degree of comorbidity occurs between depression and other mental disorders (Maser & Cloninger, 1990). While past work with depressed adults failed to demonstrate significant comorbidity with any mental disorders except substance abuse disorders (Winokur et al., 1988; Rohde et al., 1991), it has been suggested more recently that depressed adults are at risk for comorbid disorders (Kessler et al., 1996), especially anxiety-related disorders such as agoraphobia, situational phobia, panic disorder and generalized anxiety disorder (Kendler et al., 1996). Further, comorbid anxiety tends to be experienced more frequently by those adults who suffer from severe typical depression involving frequent, long episodes of severe symptoms than by those who exhibit mild typical depression.

Rohde et al. (1991) suggest that comorbid findings are much stronger and more prevalent in depressed adolescent samples than with depressed adults. Depressed adolescents are significantly more likely than expected by chance to have any one of the existing mental disorders, with the exception of bipolar disorder, in addition to their depression. With respect to the prevalence of comorbidity in depressed children and adolescents, Simonoff et al. (1997) found that approximately 77% of depressive subjects demonstrated one other comorbid mental disorder, while 27% of subjects displayed two or more comorbid disorders. Depression in children and adolescents is significantly comorbid with many anxiety-related disorders such as separation anxiety, simple phobia, social phobia, agoraphobia and overanxious disorder (Maser & Cloninger, 1990; Hewitt et al., 1997; Simonoff et al., 1997). Sex differences exist, as depressed males are more likely to demonstrate comorbid oppositional defiant disorder and conduct disorder, while depressed females are more likely to exhibit comorbid eating disorders (Rohde et al., 1991). Research is inconsistent regarding the likelihood of comorbidity between depression and attention deficit hyperactivity disorder in children and adolescents, with some suggesting moderate correlations (Hewitt et al., 1997) and some demonstrating a lack of association (Simonoff et al., 1997).

In terms of timing of onset of depression and comorbid mental disorders in childhood and adolescence, depression is significantly more likely to follow all comorbid disorders except for eating disorders (Rohde et al., 1991; Graber et al., 1994; Attie & Brooks-Gunn, 1995). Anxiety, the disorder most commonly comorbid with child and adolescent depression, tends to precede depression (Angst et al., 1990) approximately 85.1% of the time (Rohde et al., 1991). Rutter et al. (1993) assert that the mechanisms which underlie comorbidity may differ according to comorbid associations. For example, some comorbid disorders may be manifestations of the same genetic disposition, others may be the result of common environmental risk factors, and still other comorbid disorders may reflect both genetic and environmental mediation. Just as genetic disposition and family environment must be considered when examining child and adolescent depression, such factors should not be ignored when investigating depression and its comorbidity with other mental disorders, as well as the timing of onset of such disorders.

Continuity in physiological bases of depression across developmental stages

Physiological bases of clinical depression and other forms of psychopathology have long been postulated, and research continues at a rapid pace. Even environmentally focused theories must take into account physiological change, because environmental events are mediated by the brain. Regardless of the contribution of environmental and physiological events to its onset, biological dysregulation occurs once a depressive episode is triggered. Akiskal & McKinney (1973) have termed this the final common pathway model. Shelton et al. (1991) describe biological dysregulation following the onset of depression as taking 'a life of its own', which further influences behaviour, thought, mood and physiological patterns.

Theories differ in the amount of weight they place on the centrality of physiological processes in the emergence of depression and in the recovery from an episode. Physiological processes may be: (1) a response to environmental events, with biological dysregulation a result of psychosocial factors; (2) different prior to the occurrence of any environmental event for those individuals who go on to have a depressive episode; or (3) a reflection of a genetic susceptibility to experiencing the biological dysregulation associated with depression. To complicate matters further, different subtypes of depression probably have some common and some different physiological precursors and concomitants. The same is true for disorders that often co-occur with depression.

In this section, evidence is reviewed for children, adolescents and adults in several areas: biological dysregulation in the hypothalamic–pituitary axes, neurotransmitter deficits and links with the hypothalamic–pituitary axes, and other possible physiological influences. Data on children are included since any differences seen in physiological responses of children and adolescents might be due to the dramatic changes in the hypothalamic–pituitary–gonadal (HPG) and hypothalamic–pituitary–adrenal (HPA) axes which are a part of puberty. Whenever possible, reference is made to whether younger or older adolescents were studied. If changes in the neuroendocrine system at puberty influence the patterning of biological dysregulation associated with puberty, it is likely that older adolescents, having completed the pubertal process to a large extent, will evidence physiological patterns more similar to adults than will younger adolescents in the midst of puberty.

All of this research focuses on individuals with clinical depression; in contrast, research on psychological mechanisms considers both clinical depression and depressed affect. Additionally, no unique mechanisms have been proposed for adolescent clinical depression relative to adult depression.

Physiological markers of depression

Biological studies have the potential to provide information on the aetiology of various subtypes of depression, but can only do so with the use of specific comparative and longitudinal methodologies. Much of the current research is not designed to address aetiology; rather, it is concentrated on demonstrating associations between depression and neuroendocrine dysregulation. Consequently, even though literally hundreds of studies have been published on the physiological concomitants of depression and affective disorder, little evidence has been found for the existence of physiological markers for depression (Puig-Antich, 1986; Gold et al., 1988). No physiological test exists that provides a reliable diagnosis of depression. Consequently, the term 'marker' must be interpreted with caution.

The concept of physiological markers is a useful way to think about physiological influences upon psychopathology in general and depression in particular. Distinguishing between state and trait physiological markers allows for a separation of instances of biological dysregulation that are concomitant versus predictive. State markers are those which occur during a depressive episode but not at other times. Trait markers are those which differentiate individuals who are depressed from those who are not across depressive episodes, recovery and illness-free phases.

Several possible explanations for a continuing abnormality in a physiological marker after recovery from a depressive episode must be ruled out before assuming that a true trait marker has been demonstrated (Puig-Antich, 1986). First, the timing of assessment is critical, since recovery in a physiological marker might continue during and past the recovery period of the episode. Second, a physiological marker might appear in the first depressive episode, and remain different thereafter. This would not be an example of a true trait marker because the abnormality was not present *prior to* the onset of any depressive episode. Third, a physiological marker may be generally associated with psychopathology or affective disorder, not depression *per se*.

Additionally, studies need to follow individuals for a long enough time, using repeated clinical and physiological assessment, in order to rule out the possibility that physiological markers are not due to lags and leads in biological dysregulation, which no doubt occur. At the very minimum, studies of individuals who are depressed and those who are not must be conducted, seeing the depressed individuals during recovery as well as during the depressive episode. Most studies do not meet this minimal requirement. Additionally, given the expense of obtaining a sample prior to the onset of any depressive episode – a criterion necessary to rule out the second factor above – prospective studies of offspring of depressed parents are recommended.

Finally, studies should compare not only individuals who are depressed and those who are not, but also those individuals who have another disorder. This is particularly important given the high degree of comorbidity that occurs between depression and other forms of psychopathology (Maser & Cloninger, 1990). Similar arguments could be made for the study of different subtypes of depression, although the lack of agreement on what symptoms constitute a subtype and the historical changes in definitions of what symptoms constitute a subtype make it difficult to review the extant literature. Future research on physiological mechanisms must however pay more attention to putative subtypes and the timing of depressive episodes (Puig-Antich, 1986).

There are three areas providing clues that physiological differences may exist: (1) variability in response to different treatment modalities, including lack of effects in adolescents; (2) the possibility that physiological markers might differ for depressed individuals who are suicidal and those who are not; and (3) the speculation that physiological abnormalities may be more likely for those with a greater genetic risk for depression (i.e. offspring of depressed parents who exhibit their first depressive episode as children or adolescents, or bipolar versus unipolar depressed individuals). If true physiological markers are discovered, approaches might allow for the identification of individuals at risk for depression (especially in families with a history of affective disorder) and for specifying treatment.

Dysregulation in the hypothalamic–endocrine systems

The bulk of the literature on physiological bases of depression focuses on the limbic system, specifically the hypothalamus–pituitary axes. Those involving the adrenal (HPA), the thyroid (HPT), the gonadal (HPG) and the somatotropic (HPS) axes have been studied, with all systems exhibiting varying degrees of dysregulation in association with depression. Additionally, sleep architecture changes and melatonin secretion have been the subject of study, with alterations occurring in many depressed individuals. All of this research supports the general notion that biological dysregulation occurs during episodes of depression and, in a few cases, during recovery periods as well. But research is needed that examines the correlations among biological indicators during episodes of depression and subsequent recovery. In addition, the identification of links between behavioural manifestations and types of biological dysregulation would be valuable.

Several endocrine systems are involved in depression. In all cases, a releasing hormone in the hypothalamus moves to the pituitary gland and influences the release there of a stimulating hormone. This hormone then stimulates the release of a hormone by the particular gland in question (thyroid, adrenal, gonad). This hormone is secreted into circulation, where it acts to inhibit the production of the releasing and stimulating hormone at the hypothalamic and pituitary levels (Shelton et al., 1991).

Gonads develop during fetal growth. In males, androgens are secreted by the gonads, initiating a process that results in male internal and external sex organs and affects the HPG axis. In the absence of androgens the sex organs are female in appearance (Money & Erhardt, 1972). In the first few months of life, the levels of circulating hormones increase for what appears to be a short period of time (in males and probably in females as well). For the rest of the preschool period, levels of sex steroid hormones are quite low (Reiter, 1987). Sex steroids are due to the suppression of gonadotrophin-releasing hormone production and secretion (Reiter & Grumbach, 1982).

During middle childhood, sex steroid levels begin to increase (Kaplan et al., 1976). The process that triggers these increases is not well understood. Two relatively independent processes occur. The first is adrenarche, which occurs when the adrenal gland begins producing androgens in both boys and girls. The second is gonadarche, which occurs a few years after adrenarche. The HPG axis is reactivated. A release on the inhibition by the increase in steroid hormones, which is probably mediated by the central nervous system, accounts for the increase in gonadotrophin secretion. Large increases in gonadal and adrenal sex steroids occur for both boys and girls (see Brooks-Gunn and Reiter, 1990 for a review).

These changes occur prior to the onset of secondary sexual characteristics. Increases in gonadotrophins (luteinizing hormone and follicle-stimulating hormone) occur as the HPG axis is reactivated. Additionally, the pituitary secretes these gonadotrophins in pulsatile patterns, such that bursts seem to influence the gonads, which then increase production of androgens and oestrogens (Boyar et al., 1972). Physical changes associated with puberty follow, as does the maturation of the gonads (ova in females, sperm in males). The pulsatile secretion of the gonadotrophins occurs during sleep.

Two questions are relevant to our focus on depression in adolescents. The first has to do with whether the early physiological changes of adrenarche and gonadarche have any effect on children's behaviour, in this case depressed affect. To our knowledge, research has not looked at physiological changes and behaviour in middle childhood, either in terms of overall levels of sex steroid activity or the onset of pulsatile secretions. The second has to do with children diagnosed with clinical depression. No work has looked at whether childhood episodes are associated with early physiological pubertal changes (although Graber & Brooks-Gunn are currently conducting such a study). Interestingly, research with young women who have anorexia nervosa suggests that gonadotrophin output often reverts to prepubertal patterns (i.e. nighttime pulsatile secretions; cortisol secretion is also affected: Boyar et al., 1977; Katz et al., 1978). With weight gain and recovery, gonadotrophin secretions return to postpubertal secretory patterns. Given the fact that sleep architecture seems to be affected in some youth with depressive disorders, and that gonadotrophin secretion changes are first seen at night, comparable research with clinically depressed children and young adolescents might prove fruitful.

Hypothalamic–pituitary–adrenal axis

Proportionately more research has focused on the HPA axis than other hypothalamic–pituitary axes. Generally, dysregulation in the HPA axis occurs during depressive episodes in adults, as evidenced by cortisol hypersecretion and responses to challenges of cortisol secretion in some, but not all, depressed adults.

Adults who are depressed are more likely to secrete more cortisol over 24 hours, to have more secretory sessions, and to secrete in the late evening and early morning, thus having the usually diurnal secretory pattern broken (Sachar, 1975; Asnis et al., 1985; Pepper & Krieger, 1985; Sachar et al., 1985). It has been estimated that 30–50% of adults with endogenous depression hypersecrete (Sachar et al., 1973; Jarrett et al., 1983). Within the adult age range, depressed individuals who are older may be more likely to hypersecrete, while this is not true in nondepressed individuals (Asnis et al., 1981). Hypersecretion tends to disappear with recovery (Greden et al., 1983). However, it has also been suggested that hypersecretion may interfere with recovery processes. Research with inpatient depressed adults suggests that there is an inverse relationship between HPA activity level in adults and response to cognitive behavioural psychotherapy (Thase et al., 1996). Specifically, higher levels of cortisol secretion are associated with lower responsiveness to cognitive behavioural treatment. The authors hypothesize that sustained elevated levels of cortisol may cause hippocampal cell death and cortical atrophy, which may impair adult hypersecreters' ability to use the cognitive methods of therapy.

In contrast, much research suggests that depressed children and adolescents are less likely to hypersecrete cortisol than adults (Klee & Garfinkel, 1984; Puig-Antich, 1987; Kutcher & Marton, 1989; Dahl et al., 1991b; Birmaher et al., 1996). Although some subgroups of depressed youth (e.g. melancholics and suicidal youth) may have higher baseline cortisol levels than normal controls, some have found no significant difference in the cortisol secretions of depressed versus nondepressed youth (Birmaher et al., 1996). Evidence is inconclusive when researchers look specifically at the time of day of cortisol measurement in depressed subjects. It has been demonstrated that cortisol secretion is higher at the beginning of sleep for depressed than nondepressed adolescents (Dahl et al., 1991a), with this elevation being most pronounced for depressed adolescents who are suicidal (Kutcher et al., 1991; Dahl et al., 1992), while others demonstrate that depressed children have lower cortisol secretions than normal controls during the first 4 hours after sleep onset (De Bellis et al., 1996).

Recent researchers suggest that the above findings relied on single samples of plasma levels taken from inpatient subjects, and that when multiple samples of cortisol are attained through saliva collection, a procedure that is as sensitive as, and also less invasive than, blood collection (Foreman & Goodyer, 1988), evening cortisol hypersecretion is associated with depression in childhood and adolescents (Goodyer et al., 1996; Herbert et al., 1996). Morning hyposecretion of dehydroepiandrosterone (DHEA), another HPA hormone, has also been associated with depression in childhood and adolescence, and exerts a risk effect on the likelihood of depression that is independent of that which is exerted by evening cortisol hypersecretion (Goodyer et al., 1996). Researchers have examined the association of childhood and adolescent depression to the ratio of cortisol to DHEA as a more sensitive index of abnormal cortisol levels (Goodyer et al., 1998). It is suggested that the cortisol/DHEA ratios found during evening and midnight measurements are significantly higher than those found at other times during the day. Further, the higher evening and midnight cortisol/DHEA ratios are significantly associated with depression, and are predictive of persistent depression that lasts at least 36 weeks after the initial assessment.

Goodyer and colleagues (1998) conclude that the brain's exposure to abnormal ratios of cortisol/DHEA during the hours at the end of the day may impede children's and adolescents' recovery from depression. Given findings with adults and the potentially poor effects of hypersecretion on cognition, research is needed to examine secretion and cognition patterns in children; such studies may provide insights into more effective treatment strategies with children. (See Chapter 8 for a discussion of cortisol and DHEA as precursors of major depression and Chapter 6 for the possible relative effects of DHEA and sex hormones on depression. A full account of the neuroendocrine issues in depression is given in Chapter 9.)

The provocative test most often used in this type of research involves giving a dose of dexamethasone to see whether cortisol is suppressed. Nonsuppression may be more likely to occur in depressed adults than nondepressed adults. The estimates of nonsuppression vary greatly, however. Most studies report that between 30% and 70% of adults during a depression episode do not suppress cortisol, as compared to less than 15% of adults who have not been depressed (Amsterdam et al., 1982; Rabkin et al., 1983; Kutcher & Marton, 1989). Nonsuppression rates related to depression are lower during recovery periods; dexamethasone escape during recovery may be predictive of the onset of another depressive episode (Greden et al., 1983). First-degree relatives of adults with depression tend to suppress significantly less cortisol than normal controls (and suppress significantly more cortisol than depressed individuals), even though these relatives have no current or lifetime DSM-III-R diagnosis (American Psychiatric Association, 1987) of a psychiatric disorder (Holsboer et al., 1995). Long-term follow-up is needed to see whether or not the premorbid HPA abnormality indicates increased vulnerability to the development of an affective disorder.

Estimates for dexamethasone nonsuppression are similar or, more likely, lower for adolescents, with most studies falling within the 30–50% range for depressed inpatients (Crumley et al., 1982; Extein et al., 1982; Robins et al., 1982; Targum & Capodanno, 1983). Examining the dexamethasone suppression test (DST) results from four adolescent studies yielded a sensitivity estimate of 32% and a specificity of 67% (Kutcher & Marton, 1989) – not high enough for use as a diagnosis but similar to what is reported for adults. Little evidence is available on dexamethasone suppression during recovery in adolescents.

Studies using DST for children report mixed findings (Klee & Garfinkel, 1984; Livingston et al., 1984; Weller et al., 1984; Puig-Antich, 1987; Pfeffer et al., 1989; Naylor et al., 1990). Some studies report evidence of dexamethasone nonsuppression in depressed children (Puig-Antich, 1987; Pfeffer et al., 1989; however, see Birmaher et al., 1992, who found no evidence of 24-hour cortisol or DST responses discriminating among several groups of 6–12-year-olds – outpatients with major depressive disorder, nonaffectively disturbed psychiatric controls and normal controls). Mixed findings may be due in part to initial plasma dexamethasone levels for DST suppressors and nonsuppressors and possibly DST dose by weight differences across studies (Naylor et al., 1990).

Research has examined the association between basal pituitary–adrenal hormone levels at rest and individual differences in the psychological functioning of adults (Zorrilla et al., 1995). Adult self-reports of higher self-esteem and a higher degree of hardiness, all proposed buffers against depressive symptoms, are associated with higher basal levels of cortisol and β-endorphin – two indicators of hypothalamic–pituitary–adrenal activity. It is suggested that this relatively high level of cortisol and β-endorphin may reduce stress responsiveness, which may protect the individuals from the affective disruption (e.g. depression and emotional lability) associated with stress-related glucocorticoid increase. Further research is needed in this area to examine this notion.

Hypothalamic–pituitary–somatotropic axis

Most of the studies of secretion of growth hormone (GH) have focused on children, given that GH is highly age-related. GH is secreted mostly at night in children prior to puberty. After puberty, GH secretion occurs more evenly during the day and night (Finkelstein et al., 1972). It has been suggested that daytime and nighttime secretion might be under the control of different neurotransmitter systems (Mendelson, 1982). Studies to date that examine nocturnal GH secretions in depressed children and adolescents demonstrate inconsistent results. While some findings suggest there is no significant difference in the nocturnal GH secretions of prepubertal depressed children and normal controls (Dahl et al., 1992; DeBellis et al., 1995), other researchers have found that nighttime GH secretions of depressed youth are blunted as compared to controls (Kutcher et al., 1991), with blunting being more pronounced for depressed girls (De Bellis et al., 1996) or suicidal youth (Dahl et al., 1992). Still other researchers suggest that depressed children hypersecrete GH during sleep as compared to nondepressed controls (Puig-Antich et al., 1984b). Further, depressed children who report at least one stressful life event (e.g. death of a parent) secrete more GH during sleep than both depressed children without a stressful life event and nondepressed controls. Future investigations of nocturnal GH secretions of depressed youth should include a more comprehensive examination of stressful life events (including the timing, severity and duration of stressors) and their impact on GH activity.

Hypothalamic–pituitary–thyroid axis

There is some evidence that thyroid-stimulating hormone (TSH) may be lower in depressed than nondepressed adult patients (Amsterdam et al., 1979; Extein et al., 1980). Much of the past research examining children and adolescents suggests that the level of TSH is similar for depressed and nondepressed youth (Khan, 1987; Puig-Antich, 1987; Brambilla et al., 1989; Garcia et al., 1991). This has recently been supported for female children and adolescents, but not for males; pre- and early pubertal boys with depression have significantly lower levels of TSH than normal controls (Dorn et al., 1997).

Research examining the thyroid hormone thyroxine (T_4) yields inconsistent findings. Similar to findings with depressed adults, some research suggests that T_4 levels are higher in depressed adolescents than in a normal control group (Sokolov et al., 1994). However, other research suggests that depressed adolescents have lower concentrations of T_4 than do normal controls (with concentrations of T_4 still within the normal range: Dorn et al., 1996). This was supported for pre- and early pubertal depressed boys, but not for girls (Dorn et al., 1997). Depressed youth tend to have significantly lower levels of another thyroid hormone called triiodothyronine (T_3) than normal counterparts, with levels still within the normal range (Dorn et al., 1997). A low level of T_3 is associated with hypothyroidism, which is associated with depression (Rose, 1985).

Hypothalamic–pituitary–gonadal axis

Little research has focused on the HPG axis and its role in depression; this is surprising given the interest in gender differences in depression in the pubertal and postpubertal years. It has been hypothesized that low levels of oestrogen are associated with depressive symptoms in adult women (Benedek, 1952; Melges & Hamburg, 1977; Buchanan et al., 1992). Studies have focused on menarche, menstruation, pregnancy and menopause, typically with respect to depressive symptoms, not clinical depression *per se*.

Pubertal studies using menarche as a marker usually do not report an increase in depressive affect or negative affect (Brooks-Gunn & Ruble, 1983; Brooks-Gunn, 1984). However, increases in oestrogen, specifically during the most rapid period of increase during puberty, have been associated with nonlinear increases in depressive symptoms in one study (Brooks-Gunn & Warren, 1989; Warren & Brooks-Gunn, 1989); the increases in depressive symptoms occurred with the most rapid increase in hormones. Nevertheless, the magnitude of these effects was small; oestradiol accounted for about 1% of the variance while life events occurring in the past 6 months accounted for 8% of the variance in depressive symptoms. However, these increases were predictive of depressive affect a year later, even controlling for initial depressive symptom scores (Paikoff et al., 1991b). Another study, using levels of oestrogen rather than categories of oestrogen functioning, and only looking at nonlinear effects, did not report associations between oestradiol and depressive symptoms (Susman et al., 1987b, 1998). In addition, in a unique study that used an experimental design to examine the effects of hormone replacement on mood and depressive symptoms in young adolescents with delayed pubertal development, oestrogen had a small effect on the withdrawn behaviour in girls but not on depressive symptoms *per se* (Susman et al., 1987a).

Surprisingly, given the prevalence in the clinical literature of discussions of pre- and postpubertal depression, few studies actually measure pubertal status relative to depression. Rutter (1980, 1986) found some evidence that boys were more likely to be diagnosed with depression if they were later in puberty compared to those prior to or just beginning the process.[3] Later work (involving medical second review) does not confirm this hypothesis (Angold & Rutter, 1992). Angold et al. (1998) found that girls had higher rates of depression than boys once they were in mid to late pubertal development, and that gender differences in rates of depression were less pronounced prepubertally and in the early phases of puberty. Further research in the area suggests that there are significant effects for pubertal hormone (oestrogen and testosterone) levels in the onset of negative affect (Brooks-Gunn & Warren, 1989) and depression (Warren & Brooks-Gunn, 1989) in adolescent girls, and that hormonal effects are independent of age and pubertal morphological status (Angold et al., 1999). Morphological status is more a marker for the hormonal changes that underlie them than a predictor of adolescent female depression *per se* (see Chapter 6).

Most studies have focused on the occurrence of negative moods and various phases of the menstrual cycle, with more negative moods being hypothesized during times of low oestrogen concentrations or falling oestrogen concentrations. Research does not support this hypothesis when cognitive and social attributions are controlled (Ruble & Brooks-Gunn, 1979, 1987). Another line of research actually measures oestrogen concentration. Two studies report that oestrogen levels and the ratio of oestrogen to progesterone were higher in the premenstrual phase for those women who reported premenstrual symptoms, including negative affect (Backstrom et al., 1976; Munday et al., 1981). At first glance, these findings do not fit with the prediction that cycle plans characterized by low oestrogen production are linked to negative moods. The effect could be due to an abnormality in hormonal functioning in women who report premenstrual symptoms rather than actual levels (Dinnerstein et al., 1984). The findings of increased depressive effect as hormone levels rise during puberty also do not accord with beliefs about low oestrogen and depressed mood.

Dysregulation in sleep patterns

Diurnal rhythms are expressed in neuroendocrine activity, sleep–wake cycles and body temperature (Wehr & Goodwin, 1981). These rhythms are regulated by two oscillators, which exhibit dysregulation during depressive episodes probably due to central nervous system hyperarousal (Gold et al., 1986, 1988; Sack et al., 1987). Depression appears to impair the sleep onset mechanism, rendering sleep disturbance a possible physiological marker (Reynolds et al., 1987).

Sleep architecture has been studied extensively in adults who are depressed, with the findings indicating disturbance such as decreased rapid eye movement (REM) latency, increased electrical activity during REM and sleep onset delays (Reynolds et al., 1987). During periods of recovery, sleep rhythms return to normal for some but not all patients. Continuation of sleep dysregulation is probably predictive of recurrence (Giles et al., 1987).

Over the past two decades, there has been significant research activity on the question of sleep regulation in depressed children and adolescents (Puig-Antich et al., 1984a,b,c,d). Four studies comparing the expression of sleep abnormalities in prepubertal depressed children and normal controls have demonstrated inconsistent evidence, with much of it suggesting no significant group differences in sleep variables (Dahl et al., 1991a; Puig-Antich et al., 1982; Young et al., 1982). However, reduced REM latency has been demonstrated in inpatient depressed children (Emslie et al., 1990) and in response to the infusion of arecoline, a cholinergic agonist, in outpatient depressed children (Dahl et al., 1994). Regardless of these suggested sleep abnormalities, depressed children tend to demonstrate better sleep efficiency as compared to normal controls (Puig-Antich et al., 1983; Emslie et al., 1990).

Among nine published studies comparing the expression of sleep abnormalities in depressed adolescents versus normal controls (Lahmeyer et al., 1983; Goetz et al., 1987; Appleboom-Fondu et al., 1988; Dahl et al., 1990, 1996; Kahn & Todd, 1990; Kutcher et al., 1992; Emslie et al., 1994; Riemann et al., 1995), three suggested that depressed adolescents, like their prepubertal counterparts, demonstrate reduced REM latency. Unlike findings with depressed children, however, two of the eight studies reported decreased sleep efficiency in depressed adolescents. Dahl et al. (1992) proposed the interesting hypothesis that sleep is protected in children (Carskadon & Dement, 1987), with the developmental changes of puberty reducing this protection.

It now appears that there is dysregulation in the sleep onset mechanism of depressed adolescents, as depressed adolescents have significantly elevated levels of cortisol at sleep onset (Rao et al., 1996), and demonstrate significantly prolonged sleep latency when compared to nondepressed controls during several baseline nights of sleep (Dahl et al., 1996). Sleep latency differences have also been observed during recovery sleep, with depressives demonstrating significantly more prolonged sleep latencies than normal controls (Dahl et al., 1996). Research also suggests that the sleep onset mechanism is impaired in suicidal adolescents – blunting GH, increasing cortisol and increasing sleep latency (Dahl et al., 1992). Further, normal age-related changes in sleep features appear to be accelerated in depressed patients at all ages (Knowles & MacLean, 1990).

Biological dysregulation in the neurotransmitter systems

The neurotransmitter systems, specifically the serotonergic, the cholinergic and the noradrenergic systems, have also been investigated. Activity, in all three has been implicated in depression, with current research testing the notion that patterns of dysregulation in different systems are associated with different subtypes of depression (Gold et al., 1986; Shelton et al., 1991). Simple notions of deficit theories have been abandoned given the fact that interactions occur among neurotransmitter systems, among hypothalamic–pituitary systems, and between the two systems as well as between different substrates of the brain. Additionally, neurotransmitter activity is regulated at multiple levels, including synthesis, packaging and storage, release, reuptake, metabolism, and postsynaptic receptor responsiveness (Gold et al., 1988). Thus, current studies attempt to determine the level at which neurotransmitter dysregulation associated with depression occurs. For example, postsynaptic receptor responsiveness has been implicated in depression, which was suspected given the lag time between pharmacological treatment and response in adults.

Links between all hypothalamic–pituitary axes and neurotransmitter systems are being demonstrated at an ever-increasing pace. These studies will provide much needed specific information on which neurotransmitter systems are affected in different subtypes of depression. This new generation of studies should result in more effective treatment, since specification of dysregulation in particular neurotransmitter systems provides the information necessary to determine which pharmacological agent, or mix of agents, will be effective for an individual. Presently, it is very difficult, if not impossible, to know *a priori* how any individual will respond to a particular antidepressant drug (Joyce & Paykel, 1989).

Neurotransmitter systems have been implicated in depression for over 40 years. Current research has moved away from deficiency hypotheses to more complex models involving both presynaptic and postsynaptic events (down-regulation and effects on second messenger systems), rather than focus on the former exclusively (Vetulani & Sulser, 1975; Shelton et al., 1991). Additionally, the complexity may be characterized as an unstable or dysregulated system, rather than a deficient one (Siever & Davis, 1985).

Maturational changes in neurotransmitter activity and regulation occur, although less research has traced these changes compared to those in the hypothalamic–endocrine systems. Catecholamine systems take until adulthood to become fully functional in primates (Goldman-Rakic & Brown, 1982). In humans, short attention spans in children and the infrequency of mania in depressed children may also be indicative of an immature catecholamine system (Wender, 1971; Puig-Antich, 1987). In contrast, the serotonergic and cholinergic systems are functional prior to adulthood, at least in rats (Lidor & Molliver, 1982; Shelton et al., 1991).[4]

Generally, depression may be associated with an activated locus ceruleus–noradrenaline (norepinephrine) system. Besides the noradrenergic system, the cholinergic system may be hyperresponsive in depressed patients while γ-aminobutyric acid (GABA) and serotonin may be low (Gold et al., 1988).

A number of studies are linking neurotransmitter functioning to hypothalamic–endocrine dysregulation, typically through the study of pharmacological substances with different neurotransmitter effects. In the HPA axis, nonsuppression of cortisol to the dexamethasone test may be associated with cholinergic overactivity in some depressed individuals (Carroll et al., 1980). Noradrenergic system deficits have also been implicated, as seen in studies of administration of d-amphetamine, desmethylimipramine (DMI) and clonidine. All three tend to stimulate cortisol secretion, or result in a smaller increase in cortisol secretion, in nondepressed controls but not in depressed individuals (Sachar et al., 1973, 1985; Siever et al., 1984; Asnis et al., 1985; however, see the findings in the study of two samples by Waterman et al., 1991, with adolescents). The serotonergic system may also be involved, because when given 5-hydroxy-L-tryptophan (L-5HTP), depressed children show a blunted cortisol response relative to nondepressed controls (N. D. Ryan et al., unpublished manuscript; Dahl et al., 1991a; Birmaher et al., 1997).

In the HPS axis, dysregulation in GH in depressed individuals probably involves a functional noradrenergic deficit, as seen in studies using clonidine, (DMI) and d-amphetamine (Sachar, 1975; Langer et al., 1976; Checkley et al., 1981; Siever et al., 1982). Similar findings have been reported for a sample of adolescents with major depressive disorder and those who are suicidal compared to nondepressed controls using DMI (Ryan et al., 1994). However, no differences were found in GH response using amphetamine, with the exception of one finding in one of two samples examined (Waterman et al., 1991). As Ryan et al. (1988) point out, the serotonergic system is probably also involved (most likely in a decrease in presynaptic serotonergic activity), just as was seen in dysregulation of the HPA axis.

Drug therapy

As indicated, research on neurotransmitter systems and pharmacological treat-ment of depression are inherently linked. Tricyclic drugs do not seem to alter depression in adolescents (Petersen et al., 1993; Birmaher et al., 1996). More recent research, however, has suggested that fluoxetine (Prozac), a selective reuptake inhibitor of central nervous system presynaptically released serotonin, is effective in treating depressive symptoms in children, adolescents and adults. Fluoxetine has become the most widely prescribed antidepressant medication since 1988 due to its effectiveness and lack of side-effects relative to other antidepressants (Stokes & Holtz, 1997). Specifically, research with adults has demonstrated that fluoxetine is equally as effective as tricyclic antidepressants (Fabre et al., 1991; Bowden et al., 1993; Nielsen et al., 1993), but is not associated with the side-effects found with other drugs because it lacks the cholinergic, histaminergic and α-adrenergic receptor blockades that tricyclics demonstrate (Stokes & Holtz, 1997).

Studies with adults have suggested that fluoxetine is as effective as tricyclics in treating severe depression in adult inpatients (Evans & Lye, 1992) and outpatients (Montgomery, 1989; Pande & Sayler, 1993) and is effective in double-blind trials comparing fluoxetine with a placebo among mild and moderately depressed individuals (Pande & Sayler, 1993; Orengo et al., 1996). Stokes & Holtz (1997) assert that fluoxetine may be more effective than tricyclics in treating severely depressed individuals with suicidal ideation and intent. Suicidal behaviour is associated with low serotonin activity (Murphy & Kelleher, 1994), which is thought to be alleviated by the fluoxetine-induced enhancement of central serotonin neurotransmission (Stokes & Holtz, 1997). Some reports of increased suicidal tendencies and aggression have been re-ported as side-effects of antidepressants (Teicher et al., 1990), but this finding is lower for fluoxetine than tricyclics (Beasley et al., 1992).

Of particular note is that recent research has demonstrated the relative effectiveness of fluoxetine in treating depression in children and adolescents (Birmaher, 1998). Specifically, eight out of nine adolescents with major depress-ion were much improved or very much improved by 24 weeks of fluoxetine treatment (Colle et al., 1994). Further, five of the eight adolescents were able to stop taking fluoxetine 6–9 months after treatment began due to sustained improvement in mood, and two of those five remained well at 12-month follow-up. Similar effectiveness of fluoxetine treatment was demonstrated by Emslie et al. (1997), who found no difference in response rates of those 12 years old and below, and those 13 years old and above. Further, suicidal thoughts decreased significantly with fluoxetine treatment, and depression-related sleep difficulties were improved slightly more by fluoxetine than placebo (Simeon et al., 1990). This work not only holds promise for continued improvement in the treatment of children and adolescents with depression and related problems but also adds insight into physiological systems that may be at the root of depressive experiences, if not the cause.

Possible physiological concomitants of depression

Work is beginning to focus on brain function other than the neuroendocrine systems. A particularly intriguing hypothesis involves the notion of kindling, which 'refers to the eventual development of motor seizures to repeated electrical stimulation of the brain with current which was originally insufficient to produce overt behavioral effects' (Munoz, 1989; Munoz et al., 1993). The fact that subsequent depressive episodes often occur with shorter and shorter latencies might be due to such a kindling phenomenon (Post et al., 1984). The biological changes that occur during the first few episodes might sensitize the organism to experience biological dysregulation more easily (i.e. in the face of a less potent environmental and/or biological event). Consequently, early depressive episodes may predispose the individual to be more susceptible to subsequent episodes.

Timing and sequencing of pubertal events

Generally, the evidence to date is not clear as to whether the biological underpinnings – or at least concomitants – of clinical depression differ dramatically across the life span. The next generation of neuroendocrinological studies may yield more age-related differences.

Adolescents differ from children cognitively, socially and emotionally, not just physiologically as indicated by their acquisition of a reproductively mature body. However, we believe that the more physiological approaches to the study of depression during adolescence would be enhanced by a consideration of the context in which such changes occur. As stated in the introduction, the transition to adolescence brings with it a plethora of challenges in every realm of development. It has been hypothesized that the confluence of events, many of them novel, accounts in part for the rise in rates of clinical depression and depressed mood. Several studies have documented that the number of potentially stressful life events (in the peer, school and family realms) is higher during the young adolescent period than earlier or later (Compas, 1987; Brooks-Gunn, 1991; Paikoff & Brooks-Gunn, 1991; Ge et al., 1994; Compas et al., 1998). These events probably influence depressive symptoms via their effect on daily stress levels (Compas et al., 1989). The increase in life events over time is the strongest predictor of depressed symptom scores, and *changes* in these scores, as seen in one study measuring life events and girls' depression for 4 years (Brooks-Gunn, 1991; Ge et al., 1994; see also Simmons et al., 1987 for a similar finding looking at life events cross-sectionally). Interestingly, timing of puberty, but not tempo or current status, was associated with depressive symptoms, such that being an early maturer was a risk factor.[5] However, like the findings using hormonal levels rather than pubertal timing, social life events accounted for much more of the variance than pubertal timing (Brooks-Gunn, 1991). In a recent epidemiological study, pubertal timing has been linked to higher lifetime prevalence of depression in adolescent girls but not boys, as well as other disorders (Graber et al., 1997); similar findings for girls have also been reported for elevated depressive symptoms (Hayward et al., 1997). These studies have documented links to timing but as yet have not identified mechanisms through which the experience of timing translates into poor mental health, especially for girls.

The occurrence of life events may help to explain the gender differentials emerging during the middle of adolescence; girls experience more stressful events than boys in the first half of adolescence, which is directly associated with their higher depressed affect scores (Petersen et al., 1991). Girls may also perceive and even experience a particular event as more stressful than boys, adding further to the burden of multiple life events. For example, boys, being given more freedom at an earlier age than girls, may be able to manage stressful family events by relying on friends. Girls may be less likely to rely on peers as an 'arena of comfort' (Simmons et al., 1987). At the same time, girls (and boys) who have peers as an 'arena of comfort' when family relationships are strained show less depressive symptoms (Colten & Gore, 1991). If puberty heralds an intensification of gender roles, as has been suggested (Hill & Lynch, 1983), then girls may experience certain gender-linked events differently, and more negatively, than boys (not dating, being perceived as unattractive: Faust, 1983; Duke-Duncan et al., 1985; Gargiulo et al., 1987; Attie et al., 1990).

Boys' and girls' experiences and behavioural repertoires prior to adolescence may also play a role. For example, the Blocks have followed a cohort of children from the preschool to the young adult years. Preschool predictors of boys' depressive symptoms at age 18 years included being aggressive, self-aggrandizing and undercontrolled, while predictors for girls were being intropunitive, oversocialized and overcontrolled (Block & Gjerde, 1990). These characteristics are reminiscent of early sex role stereotypes (Block, 1973; Brooks-Gunn & Matthews, 1979). Perhaps many of the negative effects of rigid role expectations and sex role socialization do not become evident until the young adolescent years, when pubertal changes, and society's responses to them, render gender, and the different experiences and trajectories for males and females, highly salient. Such results suggest that continuities exist between early personality and emotional state, but that the creation of developmental trajectories may be quite gender-specific. Whether the same is true for children reared in different social and economic contexts is not known, although highly probable (Spencer & Dornbusch, 1990).

The point here is that research needs to consider physiological, social and emotional changes of the pubertal period simultaneously. Additionally, potential interactions among these domains must be modelled if we are to understand the increase in depressive affect and clinical depression during the adolescent years. Focusing on physiological change in the absence of other changes or without considering the ecosystems in which the youth resides will probably yield little understanding of the onset of both types of depression, as well as the developmental trajectories of children or youth who experience depression.

Continuity in depression across generations

A physiological and environmental process

Family aggregation of affective disorders has been demonstrated in studies of children, adolescents and adults (Andreasen et al., 1977; Gershon et al., 1982; Weissman et al., 1984; Hammen, 1991). Estimates of lifetime morbidity risks in first-degree relatives of probands with major depression for adults range from 0.18 to 0.30 (Gershon et al., 1982; Puig-Antich, 1986), with this number increasing when probands' depression is of prepubertal onset (Harrington et al., 1997). Twin studies suggest that monozygotic twins are four to five times more likely to exhibit concordance for major depression than dizygotic twins (Kendler et al., 1986; Wender et al., 1986). More recently, research examining maternal and paternal ratings of their twins suggests a genetic component of depressive symptomatology which accounts for approximately 60% of the variance (Eaves et al., 1997).

Researchers have divided symptoms of major depression into three clinically significant depressive syndromes: mild typical, severe typical and atypical depression (Kendler et al., 1996; Sullivan et al., 1998). Mild typical and severe typical depression are distinguishable, in part, in terms of the length of depressive episodes, the severity of depressive symptoms and the risk associated with future major depressive episodes. Specifically, severe typical depression is marked with longer episodes of more severe symptoms and has a higher associated risk of future major depressive episodes. Atypical depression, like mild typical depression, is associated with relatively shorter episodes of moderate depressive symptoms, but is different from the other forms of depression with respect to its association with significant weight changes. Specifically, atypical depressives are more likely to experience increased appetite and to be significantly overweight than those who exhibit typical depressive symptoms. Research suggests that female twins tended to have the same type of depressive syndrome as each other more often than would be expected by chance, and that further, this resemblance was stronger for monozygotic over dizygotic twins (Kendler et al., 1996). The finding that family aggregation is higher for those individuals with more severe and frequent episodes has been suggested in the past (Nurnberger & Gershon, 1984).

Family aggregation is higher for bipolar than unipolar depression (Mendlewicz, 1988), which might be indicative of different biological substrates being involved or different temporal patterns of biological influence. A tantalizing hypothesis has been put forth by Kendler and colleagues (1986). They believe that there may be genetic transmission for 'distress' broadly construed, with the form this distress takes being influenced by the precipitation of environmental events expressed by an individual. The two types of distress considered are anxiety and depression, which are not only often present in the same individuals, but are both characterized by dysregulation in the HPA axis (Butler & Nemeroff, 1990; Maser & Cloninger, 1990).

Generally, aggregation is higher in children than in adolescents, and in adolescents than in adults. Comparing age-corrected lifetime morbidity risks across studies in first-degree relatives of probands with major depression (since most studies do not include children, adolescents and adults), rough estimates are about 0.50 for children, 0.35 for adolescents, and 0.18 to 0.30 for adults (Gershon et al., 1982; Weissman et al., 1984; Puig-Antich, 1987). Thus, the genetic loading for childhood and adolescent depression may be higher than that for depression which first occurs in adulthood.

In addition, current longitudinal studies of childhood and adolescent onset of depression suggest that early onset may be associated with more frequent and severe depressive episodes (M. Strober, unpublished paper; Kovacs et al., 1984a, 1984b). Looking at the timing of onset of depression within one study, Weissman et al. (1987) report that individuals with an onset prior to age 20 were more likely to have family members who were depressed than those whose first episode was reported to occur after age 20.

Recent work complements the above findings regarding the influence of genetics in depression by adding an examination of adolescent twins' gender differences in liability to experience both depressive symptoms and the negative past-year life events that are associated with them. Silberg and colleagues (1999) suggest that girls tend to demonstrate significantly more increasing levels of depression through adolescence than boys, as well as more of a predisposition to experience negative life events than boys. The researchers concluded that, whereas increasing levels of depression in adolescent boys are largely associated with the experiencing of negative life events, the comparatively greater prevalence of depression in adolescent females seems to be largely explained by the influence of genetics.

Parental psychopathology itself is also accompanied by negative familial conditions – marital conflict, family conflict, other aspects of psychopathology and possibly other life stressors (Downey & Coyne, 1990). Consequently, what might at first glance seem to be heritable might also be environmental. An elegant study was conducted on the children of parents with psychiatric diagnoses of schizophrenia or major affective disorder, a history of child abuse or neglect (reported to child protective services), or both (Downey & Walker, 1992). Problem behaviours, both depression and aggression, were highest in children whose parents had a history of both abuse/neglect and psychopathology, and lowest in those whose parents had no history of abuse/neglect but had a clinical diagnosis of psychopathology. Using child-level variables to classify children into high-, average- and low-risk groups (based on self-esteem, interpersonal problem-solving, early developmental difficulties, intelligence) explains a significant amount of the variance in behaviour problems (more so for depression than aggression). Children at double jeopardy (high-risk in child and family characteristics) were much more likely to exhibit depressed symptomatology.

Recent research suggests that interpersonal traumas (e.g. molestation, rape, kidnapping and physical assault), loss events (e.g. parent death, parental divorce/separation), and other adversities (e.g. involvement in an accident, or witnessing trauma) experienced during childhood predict psychopathology, especially mood disorders, later in life (Kessler et al., 1997). In addition to predicting depressive symptomatology, research also suggests that environmental factors influence the time it takes women to recover from depressive episodes (Kendler et al., 1997). Specifically, low family income, low parental protectiveness, parental separation, high levels of neuroticism and the presence of severe life events significantly predict slower time to recovery early in depressive episodes. Late in depressive episodes, however, severe life events, infrequent contact with relatives, infrequent attendance at clubs and genetic risk for depression significantly predict slower time to recover.

Findings such as these speak to the importance of examining other characteristics of the family environment and, more specifically, other aspects of parental behaviour and psychopathology than just the existence of affective disorders (Hammen, 1991). For example, Mitchell and colleagues (1989) found that depressed children (aged 7–12) of affectively disordered mothers had mothers who reported more drug abuse and suicide attempts than a comparable sample of adolescents. And, in a study of children of unipolar, bipolar, medically ill and nonill mothers, chronic strain and current depressive symptoms of the mother were more predictive of the children's depressive symptomatology than maternal history of affective disorder (Hammen et al., 1987). The early onset of clinical depression in childhood, therefore, may be due to the co-occurrence of other forms of psychopathology in conjunction with an affective disorder.[6]

The negative influence of a depressed parent is not specific to depression. Children and adolescents of parents with an affective disorder show symptoms beyond the depressive spectrum, including neurotic illness, neurotic behaviour disturbance, sociopathy and criminal activities (Beardslee et al., 1983; Beardslee et al., 1985; Hammen, 1991).

In summary, continuity across generations is seen. However, it is often more general to psychopathology than to depression, and it may be due to more than parental psychopathology *per se*, rather than depression. Whether familial aggregation is more generally associated with psychopathology or with clinical depression would possibly alter beliefs about the primacy of physiological processes in the aetiology of childhood and adolescent depression.

Physiological and environmental pathways to depression

Perhaps the largest unanswered question in the childhood and adolescent depression literature has to do with whether continuity exists between more and less severe forms of depression. While excellent prospective work has been conducted, most of it focuses on charting the developmental course of depressive symptomatology in a nonclinical sample of adolescents, following a sample of offspring of affectively disordered parents (and perhaps comparison groups of abusing or medically ill parents), or watching a sample of clinical patients *vis-à-vis* relapse. Little work considers what predisposes some youth or children who exhibit depressive symptomatology to go on to have a clinical episode while others do not. Who is vulnerable and who is not? What are the family-level and child-level factors that protect children and youth from depression? We do not even know if a history of depressed mood is a risk factor for the onset of a major affective disorder. Perhaps the best samples in which to look for links between depressed mood and clinical depression are those focusing on children of affectively disordered parents. Several investigators have followed families for a decade or more (Weissman et al., 1987, 1997, 1999; Hammen, 1991).

Almost no work has explored possible similarities and differences in the onset and course of clinical depression and depressed mood *vis-à-vis* physiological processes. Additionally, the more biologically oriented research has focused on the clinically depressed. Little research has focused on those with less severe forms of depression.

Whether biological dysregulation occurs in adolescents without a clinical condition but with severe depressive symptoms is unexplored. Of particular interest is whether a subset of youth with depressed mood may exhibit physiological concomitants and, if so, whether such youth are more likely to go on to experience a clinical episode. Until normative studies of adolescents include physiological measures, this potentially fruitful approach to identifying youth at risk for clinical depression and depressed youth who go on to have a clinical episode will not be realized.

REFERENCES

Akiskal, H. S. & McKinney, W. T. Jr (1973). Depressive disorders: toward a unified hypothesis. *Science*, **182**, 20–9.

American Psychiatric Association (1987). *Diagnostic and Statistical Manual of Mental Disorders*, 3rd edn revised. Washington, DC: American Psychiatric Association.

American Psychiatric Association (1994). *Diagnostic and Statistical Manual of Mental Disorders*, 4th edn. Washington, DC: American Psychiatric Association.

Amsterdam, J. D., Winokur, A., Mendels, J. et al. (1979). Distinguishing depressive subtypes of thyrotropin response to TRJ testing. *Lancet*, **2**, 904–5.

Amsterdam, J. D., Winokur, A., Caroff, S. N. & Conn, J. (1982). The dexamethasone suppression test in outpatients with primary affective disorder and healthy control subjects. *American Journal of Psychiatry*, **139**, 287–91.

Andreasen, N. C., Endicott, J., Spitzer, R. L. & Winokur, G. (1977). Family history method using diagnostic criteria. *Archives of General Psychiatry*, **34**, 1223–9.

Angold, A. (1988). Childhood and adolescent depression: I. Epidemiological aspects. *British Journal of Psychiatry*, **152**, 601–17.

Angold, A. & Rutter, M. (1992). Effects of age and pubertal status on depression in a large clinical sample. *Development and Psychopathology*, **4**, 5–28.

Angold, A., Costello, E. J. & Worthman, C. M. (1998). Puberty and depression: the roles of age, pubertal status and pubertal timing. *Psychological Medicine*, **28**, 51–61.

Angold, A., Costello, E. J., Erkanli, A. & Worthman, C. M. (1999). Pubertal changes in hormone levels and depression in girls. *Psychological Medicine*, **29**, 1043–53.

Angst, J., Vollrath, M., Merikangas, K. R. & Ernst, C. (1990). Comorbidity of anxiety and depression in the Zurich cohort study of young adults. In *Comorbidity in Anxiety and Mood Disorders*, ed. J. D. Maser & C. R. Cloninger, pp. 123–38. Washington, DC: American Psychiatric Press.

Appleboom-Fondu, J., Kerkhofs, M. & Mendlewicz, J. (1988). Depression in adolescents and young adults – polysomnographic and neuroendocrine aspects. *Journal of Affective Disorders*, **14**, 35–40.

Asnis, G. M., Sachar, E. L., Halbreich, R. et al. (1981). Cortisol secretion in relation to age in major depression. *Psychosomatic Medicine*, **43**, 235–42.

Asnis, G. M., Rabinovich, H., Ryan, N. et al. (1985). Cortisol responses to desipramine in endogenous depressives and normal controls. Preliminary findings. *Psychiatry Research*, **14**, 225–32.

Attie, I. & Brooks-Gunn, J. (1992). Developmental issues in the study of eating problems and disorders. In *The Etiology of Bulimia: the individual and familial context*, ed. J. H. Crowther, S. E. Hobfoll, M. A. P. Stephens & D. L. Tennenbaum, pp. 35–58. Washington, DC: Hemisphere.

Attie, I. & Brooks-Gunn, J. (1995). The development of eating regulation across the lifespan. In *Developmental Psychopathology*, vol. 2, ed. D. Cicchetti & D. J. Cohen, pp. 332–68. New York: John Wiley.

Attie, I., Brooks-Gunn, J. & Petersen, A. C. (1990). The emergence of eating problems: a developmental perspective. In *Handbook of Developmental Psychopathology*, ed. M. Lewis & S. Miller, pp. 409–20. New York: Plenum Press.

Backstrom, T., Wide, V., Sodergard, R. & Carstensen, H. (1976). FSH, LH, TeBG-capacity, estrogen, and progesterone in women with premenstrual tension during the luteal phase. *Journal of Steroid Biochemistry*, **7**, 473–6.

Beardslee, W. R., Bemporad, J., Keller, M. B. & Klerman, G. L. (1983). Children of parents with major affective disorder: a review. *American Journal of Psychiatry*, **140**, 825–32.

Beardslee, W. R., Keller, M. B. & Klerman, G. L. (1985). Children of parents with affective disorder. *International Journal of Family Psychiatry*, **6**, 283–99.

Beasley, C. M., Dornseif, B. E., Bosomworth, J. C. et al. (1992). Fluoxetine and suicide: a meta-analysis of controlled trials of treatment for depression. *International Clinical Psychopharmacology*, **6** (Suppl. 6), 35–57.

Benedek, T. (1952). *Psychosexual Functions in Women*. New York: Ronald Press.

Birmaher, B. (1998). Child and adolescent psychopharmacology. *Psychopharmacology Bulletin*, **34**, 35–9.

Birmaher, B., Ryan, N. D., Dahl, R. et al. (1992). Dexamethasone suppression test in children with major depressive disorder. *Journal of the American Academy of Child Adolescent Psychiatry*, **31**, 291–6.

Birmaher, B., Dahl., R. E., Perel, J. et al. (1996). Corticotropin-releasing hormone challenge in prepubertal major depression. *Biological Psychiatry*, **39**, 267–77.

Birmaher, B., Kaufman, J., Brent, D. A. et al. (1997). Neuroendocrine response to 5-hydroxy-L-tryptophan in prepubertal children at high risk of major depressive disorder. *Archives of General Psychiatry*, **54**, 1113–19.

Blazer, D., George, L. K. & Lauderman, R. (1985). Psychiatric disorders: a rural/urban comparison. *Archives of General Psychiatry*, **42**, 651–6.

Block, J. H. (1973). Conceptions of sex role: some cross-cultural and longitudinal perspectives. *American Psychologist*, **28**, 512–26.

Block, J. & Gjerde, P. F. (1990). Depressive symptomatology in late adolescence: a longitudinal perspective on personality antecedents. In *Risk and Protective Factors in the Development of Psychopathology*, ed. J. E. Rolf, A. Masten, D. Cicchetti et al., pp. 334–60. New York: Cambridge University Press.

Bowden, C. L., Schatzberg, A. F., Rosenbaum, A. et al. (1993). Fluoxetine and desipramine in major depressive disorder. *Journal of Clinical Psychopharmacology*, **13**, 305–11.

Boyar, R. M., Finklestein, J., Roffwarg, H. et al. (1972). Synchronization of augmented luteinizing hormone secretion with sleep during puberty. *New England Journal of Medicine*, **287**, 582–6.

Boyar, R. M., Hellman, L. D., Roffwarf, H. et al. (1977). Cortisol secretion and metabolism in anorexia nervosa. *New England Journal of Medicine*, **296**, 190–3.

Brambilla, F., Musetti, C., Tacchini, C., Fontanillas, J. & Guareschi-Cazzulo, A. (1989). Neuroendocrine investigation in children and adolescents with dysthymic disorders: the DST, TRH, and clonidine tests. *Journal of Affective Disorders*, **17**, 279–84.

Brooks-Gunn, J. (1984). The psychological significance of different pubertal events to young girls. *Journal of Early Adolescence*, **4**, 315–27.

Brooks-Gunn, J. (1988). Antecedents and consequences of variations in girls' maturational timing. *Journal of Adolescent Health Care*, **9**, 365–73.

Brooks-Gunn, J. (1991). How stressful is the transition to adolescence in girls? In *Adolescent Stress: Causes and Consequences*, ed. M. E. Colten & S. Gore, pp. 131–49. Hawthorne, NY: Aldine de Gruyter.

Brooks-Gunn, J. & Matthews, W. (1979). *He and She: how children develop their sex-role identity*. Englewood Cliffs, NJ: Prentice-Hall.

Brooks-Gunn, J. & Petersen, A. C. (eds) (1983). *Girls at Puberty: biological and psychosocial perspectives*. New York: Plenum Press.

Brooks-Gunn, J. & Petersen, A. C. (1984). Problems in studying and defining pubertal events. *Journal of Youth and Adolescence*, **13**, 181–96.

Brooks-Gunn, J. & Petersen, A. C. (1991). Studying the emergence of depression and depressive symptoms during adolescence. *Journal of Youth and Adolescence*, **20**, 115–19.

Brooks-Gunn, J. & Reiter, E. O. (1990). The role of pubertal processes in the early adolescent transition. In *At the Threshold: the developing adolescent*, ed. S. Feldman & G. Elliott, pp. 16–53. Cambridge: Harvard University Press.

Brooks-Gunn, J. & Ruble, D. N. (1983). The experience of menarche from a developmental perspective. In *Girls at Puberty: biological and psychosocial perspectives*, ed. J. Brooks-Gunn & A. C. Petersen, pp. 155–77. New York: Plenum Press.

Brooks-Gunn, J. & Warren, M. P. (1989). Biological contributions to affective expression in young adolescent girls. *Child Development*, **60**, 372–85.

Buchanan, C. M., Eccles, J. & Becker, J. (1992). Are adolescents the victims of raging hormones? Evidence for activational effects of hormones on moods and behavior at adolescence. *Psychological Bulletin*, **111**, 62–107.

Butler, P. D. & Nemeroff, C. B. (1990). Corticotropin-releasing factor as a possible cause of comorbidity in anxiety and depressive disorders. In *Comorbidity of Mood and Anxiety Disorders*, ed. J. D. Maser & C. R. Cloninger, pp. 413–35. Washington, DC: American Psychiatric Press.

Carskadon, M. A. & Dement, W. C. (1987). Daytime sleepiness: quantification of a behavioral state. *Neuroscience and Biomedical Reviews*, **11**, 307–17.

Carroll, B. J., Greden, J. F., Haskett, R. et al. (1980). Neurotransmitter studies of neuroendocrine pathology in depression. *Acta Psychiatrica Scandinavica*, **61**, 183–99.

Checkley, S. A., Slade, A. P. & Shur, E. (1981). Growth hormone and other responses to clonidine in patients with endogenous depression. *British Journal of Psychiatry*, **138**, 51–5.

Cicchetti, D. & Schneider-Rosen, K. (1986). An organizational approach to childhood depression. In *Depression in Young People: clinical and developmental perspectives*, ed. M. Rutter, C. Izard & P. Read, pp. 71–134. New York: Guilford.

Cicchetti, D. & Toth, S. (1991). The making of a developmental psychopathologist. In *Child Behavior and Development: training for diversity*, ed. J. H. Canter, C. C. Spiker & L. P. Lipsitt, pp. 34–72. Norwood, NJ: Ablex.

Cicchetti, D., Nucombe, B. & Garber, J. (1992). Developmental approaches to depression. *Development and Psychopathology*, **4**, 1–3.

Colle, L. M., Belair, J. F., DiFeo, M. et al. (1994). Extended open-label fluoxetine treatment of adolescents with major depression. *Child and Adolescent Psychopharmacology*, **4**, 225–32.

Colten, M. E. & Gore, S. (eds.) (1991). *Adolescent Stress: Causes and Consequences*, pp. 131–40. Hawthorne, NY: Aldine de Gruyter.

Compas, B. E. (1987). Stress and life events during childhood and adolescence. *Clinical Psychology Review*, **7**, 275–302.

Compas, B. E., Connor, J. K. & Hinden, B. R. (1998). New perspectives on depression during adolescence. In *New Perspectives on Adolescent Risk Behavior*, ed. R. Jessor, pp. 319–62. New York: Cambridge University Press.

Compas, B. E., Howell, D. C., Phares, V., Williams, R. & Ledoux, N. (1989). Parent and child stress and symptoms: an integrative analysis. *Developmental Psychology*, **25**, 550–9.

Compas, B. E., Oppendisano, G., Connor, J. K. et al. (1997). Gender differences in depressive symptoms in adolescence: comparison of national samples of clinically-referred and non-referred youth. *Journal of Consulting and Clinical Psychology*, **65**, 617–26.

Cox, M. & Brooks-Gunn., J. (eds.) (1999). *Conflict and Cohesion in Families: causes and consequences*. Mahwah, NJ: Erlbaum.

Crumley, F., Clevenger, J., Steinfink, D. et al. (1982). Preliminary report on the dexamethasone suppression test for psychiatrically disturbed adolescents. *American Journal of Psychiatry*, **139**, 1062–4.

Dahl., R. E., Puig-Antich, J., Ryan, N. E. et al. (1990). EEG sleep in adolescents with major depression: the role of suicidality and inpatient status. *Journal of Affective Disorders*, **19**, 63–75.

Dahl, R. E., Ryan, N. D., Birmaher, B. et al. (1991a). EEG sleep measures in prepubertal depression. *Psychiatry Research*, **38**, 201–14.

Dahl, R. E., Ryan, N. D., Puig-Antich, J. et al. (1991b). 24-hour cortisol measures in adolescents with major depression: a controlled study. *Biological Psychiatry*, **30**, 25–36.

Dahl, R. E., Ryan, N. D., Matty, M. K. et al. (1996). Sleep onset abnormalities in depressed adolescents. *Biological Psychiatry*, **39**, 400–10.

Dahl, R. E., Ryan, N. D., Williamson, D. E. et al. (1992). Regulation of sleep and growth hormone in adolescent depression. *Journal of the American Academy of Child and Adolescent Psychiatry*, **31**, 615–21.

Dahl, R. E., Ryan, N. D., Perel, J. et al. (1994). Cholinergic REM induction test with arecoline in depressed children. *Psychiatry Research*, **51**, 269–82.

De Bellis, M. D., Dahl, R. E., Perel, J. et al. (1995). Nighttime ACTH, cortisol, prolactin, and growth hormone secretion in prepubertal depression. *Biological Psychiatry*, **37**, 594.

De Bellis, M. D., Dahl, R. E., Perel, J. et al. (1996). Nocturnal ACTH, cortisol, growth hormone, and prolactin secretion in prepubertal adolescence. *Journal of the American Academy of Child and Adolescent Psychiatry*, **35**, 1130–8.

Dinnerstein, L., Spencer-Gardner, C., Brown, J. B., Smith, M. A. & Burrows, G. D. (1984). Premenstrual tension-hormonal profiles. *Journal of Psychosomatic Obstetrics and Gynecology*, **3**, 37–51.

Dorn, L. D., Burgess, E., Dichek, H. L. et al. (1996). Thyroid hormone concentration in depressed and nondepressed adolescents: group differences and behavior relations. *Journal of the American Academy of Child Adolescent Psychiatry*, **35**, 299–306.

Dorn, L. D., Dahl, R. E., Birmaher, B. et al. (1997). Baseline thyroid hormones in depressed and non-depressed pre- and early-pubertal boys and girls. *Journal of Psychiatric Research*, **31**, 555–67.

Downey, G. & Coyne, J. C. (1990). Children of depressed parents: an integrative review. *Psychological Bulletin*, **108**, 50–76.

Downey, G. & Walker, E. (1992). Distinguishing family-level and child-level influences on the development of depression and aggression in children at risk. *Development and Psychopathology*, **4**, 81–95.

Duke-Duncan, D., Ritter, P. L., Dornbusch, S. M., Gross, R. T. & Carlsmith, J. M. (1985). The effects of pubertal timing on body image, school behavior, and deviance. *Journal of Youth and Adolescence*, **14**, 227–35.

Eaves, L. J., Silberg, J. L., Meyer, J. M. et al. (1997). Genetics and developmental psychopathology: II. The main effects of genes and environment on behavioral problems in the Virginia twin study of adolescent behavioral development. *Journal of Child Psychology and Psychiatry*, **38**, 965–80.

Emslie, G. J., Rush, A. J., Weinberg, W. A., Rintelmann, J. W. & Roffwarg, H. P. (1990). Children with major depression show reduced rapid eye movement latencies. *Archives of General Psychiatry*, **47**, 119–24.

Emslie, G. J., Rush, A. J., Weinberg, W. A., Rintelmann, J. W. & Roffwarg, H. P. (1994). Sleep EEG features of adolescents with major depression. *Biological Psychiatry*, **36**, 573–81.

Emslie, G. J., Rush, A. J., Weinberg, W. A. et al. (1997). A double-blind, randomized, placebo-controlled trial of fluoxetine in children and adolescents with depression. *Archives of General Psychiatry*, **54**, 1031–7.

Evans, M. E. & Lye, M. (1992). Depression in the elderly physically ill: an open study of treatment with the 5-HT reuptake inhibitor fluoxetine. *Journal of Clinical Experimental Gerontology*, **14**, 297–307.

Extein, I., Pottash, A. L. C. & Gold, M. S. (1980). TRH test in depression. *New England Journal of Medicine*, **302**, 923–4.

Extein, I., Rosenberg, G., Pottash, A. L. C. & Gold, M. S. (1982). The dexamethasone suppression test in depressed adolescents. *American Journal of Psychiatry*, **139**, 1617–19.

Fabre, L. F., Scharf, M. B. & Itil, T. M. (1991). Comparative efficacy and safety of nortriptyline and fluoxetine in the treatment of major depression: a clinical study. *Journal of Clinical Psychiatry*, **52**, 62–7.

Faust, M. S. (1983). Alternative constructions of adolescent growth. In *Girls at Puberty: biological and psychosocial perspectives*, ed. J. Brooks-Gunn & A. C. Petersen, pp. 105–25). New York: Plenum Press.

Feldman, S. S. & Elliott, G. (eds) (1990). *At the Threshold: the developing adolescent*. Cambridge, MA: Harvard University Press.

Fendrich, M., Warner, V. & Weissman, M. M. (1990). Family risk factors, parental depression, and psychopathology in offspring. *Developmental Psychology*, **26**, 40–50.

Finkelstein, J. W., Roffwarg, H. P., Boyar, R. M., Kream, J. & Hellman, L. (1972). Age related change in the 24 hour spontaneous secretion of growth hormone. *Journal of Clinical Endocrinology*, **35**, 665–70.

Foreman, D. M. & Goodyer, I. M. (1988). Salivary cortisol hypersecretion in juvenile depression. *Journal of Child Psychology and Psychiatry and Allied Disciplines*, **29**, 311–20.

Friedrich, W. M., Reams, R. & Jacobs, J. (1982). Depression and suicidal ideation in early adolescents. *Journal of Youth and Adolescence*, **11**, 403–7.

Garcia, M. R., Ryan, N. D., Rabinovitch, H. et al. (1991). Thyroid stimulating hormone response to thyrotropin in prepubertal depression. *Journal of the American Academy of Child and Adolescent Psychiatry*, **30**, 398–406.

Gargiulo, J., Attie, I., Brooks-Gunn, J. & Warren, M. P. (1987). Girls' dating behavior as a function of social context and maturation. *Developmental Psychology*, **23**, 730–7.

Ge, X., Lorenz, F. O., Conger, R. D., Elder, G. H. & Simons, R. L. (1994) Trajectories of stressful life events and depressive symptoms during adolescence. *Developmental Psychology*, **30**, 467–83.

Gershon, E. S., Hanovit, J., Guroff, J. J. et al. (1982). A family study of schizoaffective, bipolar I, bipolar II, unipolar, and normal control probands. *Archives of General Psychiatry*, **39**, 1157–67.

Giles, D. E., Jarrett, R. B., Roffwarg, H. P. & Rush, A. J. (1987). Reduced REM latency: a predictor of recurrence in depression. *Neuropsychopharmacology*, **1**, 33–9.

Goetz, R. R., Puig-Antich, J., Ryan, N. et al. (1987). Electroencephalographic sleep of adolescents with major depression and normal controls. *Archives of General Psychiatry*, **44**, 61–8.

Gold, P. W., Loriauz, L., Roy, A. et al. (1986). Responses to corticotropin-releasing hormone in the hypercortisolism of depression and Cushing's disease. *New England Journal of Medicine*, **341**, 1329–35.

Gold, P. W., Goodwin, F. K. & Chrousos, G. P. (1988). Clinical and biochemical manifestations of depression: relation to the neurobiology of stress, part 1. *New England Journal of Medicine*, **319**, 348–53.

Goldman-Rakic, P. S. & Brown, R. M. (1982). Post-natal development of monoamine content and synthesis in the cerebral cortex of the rhesus monkey. *Brain Research Bulletin*, **256**, 339–49.

Goodyer, I. M. (1990). *Life Experiences, Development, and Childhood Psychopathology*. Chichester: Wiley.

Goodyer, I. M., Herbert, J., Altham, P. M. E. et al. (1996). Adrenal secretion during major depression in 8- to 16-year-olds, I. Altered diurnal rhythms in salivary cortisol and dehyd-roepiandrosterone (DHEA) at presentation. *Psychological Medicine*, **26**, 245–56.

Goodyer, I. M., Herbert, J. & Altham, P. M. E. (1998). Adrenal steroid secretion and major depression in 8- to 16-year-olds, III. Influence of cortisol/DHEA ratio at presentation on subsequent rates of disappointing life events and persistent major depression. *Psychological Medicine*, **28**, 265–73.

Graber, J., Brooks-Gunn, J., Paikoff, R. L. & Warren, M. P. (1994). Prediction of eating problems: an eight year study of adolescent girls. *Developmental Psychology*, **30**, 823–34.

Graber, J. A., Lewinsohn, P. M., Seeley, J. R. & Brooks-Gunn, J. (1997). Is psychopathology associated with the timing of pubertal development? *Journal of the American Academy of Adolescent and Child Psychiatry*, **36**, 1768–76.

Greden, J. F., Gardner, R., King, D. et al. (1983). Dexamethasone suppression tests in antidepress-ant treatment of melancholia. *Archives of General Psychiatry*, **40**, 493–500.

Greenough, W. T., Black, J. E. & Wallace, C. S. (1987). Experience and brain development. *Child Development*, **58**, 539–59.

Gunnar, M. R. & Collins, W. A. (eds) (1988). *Transitions in Adolescence*: Minnesota symposium on child psychology. Hillsdale, NJ: Erlbaum.

Hammen, C. (1991). *Depression Runs in Families*. New York: Springer-Verlag.

Hammen, C. L., Adrian, C., Fordon, D. & Jaenicke, C. (1987). Children of depressed mothers: maternal strain and symptom predictors of dysfunction. *Journal of Abnormal Psychology*, **96**, 190–8.

Harrington, R., Rutter, M., Weissman, M. et al. (1997). Psychiatric disorders in the relatives of depressed probands, I: comparison of prepubertal, adolescent and early adult onset cases. *Journal of Affective Disorders*, **42**, 9–22.

Harter, S., Marold, D. B. & Whitesell, N. R. (1992). Model of psychosocial risk factors leading to suicidal ideation in young adolescents. *Development and Psychopathology*, **4**, 167–88.

Hayward, C., Killen, J. D., Wilson, D. M. et al. (1997). Psychiatric risk associated with early puberty in adolescent girls. *Journal of the American Academy of Child and Adolescent Psychiatry*, **36**, 255–62.

Herbert, J., Goodyer, I. M., Altham, P. M. E. et al. (1996). Adrenal secretion and major depression in 8- to 16-year-olds, II. Influence of co-morbidity at presentation. *Psychological Medicine*, **26**, 257–63.

Hewitt, J. K., Rutter, M., Simonoff, E. et al. (1997). Genetics and developmental psychopathol-ogy: I. Phenotypic assessment in the Virginia twin study of adolescent behavioral development. *Journal of Child Psychology and Psychiatry*, **38**, 943–63.

Hill, J. P. & Lynch, M. E. (1983). The intensification of gender-related role expectations during early adolescence. In *Girls at Puberty: biological and psychosocial perspectives*, ed. J. Brooks-Gunn & A. C. Petersen, pp. 201–28. New York: Plenum Press.

Holsboer, F., Lauer, C. J., Schrieber, W. & Krieg, J. (1995). Altered hypothalamic–pituitary–adrenocortical regulation in healthy subjects at high familial risk for affective disorders. *Neuroendocrinology*, **62**, 340–7.

Jarrett, D. B., Coble, P. A. & Kupfer, D. J. (1983). Reduced cortisol latency in depressive illness. *Archives of General Psychiatry*, **40**, 506–11.

Joyce, P. R. & Paykel, E. S. (1989). Predictors of drug response in depression. *Archives of General Psychiatry*, **46**, 89–99.

Kahn, A. U. & Todd, S. (1990). Polysomnographic findings in adolescents with major depression. *Psychiatry Research*, **33**, 313–20.

Kaplan, S. L., Grumbach, M. M. & Aubert, M. L. (1976). The ontogenesis of pituitary hormones and hypothalamic factors in the human fetus: maturation of the central nervous system regulation of anterior pituitary function. *Recent Progress in Hormone Research*, **32**, 161–243.

Katz, J. L., Boyar, R. M., Roffwarg, H., Hellman, L. & Weiner, H. (1978). Weight and circadian luteinizing hormone secretory pattern in anorexia nervosa. *Psychosomatic Medicine*, **40**, 549–67.

Kazdin, A. (1990). Childhood depression. *Journal of Child Psychology and Psychiatry*, **31**, 121–60.

Kendler, K. S., Heath, A., Martin, N. G. & Eaves, L. J. (1986). Symptoms of anxiety and depression in a volunteer twin population. *Archives of General Psychiatry*, **43**, 213–21.

Kendler, K. S., Eaves, L. J., Walters, E. E. et al. (1996). The identification and validation of distinct depressive syndromes in a population-based sample of female twins. *Archives of General Psychiatry*, **53**, 391–9.

Kendler, K. S., Walters, E. E. & Kessler, R. C. (1997). The prediction of length of major depressive episodes: results from an epidemiological sample of female twins. *Psychological Medicine*, **27**, 107–17.

Kessler, R. C., McGonagle, K. A., Zhao, S. et al. (1994). Lifetime and 12-month prevalence of DSM-III-R psychiatric disorders in the United States: results from the national comorbidity survey. *Archives of General Psychiatry*, **51**, 8–19.

Kessler, R. C., Nelson, C. B., McGonagle, K. A. et al. (1996). Comorbidity of DSM-III-R major depressive disorder in the general population: results from the U.S. national comorbidity survey. *British Journal of Psychiatry*, **168**, 17–30.

Kessler, R. C., Davis, C. G. & Kendler, K. S. (1997). Childhood adversity and adult psychiatric disorder in the US national comorbidity survey. *Psychological Medicine*, **27**, 1101–19.

Khan, A. (1987). Heterogeneity of suicidal adolescents. *Journal of the American Academy of Child and Adolescent Psychiatry*, **26**, 92–6.

Klee, S. H. & Garfinkel, B. D. (1984). Identification of depression in children and adolescents: the role of the dexamethasone suppression test. *Journal of the American Academy of Child and Adolescent Psychiatry*, **23**, 410–15.

Knowles, J. B. & MacLean, A. W. (1990). Age-related changes in sleep in depressed and healthy subjects: a meta-analysis. *Journal of Neuropsychopharmacology*, **3**, 251–9.

Kovacs, M., Feinberg, T. L., Crouse-Novak, M. A., Paulauskas, S. L. & Finkelstein, R. (1984a). Depressive disorders in childhood. I. A longitudinal prospective study of characteristics and recovery. *Archives of General Psychiatry*, **41**, 229–37.

Kovacs, M., Feinberg, T. L., Crouse-Novak, M. A. et al. (1984b). Depressive disorders in childhood. II. A longitudinal study of the risk for a subsequent major depression. *Archives of General Psychiatry*, **41**, 643–9.

Kutcher, S. P. & Marton, P. (1989). Parameters of adolescent depression, a review. *Psychiatric Clinics of North America*, **12**, 895–918.

Kutcher, S., Malkin, D., Kutcher, S. et al. (1991). Nocturnal cortisol, thyroid stimulating hormone, and growth hormone secretory profiles in depressed adolescents. *Journal of the American Academy of Child and Adolescent Psychiatry*, **30**, 407–13.

Kutcher, S., Williamson, P., Szalai, J. & Marton, P. (1992). REM latency in endogenously depressed adolescents. *British Journal of Psychiatry*, **161**, 399–402.

Lahmeyer, H. W., Poznanski, E. O. & Bellur, S. N. (1983). EEG sleep in depressed adolescents. *American Journal of Psychiatry*, **140**, 1150–3.

Langer, G., Heinze, G., Rin, B. & Matussek, N. (1976). Reduced growth hormone response to amphetamine in endogenous depressive patients. *Archives of General Psychiatry*, **33**, 1471–5.

Lerner, R. M. & Foch, T. T. (1987). *Biological–Psychosocial Interactions in Early Adolescence: a life-span perspective*. Hillsdale, NJ: Lawrence Erlbaum.

Lewinsohn, P. M., Rohde, P., Seeley, J. R. & Hops, H. (1991). Comorbidity of unipolar depression: I. Major depression with dysthymia. *Journal of Abnormal Psychology*, **100**, 205–13.

Lewinsohn, P. M., Rohde, P., Seeley, J. R. & Fischer, S. A. (1993). Age-cohort changes in the lifetime occurrence of depression and other mental disorders. *Journal of Abnormal Psychology*, **102**, 110–20.

Lidor, H. G. & Molliver, M. E. (1982). An immunohistochemical study of serotonin neuron development in the rat: ascending pathways and terminal fields. *Brain Research Bulletin*, **8**, 389–430.

Livingston, R., Reis, C. J. & Ringdahl, I. C. (1984). Abnormal dexamethasone suppression test results in depressed and nondepressed children. *American Journal of Psychiatry*, **141**, 106–7.

Maser, J. D. & Cloninger, C. R. (eds) (1990). *Comorbidity of Mood Anxiety Disorders*. Washington, DC: American Psychiatric Press.

McAnarney, E. R. & Levine, M. (1988). *Early Adolescent Transitions*. New York: Health Publication.

Melges, F. T. & Hamburg, D. A. (1977). Psychological effects of hormonal changes in women. In *Human Sexuality in Four Perspectives*, ed. F. A. Beach, pp. 269–95. Baltimore: Johns Hopkins University Press.

Mendelson, M. (1982). Psychodynamics of depression. In *Handbook of Affective Disorders*, ed. E. Paykel, pp. 162–74. New York: Guilford Press.

Mendlewicz, J. (1988). Genetics of depression and mania. In *Depression and Mania*, ed. A. Georgotas & R. Cancro, pp. 196–212. New York: Elsevier.

Mitchell, J., McCauley, E., Burke, P., Calderon, R. & Schloredt, K. (1989). Psychopathology in parents of depressed children and adolescents. *Journal of the American Academy of Child and*

Adolescent Psychiatry, **28**, 352–7.

Money, J. & Erhardt, A. A. (1972). *Man and Woman, Boy and Girl*. Baltimore: Johns Hopkins University Press.

Montgomery, S. A. (1989). The efficacy of fluoxetine as an antidepressant in the short and long term. *International Clinical Psychopharmacology*, **4** (Suppl. 1), 113–19.

Munday, M. R., Brush, M. G. & Taylor, R. W. (1981). Correlations between progesterone, estradiol, and aldosterone levels in the premenstrual syndrome. *Clinical Endocrinology*, **14**, 1–9.

Munoz, R. F. (1989). Prevention of depression: training issues for research and practice. In *Proceedings of the Boulder Symposium on Clinical Psychology: Depression*, ed. B. Bloom & K. Schlesinger.

Munoz, R. F., Ying, Y. W., Perez-Stable, E. J. & Miranda, J. (1993). *The Prevention of Depression: research and practice*. Baltimore: Johns Hopkins University Press.

Murphy, B. & Kelleher, M. J. (1994). Does fluoxetine induce suicidal thoughts? *Irish Journal of Psychological Medicine*, **11**, 99–100.

Naylor, M. W., Greden, J. F. & Alessi, N. E. (1990). Plasma dexamethasone levels in children given the dexamethasone suppression test. *Biological Psychiatry*, **27**, 592–600.

Nielsen, B. M., Behnke, K., Arup, P. et al. (1993). A comparison of fluoxetine and imipramine in the treatment of outpatients with major depressive disorder. *Acta Psychiatrica Scandinavica*, **87**, 269–72.

Nolen-Hoeksema, S. & Girgus, J. S. (1994). The emergence of gender differences in depression during adolescence. *Psychological Bulletin*, **115**, 424–43.

Nurnberger, J. I. & Gershon, E. S. (1984). Genetics of affective disorders. In *Neurobiology of Mood Disorders*, ed. R. M. Post & J. C. Ballenger, pp. 76–101. Baltimore: Williams & Wilkins.

Orengo, C. A., Kunik, M. E., Molinari, V. & Workman, R. H. (1996). The use and tolerability of fluoxetine in geropsychiatric inpatients. *Journal of Clinical Psychiatry*, **57**, 12–16.

Paikoff, R. & Brooks-Gunn, J. (1991). Do parent–child relationships change during puberty? *Psychological Bulletin*, **110**, 47–66.

Paikoff, R. L., Brooks-Gunn, J. & Carlton-Ford, S. (1991a). Effect of reproductive status changes upon family functioning and well-being of mothers and daughters. *Journal of Early Adolescence*, **11**, 201–20.

Paikoff, R. L., Brooks-Gunn, J. & Warren, M. P. (1991b). Effects of girls' hormonal status on depressive and aggressive symptoms over the course of one year. *Journal of Youth and Adolescence*, **20**, 191–215.

Pande, A. C. & Sayler, M. E. (1993). Severity of depression and response to fluoxetine. *International Clinical Psychopharmacology*, **8**, 243–5.

Pepper, G. & Krieger, D. (1985). Hypothalamic–pituitary–adrenal abnormalities in depression: their possible relation to central mechanisms regulating ACTH release. In *Neurobiology of Mood Disorders*, ed. R. M. Post & J. C. Ballanger, pp. 245–70. Baltimore: Williams & Wilkins.

Petersen, A. C., Sarigiani, P. A. & Kennedy, R. E. (1991). Adolescent depression: why more girls? *Journal of Youth and Adolescence*, **20**, 247–71.

Petersen, A. C., Kennedy, R. E. & Sullivan, P. (1992). Coping with adolescence. In *Adolescent Stress: causes and consequences*, ed. M. E. Colten & S. Gore, pp. 93–110. New York: Aldine de

Gruyter.

Petersen, A. C., Compas, B., Brooks-Gunn, J. et al. (1993). Depression in adolescence. *American Psychologist*, **48**, 155–68.

Pfeffer, C. R., Stokes, P., Weiner, A. et al. (1989). Psychopathology and plasma cortisol responses to dexamethasone in prepubertal psychiatric inpatients. *Biological Psychiatry*, **267**, 677–89.

Post, R. M., Rubinow, D. R. & Ballenger, J. C. (1984). Conditioning, sensitization, and kindling: implications for the course of affective illness. In *Neurobiology of Mood Disorders*, ed. R. M. Post & J. C. Ballenger, pp. 432–66. Baltimore: Williams & Wilkins.

Puig-Antich, J. (1986). Psychobiological markers: effects of age and puberty. In *Depression in Young People: clinical and developmental perspectives*, ed. M. Rutter, C. E. Izard & P. B. Read, pp. 341–82. New York: Guilford.

Puig-Antich, J. (1987). Sleep and neuroendocrine correlates of affective illness in childhood and adolescence. *Journal of Adolescent Health Care*, **8**, 505–29.

Puig-Antich, J., Goetz, R., Hanlon, C. et al. (1982). Sleep architecture and REM sleep measures in prepubertal major depressives during an episode. *Archives of General Psychiatry*, **39**, 932–9.

Puig-Antich, J., Goetz, R., Hanlon, C. et al. (1983). Sleep architecture and REM sleep measures in prepubertal major depressives: studies during recovery from a major depressive episode in a drug free state. *Archives of General Psychiatry*, **40**, 187–92.

Puig-Antich, J., Davies, M., Novacenko, H. et al. (1984a). Growth hormone secretion in prepubertal major depressive children. III. Response to insulin induced hypoglycemia in a drug-free, fully recovered clinical state. *Archives of General Psychiatry*, **41**, 471–5.

Puig-Antich, J., Goetz, R., Davies, M. et al. (1984b). Growth hormone secretion in prepubertal major depressive children. II. Sleep related plasma concentrations during a depressive episode. *Archives of General Psychiatry*, **41**, 463–6.

Puig-Antich, J., Goetz, R., Davies, M. et al. (1984c). Growth hormone secretion in prepubertal major depressive children. IV. Sleep related plasma concentrations in a drug-free fully recovered clinical state. *Archives of General Psychiatry*, **41**, 479–83.

Puig-Antich, J., Novacenko, H., Davies, M. et al. (1984d). Growth hormone secretion in prepubertal major depressive children. I. Sleep related plasma concentrations during a depressive episode. *Archives of General Psychiatry*, **41**, 455–60.

Rabkin, J., Quitkin, F., Stewart, J., McGrath, P. & Puig-Antich, J. (1983). Dexamethasone suppression test with mild to moderately depressed outpatients. *American Journal of Psychiatry*, **140**, 926–8.

Rao, U., Dahl, R. E., Ryan, N. D. et al. (1996). The relationship between longitudinal clinical course and sleep and cortisol changes in adolescent depression. *Biological Psychiatry*, **40**, 474–84.

Reinherz, H. Z., Stewart-Berghauer, G., Pamkiz, B., Frost, A. Z. & Moeykens, B. A. (1989). The relationship of early risk and current mediators to depressive symptomatology in adolescence. *Journal of the American Academy of Child and Adolescent Psychiatry*, **28**, 942–7.

Reiter, E. O. (1987). Neuroendocrine control processes. *Journal of Adolescent Health Care*, **8**, 479–91.

Reiter, E. O. & Grumbach, M. M. (1982). Neuroendocrine control mechanisms and the onset of puberty. *Annual Review of Physiology*, **44**, 595–613.

Reynolds, C. F., Gillen J. C. & Kupfer, D. J. (1987). Sleep and affective disorders. In *Psychopharmacology: the third generation of progress*, ed. H. Y. Meltzer, pp. 647–54. New York: Raven Press.

Riemann, D., Kammerer, J., Low, H. & Schmidt, M. H. (1995). Sleep in adolescents with primary major depression and schizophrenia: a pilot study. *Journal of Child Psychology and Psychiatry*, **36**, 313–26.

Roberts, R. E., Lewinsohn, P. M. & Seeley, J. R. (1991). Screening for adolescent depression: a comparison of depression scales. *Journal of the American Academy of Child and Adolescent Psychiatry*, **30**, 58–66.

Robins, D. R., Alessi, N. E. & Yanchyschyn, G. W. (1982). Preliminary report on the dexamethasone suppression test in adolescents. *American Journal of Psychiatry*, **14**, 1414–18.

Rohde, P., Lewinsohn, P. M. & Seeley, J. R. (1991). Comorbidity of unipolar depression: II. Comorbidity with other mental disorders in adolescents and adults. *Journal of Abnormal Psychology*, **100**, 214–22.

Rose, R. M. (1985). Psychoneuroendocrinology. In *Williams Textbook of Endocrinology*, ed. J. D. Wilson & D. W. Foster, 7th edn. Philadelphia: W. B. Saunders.

Ruble, D. N. & Brooks-Gunn, J. (1979). Menstrual symptoms: a social cognition analysis. *Journal of Behavioral Medicine*, **2**, 171–94.

Ruble, D. N. & Brooks-Gunn, J. (1987). Perceptions of menstrual and premenstrual symptoms: self definitional processes at menarche. In *Premenstrual Syndrome: ethical and legal implications in a biomedical perspective*, ed. B. E. Ginsberg & B. F. Carter, pp. 237–51. New York: Plenum Press.

Rutter, M. (1980). The long-term effects of early experience. *Developmental Medicine and Child Neurology*, **22**, 800–15.

Rutter, M. (1986). The developmental psychopathology of depression: issues and perspectives. In *Depression in Young People: developmental and clinical perspectives*, ed. M. Rutter, C. E. Tizard & P. B. Read, pp. 3–32. New York: Guilford Press.

Rutter, M., Graham, P., Chadwick, O. F. D. & Yule, W. (1976). Adolescent turmoil: fact or fiction? *Journal of Child Psychology and Psychiatry*, **17**, 35–56.

Rutter, M., Izard, C. E. & Read, P. B. (eds) (1986). *Depression in Young People: developmental and clinical perspectives*. New York: Guilford.

Rutter, M., Simonoff, E. S. & Silberg, J. L. (1993). Whither behavior genetics? A developmental psychopathology perspective. In *Nature, Nurture and Psychology*, ed. R. Plomin & G. E. McClearn, pp. 433–56. Washington, DC: APA Books.

Ryan, N. D., Puig-Antich, J., Rabinovich, H. et al. (1988). Growth hormone response to desmethylimipramine in depressed and suicidal adolescents. *Journal of Affective Disorders*, **15**, 323–37.

Ryan, N. D., Dahl, R. E., Birmaher, B. et al. (1994). Stimulatory tests of growth hormone secretion in prepubertal major depression: depressed versus normal children. *Journal of the American Academy of Child and Adolescent Psychiatry*, **33**, 824–33.

Sachar, E. J. (1975). Neuroendocrine abnormalities in depressive illness. In *Topics in Psychoendocrinology*, ed. E. J. Sachar, pp. 182–201. New York: Grune & Stratton.

Sachar, E. J., Hellman, L., Roffwarg, H. P. et al. (1973). Disrupted 24-hour pattern of cortisol secretion in psychotic depression. *Archives of General Psychiatry*, **28**, 19–25.

Sachar, E., Puig-Antich, J. & Ryan, N. (1985). Three tests of cortisol secretion in adult endogenous depressives. *Acta Psychiatrica Scandinavica*, **71**, 1–8.

Sack, D. A., Rosenthal, N. E., Parry, B. L. & Wehr, T. A. (1987). Biological rhythms in psychiatry. In *Psychopharmacology: the third generation of progress*, ed. H. T. Meltzer, pp. 669–85. New York: Raven Press.

Shelton, R. C., Hollon, S. D., Purdon, S. E. & Loosen, P. T. (1991). Biological and psychological aspects of depression. *Behavior Therapy*, **22**, 201–28.

Siever, L. J. & Davis, K. L. (1985). Overview: toward a dysregulation hypothesis of depression. *American Journal of Psychiatry*, **142**, 1017–31.

Siever, L. J., Uhde, T. W., Silberman, E. K. et al. (1982). The growth hormone response to clonidine as a probe of noradrenergic receptor responsiveness in affective disorder patients and controls. *Psychiatry Research*, **6**, 171–83.

Siever, L. J., Uhde, T. W., Jimerson, D. C. et al. (1984). Plasma cortisol responses to clonidine in depressed patients and controls. *Archives of General Psychiatry*, **41**, 63–71.

Silberg, J., Pickles, A., Rutter, M. et al. (1999). The influence of genetic factors and life stress on depression among adolescent girls. *Archives of General Psychiatry*, **56**, 225–32.

Simeon, J. G., Dinicola, V. Ferguson, H. B. & Copping, W. (1990). Adolescent depression: a placebo-controlled fluoxetine treatment study and follow-up. *Progress in Neuropsychopharmacology and Biological Psychiatry*, **14**, 791–5.

Simmons, R. G., Burgeson, R. & Carlton-Ford, S. (1987). The impact of cumulative change in early adolescence. *Child Development*, **58**, 1220–34.

Simonoff, E., Pickles, A., Meyer, J. M. et al. (1997). The Virginia twin study of adolescent behavioral development. *Archives of General Psychiatry*, **54**, 801–8.

Sokolov, S. T. H., Kutcher, S. P. & Joffe, R. T. (1994). Basal thyroid indices in adolescent depression and bipolar disorder. *Journal of the American Academy of Child and Adolescent Psychiatry*, **33**, 469–75.

Spencer, M. B. & Dornbusch, S. M. (1990). Ethnicity and adolescence. In *At the Threshold: the developing adolescent*, ed. S. Feldman & G. Elliott, pp. 123–46. Cambridge: Harvard University Press.

Sroufe, A. & Rutter, M. (1984). The domain of developmental psychopathology. *Journal of Child Development*, **55**, 17–29.

Stokes, P. E. & Holtz, A. (1997). Fluoxetine tenth anniversary update: the progress continues. *Clinical Therapeutics*, **19**, 1135–250.

Sullivan, P. F., Kessler, R. C. & Kendler, K. S. (1998). Latent class analysis of lifetime depressive symptoms in the national comorbidity survey. *American Journal of Psychiatry*, **155**, 1398–406.

Susman, E. J., Inoff-Germain, G., Nottelmann, E. D. et al. (1987a). Hormones, emotional dispositions, and aggressive attributes in young adolescents. *Child Development*, **58**, 1114–34.

Susman, E. J., Nottelmann, E. D., Inoff-Germain, G., Dorn, L. D. & Chrousos, G. P. (1987b). Hormonal influences on aspects of psychological development during adolescence. *Journal of Adolescent Health Care*, **8**, 492–504.

Susman, E. J., Finkelstein, J. W., Chinchilli, V. M. et al. (1998). The effect of sex hormone replacement therapy on behavior problems and moods in adolescents with delayed puberty. *Journal of Pediatrics*, **133**, 521–5.

Targum, S. & Capodanno, A. (1983). The dexamethasone suppression test in adolescent psychiatric inpatients. *American Journal of Psychiatry*, **140**, 589–92.

Teicher, M. H., Glod, C. & Cole, J. O. (1990). Emergence of intense suicidal preoccupation during fluoxetine treatment. *American Journal of Psychiatry*, **147**, 207–10.

Thase, M. E., Dubé, S., Bowler, K. et al. (1996). Hypothalamic–pituitary–adrenocortical activity and response to cognitive behavioral therapy in unmedicated, hospitalized depressed patients. *American Journal of Psychiatry*, **153**, 886–91.

Vetulani, J. & Sulser, F. (1975). Action of various antidepressant treatments reduces reactivity of noradrenergic cyclic AMP-generating system in limbic forebrain. *Nature*, **257**, 495–6.

Warren, M. P. & Brooks-Gunn, J. (1989). Mood and behavior at adolescence: evidence for hormonal factors. *Journal of Clinical Endocrinology and Metabolism*, **69**, 77–83.

Waterman, G. S., Ryan, N. D., Puig-Antich, J. et al. (1991). Hormonal responses to examphetamine in depressed and normal adolescents. *Journal of the American Academy of Child and Adolescent Psychiatry*, **30**, 415–22.

Watson, D. & Kendall, P. C. (1989). Common differentiating features of anxiety and depression: current findings and future directions. In *Anxiety and Depression: distinctive and overlapping features*, ed. P. C. Kendall & D. Watson, pp. 493–508. New York: Academic Press.

Watson, D. & Tellegen, A. (1985). Toward a consensual structure of mood. *Psychological Bulletin*, **98**, 219–35.

Wehr, T. A. & Goodwin, F. K. (1981). Biological rhythms and psychiatry. In *American Handbook of Psychiatry*, ed. S. H. Arieti & K. H. Brodie, pp. 46–74. New York: Basic Books.

Weissman, M. M., Gershon, E. S., Kidd, K. K. et al. (1984). Psychiatric disorders in the relatives of probands with affective disorders. *Archives of General Psychiatry*, **41**, 13–21.

Weissman, M. M., Gammon, D., John, K. et al. (1987). Children of depressed parents: increased psychopathology and early onset of major depression. *Archives of General Psychiatry*, **44**, 847–53.

Weissman, M. M., Warner, B., Wickramaratne, P., Moreau, D. & Olfson, M. (1997). Offspring of depressed parents: 10 years later. *Archives of General Psychiatry*, **54**, 932–40.

Weissman, M. M., Wolk, S., Goldstein, R. B. et al. (1999). Depressed adolescents grown up. *Journal of the American Medical Association*, **281**, 1707–13.

Weller, E. B., Weller, B. Z., Fristad, M. A. & Preskorn, S. H. (1984). The dexamethasone suppression test in hospitalized prepubertal depressed children. *American Journal of Psychiatry*, **141**, 290–1.

Wender, P. H. (1971). *Minimal Brain Dysfunction in Children*. New York: Wiley-Interscience.

Wender, P. H., Kety, S. S., Rosenthal, P. et al. (1986). Psychiatric disorders in the biological and adoptive families of adopted individuals with affective disorder. *Archives of General Psychiatry*, **43**, 923–9.

Winokur, G., Black, D. W. & Nasrallah, A. (1988). Depressions secondary to other psychiatric disorders and medical illness. *American Journal of Psychiatry*, **145**, 233–7.

Young, W., Knowles, J. B., MacLean, A . W., Boag, L. & McConville, B. J. (1982). The sleep of childhood depressives: comparison with age-matched controls. *Biological Psychiatry*, **17**, 1163–9.

Zorrilla, E. P., DeRubeis, R. J. & Redei, E. (1995). High self-esteem, hardiness and affective stability are associated with higher basal pituitary–adrenal hormone levels. *Psychoneuroendocrinology*, **20**, 591–601.

Acknowledgement

The authors were supported by grants from the National Institute of Child Health and Development (NICHD) and the National Institute of Mental Health–Administration for Children, Youth, and Family (NIMH–ACYF) Consortium on Mental Health. We would also like to acknowledge Julia Graber for her support and critical reading of the manuscript, and Andrea Bastiani Archibald for searching the literature.

NOTES

1 Depressed symptoms are often distinguished from depressive mood in terms of duration, severity and number of symptoms. From a methodological point of view, behaviour problem checklists are the main source of research information on depressive symptomatology. These scales include a large number of symptoms, include either severity or duration ratings (or sometimes a combination of the two), and include behaviours representing internalizing and externalizing dimensions. Symptoms include sadness, crying, moody, low appetite, sleep disturbances, feelings of worthlessness, guilt and loneliness. Estimates of the number of youth with depressive symptomatology are variable, in part because of the lack of a consensus about criteria. However, based on the review by Angold (1988), about one-sixth of youth at any point of time might be characterized as having depressed symptomatology (Petersen et al., 1992). It is important to note that studies of risk factors do not differentiate between depressed mood and symptomatology. Consequently, the distinction is not made in the rest of this chapter.

2 However, a review of 10 recent studies suggests that the rate for teenagers might be higher (Petersen et al., 1992, 1993).

3 Pubertal timing, that is, whether one develops earlier or later than one's peers, is more likely to be associated with depressive symptoms in girls than pubertal status. Early-developing girls report more depressed affect than those who are average or late developers (Brooks-Gunn, 1988, 1991; Petersen et al., 1991; Graber et al., 1997).

4 Brain cell growth also occurs during childhood and adolescence (Greenough et al., 1987).

5 Timing of maternal reproductive status is also associated with adolescent girls' depressive symptoms (Paikoff et al., 1991a).

6 On a more general level, low family cohesion and expression seem to be associated with

depressive symptoms (Friedrich et al., 1982; Reinherz et al., 1989). Parents in such families tend to show a low degree of commitment and support for their children as well as low communication. Low parental commitment is associated with depressive symptoms and low self-esteem (Harter et al., 1992). And low family cohesion, when accompanied by stress, results in pronounced depressive symptoms among children (Friedrich et al., 1982; Cox & Brooks-Gunn, 1999).

5

Childhood depression: clinical phenomenology and classification

Israel Kolvin and Hartwin Sadowski

The concept of depression in childhood

Contribution of adult psychiatry to the concept of depression in childhood

Research into the nature and characteristics of depression in adults has provided an important framework for wider investigations of depression. In a
clinical sense, the term 'depression' denotes an illness characterized by a change
in mood that is persistent and sufficiently severe for it to be labelled a disorder.
In adult psychiatry, much research attention has focused on the classification of
depression. Two major distinctions have emerged: first, between bipolar and
unipolar affective disorders and second, between psychotic (or endogenous)
and neurotic (or reactive) depression (Paykel & Priest, 1992; Ramana & Paykel,
1992).

Using multivariate analysis methods, the Newcastle school asserted that two
separate depressive syndromes could be distinguished in adult patients: neurotic (reactive) and psychotic (endogenous) (Kiloh & Garside, 1963; Carney et
al., 1965). The distinctions within unipolar depression have not been replicated
(Kendell, 1968, 1975). The term 'endogenous' has, however, come to reflect,
clinically, a more severe and persistent depressive disorder, possibly unrelated
to environmental adversities (diagnostic criteria include somatic symptoms of
anorexia or weight loss; insomnia; early-morning wakening; diurnal variation
of mood; severe guilt; hopelessness and psychomotor retardation or agitation;
Ramana & Paykel, 1992). By contrast, neurotic or reactive depression is
considered clinically to be a milder disorder and possibly reactive to environmental adversities (accompanied by anxiety, initial insomnia, self-pity rather
than self-blame, and complaints of anorexia rather than complaints of weight
loss; Ramana & Paykel, 1992).

The earlier work on the classification of depression in adulthood concerning
the relationship between endogenous and neurotic depression has given way to
addressing not only the distinction and relationship between major depressive

disorder and dysthymia but also the superimposition of acute depressive episodes on chronic depressive disorders, i.e. the concept of 'double depression' (Keller & Shapiro, 1982; Keller et al., 1983).

Research in child psychiatry has followed in these footsteps. The focus of this chapter is the clinical phenomenology and descriptive classification of unipolar disorders of childhood. Research has confirmed that the clinical picture of affective disorders in children and adolescents resembles the presentation of affective disorders in adults (Kovacs et al., 1984a; Ryan et al., 1987; Mitchell et al., 1988; Kolvin et al., 1991). In addition, there is a focus on comorbidity of depressive disorders with other internalizing and externalizing disorders (Kovacs et al., 1984a; Mitchell et al., 1988; Kolvin et al., 1991).

Diagnostic criteria

A series of criteria for the classification of depression was subsequently proposed by Feighner and colleagues at St Louis (Feighner et al., 1972). These criteria were not dependent on the presence or absence of environmental events. Spitzer and colleagues (1978) adopted and further refined these proposals when producing the Research Diagnostic Criteria for the diagnosis of depression. For these purposes 'a diagnostic category has to be supported by specific descriptive criteria that specify characteristics that lead to making the diagnosis (inclusion criteria) and characteristics that lead to not making the diagnosis (exclusion criteria)' (Ramana & Paykel, 1992). The above are the bases of the *DSM-IV* classification, which offers strict diagnostic criteria that depend primarily on the symptoms and course of the disease; it is a system with a satisfactory interobserver reliability.

According to *DSM-IV* (American Psychiatric Association, 1994) the diagnosis of a major depressive disorder (MDD) requires the presence of at least five of nine symptoms during the same 2-week period, with one of the symptoms being depressed mood (dysphoria) for most of the day nearly every day, which can be irritable mood in children and adolescents or loss of interest or pleasure (anhedonia). The other listed nonmandatory symptoms include anhedonia, significant weight change (in children, a failure to make expected weight gains), insomnia or hypersomnia, psychomotor agitation or retardation, fatigue or loss of energy, feelings of worthlessness or inappropriate guilt, diminished ability to think or concentrate, and recurrent thoughts of death or suicidal ideation. The symptoms are not due to direct psychological effects of a substance or a general medical condition and are not accounted for by a bereavement. In addition to MDDs that are either single or recurrent, *DSM-IV* includes dysthymia and depressive disorders not otherwise specified.

Dysthymic disorder (DD), according to *DSM-IV*, mandates the experience of depressed mood for most of the day, for more days than not, for at least 2 years. For children and adolescents it allows an alternative criterion instead of depressive mood – namely, irritable mood – and also a shorter duration of at least 1 year. In addition to depressed or irritable mood, a diagnosis of dysthymic disorder requires two of the following six symptoms: (1) poor appetite or overeating; (2) insomnia or hypersomnia; (3) low energy or fatigue; (4) low self-esteem; (5) poor concentration or difficulty making decisions; and (6) feelings of hopelessness. As with MDD, the symptoms must not be due to direct physiological effects of a substance or a general medical condition, and the symptoms must cause clinically significant distress and impairment in social, occupational or other relevant areas of functioning. *DSM-IV* also specifies that, during the first year of dysthymia (for children and adolescents) there should be no evidence of MDD unless there has been a full remission of symptoms for 2 months before development of the dysthymia. After this 1 year in children and adolescents, there may be superimposed episodes of major depression, in which case both diagnoses are given.

Kovacs et al. (1994) described 'dysthymia' as predominantly characterized by gloomy and depressed mood, brooding about feeling unloved and additional manifestations of affective dysregulation, including irritability and anger. The other predominant feature is the 'cognitive' symptom of self-deprecation or negative self-esteem. As compared with MDD, dysthymia is distinguished by the virtual absence and significantly lower prevalence of anhedonia and social withdrawal; and comparatively lower rates of guilt, morbid preoccupation and impaired concentration. Practically none of the dysthymic children had reduced appetite, and few had hyposomnia and fatigue. Disobedient behaviour was the most prevalent associated feature of dysthymic disorder. Kovacs et al. (1994) see dysthymia as a persistent and chronic form of childhood depression.

In *ICD-10* (World Health Organization, 1992) there are similarly strict operationally defined diagnostic criteria. The main features have been described by Ramana & Paykel (1992) as follows: the single episode is distinguished from recurrent disorders and there is also a group of persistent affective disorders; three grades of severity are noted – mild, moderate, and severe. The term 'somatic syndrome' indicates the presence of endogenous or biological symptoms; the term 'psychotic' the presence of delusions, hallucinations or depressive stupor; finally, 'dysthymia' has been included as a persistent affective disorder.

However, in *ICD-10*, the definition and diagnostic criteria of dysthymia or mild depression are less clear and precise. *ICD-10* also states that dysthymia has much in common with the concepts of depressive neurosis and neurotic depression, and the age of onset is specified as being as early as the teenage years.

Kovacs & Devlin (1998) pointed out that the categories of depressive disorder in *DSM-IV* do not fully coincide with *ICD-10*. *DSM-IV* is more likely to view depression in relation to pattern of symptomatology and the nature of the impairment, rather than to stress-related factors. Further, *ICD-10*, although being explicit in relation to MDD and DD, has not yet given attention to the concept of 'double depressive' disorders. In these respects, *ICD-10* will need to be modified in the light of recent clinical experience and research findings.

Developmental influences

It has always been well known that misery and sadness could occur as symptoms in children of all ages. However, the notions of the negative affects of depressive disorders in childhood have only evolved over the last 20 years (Carlson & Cantwell, 1980a, b). The diagnosis of MDD and DD as specific conditions associated with impairment of function is now well accepted.

Kovacs (1986) argued that, in contrast to adults, children may not be capable of experiencing and/or reporting the symptoms thought to be representative of MDD. These include not only such characteristics as dysphoric mood and anhedonia, but especially negative cognitions of hopelessness, worthlessness and self-denigration, and feelings of guilt and self-blame. Thus, not only may many children be unable to differentiate between basic emotions, but also they may lack the ability to give an account of their presence and duration. Indeed, some authorities have argued that it is only from the age of 7 or 8 years that children can begin to reveal thoughts of self-denigration and feelings of shame (Kovacs, 1986). It was thought that despair and a sense of hopelessness did not fully surface before adolescence – a stage when formal operational thinking emerges (Verhulst, 1989). Thus, the pattern of depressive symptoms is likely to vary according to age and stage of development of the child or young adolescent, which may lead to a difference in the clinical manifestations of depression at different ages, even in the preschool years. For example, Kashani and colleagues (Kashani et al., 1984, 1987; Kashani & Carlson, 1985, 1987) reported that the symptom profiles in young children with DD appeared to differ from those in adolescents, probably reflecting the evolving language and cognitive abilities at different stages of child development. Although initially this notion was viewed with some dubiety, 10 years later the same group published more convincing empirical evidence (Kashani et al., 1997). Eight of 300 (2.7%) consecutively referred preschool children were diagnosed as having DD. Data were obtained from multiple informants. All of these preschool children presented with somatic complaints and aggressive behaviour; six of the eight showed psychomotor agitation. None of these symptoms is listed in *DSM-IV* under dysthymic disorder. In addition, none of the dysthymic disordered preschoolers experienced hopelessness, a pervasive loss of interest or brooding. Kashani et al. (1997) suggested that DD may be overlooked because of the associated symptoms (e.g. irritability, aggression, psychomotor agitation), which may be assumed to be indicative of externalizing disorders such as oppositional defiant, conduct, or attention deficit hyperactivity disorders, especially in preschool children, which may lead to an underreporting of depression at this developmental stage.

Mitchell et al. (1988) compared the phenomenology of major depression in 45 children with that in 50 adolescents. The symptom presentation did not differ according to age groups and the depressive symptoms in later age groups resembled those in adults. However, in a comparison of 95 children with 92 adolescents who met diagnostic criteria for MDD, Ryan et al. (1987) found that children were rated higher on somatic complaints, psychomotor agitation, and symptoms of phobic and separation anxiety. In contrast, adolescents were rated higher on anhedonia, hypersomnia, weight loss and gain, hopelessness and lethality of suicide attempts. Angold & Costello (1993) found higher levels of vegetative symptoms (weight loss or gain, insomnia or hypersomnia) reported by adolescent girls than by preadolescent girls (no differences were found for boys). In addition, Birmaher et al. (1996), in their review, note that endogenous-type symptoms (such as melancholia and suicidal attempts) increase with age. Other associated symptoms are childhood stage-related (such as separation anxiety, phobias, somatic complaints and behaviour problems) which occur more frequently in younger children (Carlson & Kashani, 1988; Mitchell et al., 1988; Kolvin et al., 1991).

To conclude, the picture that has emerged is that depression in childhood or adolescence resembles that of adults; the similarities are greatest between adolescents and adults, and least so in the preschool years, which probably relates to evolving conceptual and language development. Distress and negative affect may be expressed by externalizing symptomatology, especially during the preschool years.

Masked depression

The theme of one disorder masking or concealing another is not new in child psychiatry and dates from the writings of Glaser (1968), Cytryn & McKnew (1972) and Cytryn et al. (1980). These incorporate two allied concepts, the first of which is masked depression, which is depression without mood change where a wide range of symptoms – including hyperactivity, delinquency, aggressive behaviour and learning disorders – are the presenting clinical features. The second concept is that of depressive equivalents, where the characteristic features are somatic complaints, such as aches and pains which can occur in 'school phobia' (Kolvin et al., 1984). It is now known that school-age children with so-called masked depression do, in fact, show overt depressive features and may report depressed symptoms (Carlson & Cantwell, 1980a,b). The clinical features of depression may however be more basic or covert in younger children (McConville et al., 1973; Kashani & Carlson, 1985, 1987; Zeitlin, 1986). Kolvin et al. (1991) asserted that Cytryn et al. (1980) and Glaser (1968) were correct in suggesting that depression was often undetected. They did not find any evidence to support the notion that depressive conditions may manifest in a different way, but found that an important reason for depression remaining undetected and poorly delineated was inadequate systematic interviewing. There is now strong evidence that it is possible to diagnose both major depression and dysthymia in childhood and adolescence using criteria similar to those used in adults (Kovacs et al., 1984a,b; Cooper & Goodyer, 1993; Goodyer & Cooper, 1993; Kashani et al., 1997).

Thus the concept of masked depression is outdated: its basis was in a lack of systematic assessment, in poor diagnostic techniques, and in a focus on one single, predominant disorder rather than valid comorbid diagnoses.

Depression as a symptom, syndrome or disorder

Several authors have previously highlighted the distinction between depressive symptoms, syndromes and disorders in adulthood (Hamilton, 1982) and also in childhood (Carlson & Cantwell, 1980a,b; Kashani et al., 1984; Kolvin et al., 1984, 1991). In other words, sadness is not synonymous with depression. Thus, although dysphoria is commonly viewed as a necessary characteristic of depression, it is not a sufficient criterion in itself: for instance, sadness and misery are commonly observed in both clinical and nonclinical child populations. Verhulst et al. (1985) reported that parents of clinically referred children describe a high rate of depressive affect, ranging from over 20% in preschool children and over 40% of those in primary schools to 50% in those in secondary schools, with the rates for boys being marginally lower than those for girls. The respective rates in the nonreferred population were 5%, 6% and 9%, for girls; again, the rates for boys were marginally lower. Much higher rates are recorded in school population surveys in the USA.

There is some confusion about the distinction between syndromes and disorders. Nurcombe et al. (1989) have pointed out that the term 'depression' may be used to refer to a symptom of negative affect or mood; a syndrome consisting of a cluster of depressive symptoms; and a disorder reflecting a group of individuals with a set of clinical features associated with impairment of function. Others assert that the condition of a depressive disorder should be distinguished from other depressive states by differences in environmental factors, family patterns of illness, natural history, biological factors and response to treatment (Carlson & Cantwell, 1980b).

A more varied and integrating set of constructs derives from the work of Compas et al. (1993), who explore taxonomy, assessment and diagnosis of depression in adolescents. They highlight three separate hierarchical levels of depression: depressed mood, depressive syndromes and depressive disorder. Common to all three levels are a sad or depressed mood, low self-esteem and feelings of worthlessness. The three levels of depression are not based merely on progressively higher cut-offs regarding the same symptoms, but they also differ in their inclusion of symptoms of anxiety, somatic problems, concentration, and severity and duration of the symptoms included.

For *depressed mood*, the population rates vary from 15 to 40% according to definition and measurement of the depressed mood, the time frame employed and the gender of adolescence. Thus, up to 40% of youths experience transient elevations of a depressed mood resulting from diverse factors such as stressful life experiences, problematic interpersonal situations and hormonal fluctuations. For some adolescents the depressed mood will continue and develop into a *syndrome* – an anxious depressed syndrome with a 6-month period prevalence of 5–6%. This syndrome includes symptoms of anxiety that are not part of a purely depressed or sad mood.

The *depressive disorder* occurs in 1–3% of adolescents (either MDD or DD) as judged by diagnostic interviews. It includes somatic and vegetative symptoms that are not included in the depressed mood level or the depressive syndrome and involves dysregulation of somatic functioning, appetite and concentration. Compas et al. (1993) argue that depressive disorders do not explicitly include symptoms of anxiety, although symptoms are likely to accompany a diagnosis of depression.

Compas et al. (1993) suggest that adolescents with depressive disorders are a subgroup of those who are in the clinical range on measures of depressive syndromes (anxious depressed syndromes). They argue the directionality, when it is stated, is that anxiety disorders more often precede than follow depression (Kovacs et al., 1989): most of those with the depressive mood will not meet the criteria for an anxious depressed syndrome or disorder; in contrast, most of those with the syndrome or disorder will have recently experienced a significant depressed mood. Hence, Compas et al. argue that the syndrome is a subset of depressed mood, and the depressive disorder is a subset of the syndrome with a common core of negative affect. They assert that their model is corroborated by the high rates of comorbidity of depressive with anxiety disorder in adolescence (Kovacs et al., 1989).

Subclassification of depression

A crucial issue, from both a clinical and a theoretical viewpoint, is how depression in childhood should be subclassified. In adult psychiatry, this is a notoriously complex area and, even if depression in childhood is clinically similar, classification problems would be compounded by issues of child development.

There are two ways of defining depressive subsyndromes in childhood. The first is the classical clinical approach where clinical pictures are drawn, utilizing an inductive method combined with clinical judgement. In this way new subcategories of depression can be defined and complement the general profile of depression. This necessary first step needs to be validated by empirical research: for example, it has not yet been established that MDD in childhood is a homogeneous condition. The second method is a statistical approach using multivariate procedures such as exploratory factor analysis. In this method it is hypothesized that a set of variates exists that account substantially for any interrelationships between symptoms (Maxwell, 1977). Hence, theoretically, exploratory factor analysis is capable of identifying those symptoms (and perhaps other features) with greatest validity because they will be grouped in characteristic patterns. This view is consistent with the hypothesis that there is one general factor representing all the symptoms, as well as additional differentiating bipolar factors. More often, principal component analysis (PCA) is widely used for exploring a covariance structure; it is a useful technique in nonstandard situations where the data may not fit classical assumptions of multinormality (Taylor, 1979). It is hoped that the derived components will represent more basic variability in the data than in the observed variates (Maxwell, 1977). Using PCA, the first few rotated components 'often give a robust identification of major trends in the data' (Taylor, 1979). For classification purposes, varimax rotation may help to clarify which symptoms are related to particular factors or components. It is possible, however, that in the process their variances may be greatly inflated by error (Maxwell, 1977).

If the sample is of sufficient size, PCA can be complemented with a further technique: cluster analysis. Cluster procedures are a way of identifying those subsets of individuals whose behavioural features cluster together, i.e. which have much in common within each cluster, but little in common between the clusters (Aldenderfer & Blashfield, 1984). Although the cluster analysis approach is theoretically sound, there is still debate about the variability and meaning of the number of clusters still identified (Kolvin et al., 1991).

Kolvin and colleagues (1991) factor-analysed mental state data obtained from interviews using a modified version of the Kiddie-SADS (Schedule for Affective Disorders and Schizophrenia for School-age Children; see later). The subjects were clinically referred children, aged 9–16 years. Data from interviews carried out independently with both the child and its parents were used for the analysis. A number of components emerged, but only results concerning depressive syndromes are given here. The PCA revealed an 'endogenous-type' depression component composed of the features of dysphoria, anhedonia, increased fatigue and psychomotor retardation, and a depressive cognitions component accompanied by thoughts of suicide. The two emergent components overlapped extensively with those identified by Ryan et al. (1987) in their Pittsburgh study.

A further cluster analysis also identified two clusters – negative cognitions and endogenous depression – with features markedly similar to the PCA findings. The negative cognitions cluster consisted of self-denigration, hopelessness and guilt, irritability; suicide; a sense of anxiety, fear and anger; the endogenous depression cluster consisted of anhedonia; hopelessness; withdrawal; dysphoric mood, worrying, insomnia; loss of appetite; lack of energy; suicidal ideation, somatic complaints, slowing of thoughts; anxiety, and school refusal (details of these analyses are available in Kolvin et al., 1991).

Verhulst and colleagues carried out a similar factor analysis using data from the Child Behavior Checklist completed on samples of boys and girls aged 6–11 and 12–16 in a province of Holland (Verhulst et al., 1985). These authors reported the presence of an empirically derived depressive syndrome in 6–11-year-olds: the main features that emerged were those of feeling unloved, unhappy, sad, depressed mood; feelings of worthlessness; feeling persecuted; feeling lonely; worrying; fears of schools; suicidal talk; suspiciousness; feelings of guilt and obsessions. However, in the 12–16-year-old sample, the symptoms of depression seemed to vary and no distinctive depressive syndrome emerged. It would seem, therefore, that the findings from multivariate data analysis are influenced to some extent by the method by which data were obtained (such as self-rating compared with direct interview), the age and gender of the subjects, the population under scrutiny and the type of multivariate analysis that is employed.

It is important to note the similarities between cross-national studies and also with adult studies. For instance, Ryan et al. (1987) in Pittsburgh reported meaningful components (factors) that proved to be similar for both children and adolescents and that included endogenous depression and depression with negative cognitions. This pattern proved also to be the case in the Newcastle studies. However, the Dutch study (Verhulst et al., 1985) did not replicate the presence of a depressive syndrome in the senior school sample. Further, in the Pittsburgh research, cluster analysis was rather inconclusive, with the clusters not indicating any precise pattern of symptoms. However, as the Newcastle workers identified symptom clusters that proved to be discrete, it is likely that the basis of the discrepancy across these studies resides in the methods that have been employed.

The distinction between negative cognitions and endogenous depressive factors in the Pittsburgh (Ryan et al., 1987) and Newcastle (Kolvin et al., 1991) studies suggests that depression syndromes in childhood may differ in their nature and characteristics from those in adults (Kiloh & Garside, 1963; Carney et al., 1965). Thus, both the Dutch and UK child studies support the notion that a number of the depressive symptoms considered to be characteristic in adults emerge as less evident in childhood: for instance, loss of weight, diurnal variation of mood and psychomotor retardation are less pronounced in childhood than in adulthood (Verhulst, 1989; Kolvin et al., 1991). Further, whereas initial insomnia is frequently reported in childhood, terminal insomnia is reported less often (Ryan et al., 1987; Carlson & Kashani, 1988; Kolvin et al., 1991). In contrast, somatic symptoms are often reported by younger children with depression (Carlson & Kashani, 1988). It is essential that more is known about the origins, nature, duration and course of these subsyndromes in child populations.

Mixed depression – comorbidity

Comorbidity is the concurrent presence of two or more disorders greater than would be expected by chance alone. As already indicated, the pattern of nondepressive comorbid disorders (such as phobic anxiety or conduct disorder) varies between depressed children and adolescents. These comorbid conditions suggest that depression in childhood is a clinically heterogeneous phenomenon (Ryan et al., 1987; Kolvin et al., 1992).

Comorbid psychiatric disorders are common in major depressive disorders. The rates in clinical studies run from up to 70% in depressed children in North

American studies (Kovacs et al., 1984a; Ryan et al., 1987; Biederman et al., 1993, 1995), to as high as 90% in UK community and clinical studies (Kolvin et al., 1991; Goodyer et al., 1997). In the USA the most frequent comorbid diagnoses are DD, anxiety disorders and disruptive disorders (Lewinsohn et al., 1991; Angold & Costello, 1993); in the UK they consist of separation anxiety disorders (33–65%), conduct disorder (20–37%) and DD (25–50%; Kolvin et al., 1991; Goodyer et al., 1997).

Angold et al. (1999), in their review of 19 population studies of depressive disorders, reported that nine had comorbid anxiety disorders with rates of 40% or more. They make the distinction between homotypic comorbidity (which refers to continuity of the same phenomena over time) and heterotypic comorbidity (which refers to different forms of disorders over time); they also differentiate between concurrent and successive comorbidity (which are self-explanatory).

A high rate of comorbid depression in children presenting with school refusal disorder (separation anxiety disorder) has also been described (Kolvin et al., 1984). Kolvin and colleagues (1991) argued that these findings did not support the concept of a single MDD in childhood and adolescence. Indeed, such a classification may merely obscure the wider psychopathological picture of depressive disorders in this age group. This may be true even where the diagnosis is that of a conduct or phobic disorder. Hence, it is essential, whatever the predominant disorder, that the assessor should check for associated disorders. In particular, depression should be looked for in nondepressive presentations. Kolvin et al. (1991) argued that, if such an assessment is omitted, depression may simply remain undetected because of diagnostic ideology, or may be concealed by other symptoms through an inadequate technique of clinical assessment and diagnosis.

Advances in knowledge about phenomenology and relationships between depressive disorders, anxiety disorders and externalizing disorders is accumulating at a rapid pace. The studies available are not always rigorous but they are beginning to achieve a meaningful pattern covering the three major forms of comorbidity. These are:

1. comorbidity between affective disorders, such as internalizing disorder running true to form, and the distinction and relationship between major depression, dysthymia and double depression in children and adolescents;
2. comorbidity between depressive and anxiety disorders, and
3. comorbidity between depressive and externalizing disorders.

Each of these is discussed below.

Affective disorders running true to form and comorbidity

Kovacs & Devlin (1998) emphasize that one of the assumptions of studies of diagnostic validity is that disorders should run 'true to form' (Feighner et al., 1972; Kendell, 1975). In brief, a subject with a depressive disorder at some point in time is more likely to develop a subsequent episode of depression than of any other disorder; this is also true for anxiety disorders, which have a high risk for further episodes of anxiety, despite both these disorders being associated with various other comorbid psychiatric conditions. This homotype of internalizing disorders on follow-up has been documented in various epidemiological studies (McGee et al., 1992; Orvaschel et al., 1995).

In their review, Kovacs & Devlin (1998) concluded as follows: first, having had one episode of depressive or anxiety disorder represents a risk factor for further episodes of the same general type of disorder; and second, the persistent risks of illness episodes in affected children and adolescents may be in part a function of some attribute which is within a person, and which is reasonably stable during development. They hypothesize that there may well be a biological underpinning of personality and temperament which could influence the psychiatric outcome. They go on to propose that the construct of previous 'high negative emotionality' or 'negative affectivity' reflects a specific temperament–personality characteristic which consists of the poor ability to regulate negative emotion or mood. The paper provides an interesting theoretical account of the biological cognitive mechanisms that potentially complement the genetic factors to increase the probability of the recurrence of the same disorder, thereby promoting predictability.

One of the fascinating distinctions that has emerged from the recent literature relates to the concept of double depression, where both MDD and DD coexist in the same subject.

Ferro et al. (1994) studied 62 male depressive inpatients, admittedly with a higher age ceiling (6–23 years) than would be perceived as acceptable for adolescents. They made a distinction between double depression consisting of MDD and DD; MDD without DD; and DD without MDD. They reported as follows:

1. All the children in the dysthymia group had comorbid externalizing disorders and fewer comorbid anxiety disorders – the latter were more common in major depressives.
2. Both dysthymics and double depressives were the most socially impaired, and major depressives alone were the least socially impaired.
3. Suicidal behaviour, anhedonia, low self-esteem and loss of energy were more common in major and double depression than in dysthymia.

Kovacs et al. (1994) found that three-quarters of early-onset DD children had a subsequent MDD during a 3–12-year follow-up, which far outnumbered nonaffective conditions. In a study of 112 clinically referred 8–13-year-olds with a first episode of MDD or DD, Kovacs et al. (1997) followed recovery from onset and also studied baseline predictors of recovery, comparing patterns for MDD and DD and the relation between these two. They found that 86% of major depressives but only 7% of dysthymic children had recovered 2 years after onset. The median episode length of MDD was 8–9 months, with 30–40% who could be expected to recover by 6 months from onset, 70–80% by 12 months from onset and 80–95% by 18 months. In contrast, the median duration of dysthymia was nearly 4 years.

An important clinical implication of double depression is that it results in more severe and longer depressive episodes, more suicidal behaviour and greater psychosocial impairment than in the subgroups of youths with MDD alone or DD alone (Ferro et al., 1994; Kovacs et al., 1994). When MDD was superimposed on previous DD, recovery from MDD was faster than in the absence of underlying DD. Kovacs et al. (1997) suggested that this probably reflects the fact that it is easier to return to asymptomatic (dysthymia) baseline than to an entirely asymptomatic state.

Flisher (1999) has reviewed the relationship between mood disorders and suicidal behaviour in children, with the major conclusion that mood disorder is a predictor of subsequent suicidal ideation and attempts, and that both are predictors of subsequent depression. Flisher & Schaffer (1997) offer three possible explanations for these relationships: first, suicidal phenomena may be manifestations of depression; second, depression may be a manifestation of suicidal thoughts or feelings; third, both depression and suicidal phenomena may be manifestations of a third variable. Factors that distinguish depressed children or adolescents from those who do not make suicidal attempts include cognitive distortions, life stresses, sense of hopelessness, impulsivity, inability to tolerate intense negative affect or emotional distress and anger (Brent et al., 1990; Kovacs et al., 1993). However, there is not sufficient information to explain the pathways to these behaviours. For a detailed discussion of suicide and depression, see Chapter 10.

Comorbidity between depressive and anxiety disorders

Mitchell et al. (1988) reported that subjects with combined depression and anxiety were more severely depressed than those with major depression alone. There was a strong relationship between separation anxiety and depression in children and adolescents, irrespective of age or gender. Having a coexisting anxiety disorder also increases the likelihood that the depression is endogenous. Kovacs et al. (1989) reported that anxious children tend to be younger than depressed children when first diagnosed. Furthermore, there is evidence that a high level of anxiety predicts subsequent depression (Compas et al., 1993; Reinherz et al., 1993).

Cole et al. (1998) monitored 330 elementary school children and their parents ($n = 228$) and examined the temporal relationship between anxiety and depressive symptoms in children. Individual differences on measures of depression and anxiety proved remarkably stable over time. High levels of children's self-reported and parent-reported anxiety in children predicted increases in self- and parent-reported depression over time; however, high levels of reported depression in children did not predict increases in anxiety. These findings support the hypothesis that prior anxiety predisposes children and adolescents to depression. These findings do not imply that the individuals' level of depression and anxiety did not change but, rather, that each of these individuals was stable in the ranking in relation to other individuals in the sample. Furthermore, children with anxiety and depressive disorders had a relatively high likelihood of receiving a similar diagnosis later in life (Kovacs et al., 1989; Sanford et al., 1995). Cole et al. (1998) argued that, to regard such individuals as relatively symptom-free between episodes may be unwise, as the children with depressive anxiety disorders may move back and forth across a diagnostic threshold without showing substantial increases or decreases in the underlying condition. Like many other studies, the above research focuses attention on anxiety as a precursor of depression. However, the fact that high levels of self- and parent-reported depression did not predict increases in children's anxiety symptoms leads Cole et al. (1998) to argue that not only does anxiety give rise to depression but, additionally, increases in depression proved to be a precursor of a reduction in anxiety symptoms. They, therefore, suggest a model compatible with their data in which anxiety shifts into depression.

McCauley et al. (1993) examined the initial presentation and longitudinal clinical course of depression in children and adolescents over a period of 3 years. Female gender and the presence of a coexisting anxiety disorder were significantly related to the severity of the initial depression. Cole et al. (1998) point out this overlap between anxiety and depression, which has now been well documented (Bernstein et al., 1996), and led Finch et al. (1985) to hypothesize that both depression and anxiety reflect a unitary construct of negative affect rather than two distinct disorders. Further, the concurrence of depression with an anxiety disorder increases the severity and duration of depressive disorders (McCauley et al., 1993) and increases suicidal behaviour and psychosocial problems (Kovacs et al., 1989; Brent et al., 1990).

Another view put forward by Mitchell et al. (1988) is that comorbid anxiety, with major depression, may discriminate a subtype of depressed youths.

An important overlap is the extensive comorbidity between MDD and posttraumatic stress disorder (PTSD) in the various studies of psychic trauma in children (McLeer et al., 1994; Trowell et al., 1999). Some argue that PTSD precedes posttrauma depression, possibly enhancing the vulnerability of children and adolescents to the emergence of subsequent MDD.

Comorbidity between depressive and externalizing disorders

Kovacs et al. (1994) reported that conduct problems may occur as a consequence of depression and may persist after depression remits. In their follow-up, the median duration of a DD in children was nearly twice as long (6 years) if a comorbid externalizing disorder was present than it was in children without any externalizing disorders (3.7 years). Depressed subjects with an associated disruptive disorder also have a worse short-term outcome: although there are fewer recurrences of depression, there are higher rates of suicidal attempts and higher rates of adult criminality. Thus, in their review, Birmaher et al. (1996) concluded that depressed children with disruptive disorders may comprise a distinct clinical and aetiological subgroup.

Renouf et al. (1997) studied the social competence and self-esteem of 94 psychiatrically referred boys and 67 girls who had a conduct disorder, depression, or both. A repeated-measures design was used over an interval of 4.4 years; the two measures were the social competence scale of the Child Behavior Checklist and the Cooper–Smith self-esteem measure. These investigators found that either conduct disorder or a depressive disorder, during a given period, predicted subsequent lower social competence than if the child was free of these conditions. (These are similar to the findings of Asarnow & Ben-Meir, 1988; Goodyer et al., 1989; Biederman et al., 1993.) Having both disorders predicted greater impairment in social competence than having only one. Conduct disorder had a more severe and longer-term impact on children's social competence than did depression; furthermore, with depression, the adverse effect on self-esteem was transient. Renouf et al. (1997) conclude that such findings may not be replicable to younger children or older adolescents.

Diagnostic schemas

A range of diagnostic schemas have emerged from the different centres, all to a greater or lesser extent addressing the above issues. Recent work provides some information about the validity of these schemas and the extent to which they agree, or disagree, with each other. The main schemas so far are those developed in the USA by Puig-Antich & Chambers (1978) and by Weinberg et al. (1973), and in the UK by Kolvin et al. (1991).

The diagnostic schemas incorporate different criteria. For instance, in a recent study the Newcastle group used the Standard Psychiatric Interview (SPI) (Goldberg et al., 1970), which is a semistructured schedule designed to study psychiatric disorders in adults in a community setting. It has a number of precise probes as well as clearcut definition of symptoms and can provide ratings on a range of clinical disorders. For these purposes it was appropriately modified by the inclusion of an introductory interview: interviewers were encouraged to use phraseology and concepts appropriate to the child's cognitive level and stage of psychological development, and in this way to accommodate the different abilities of children to give accounts about themselves. These workers reported that the instrument showed satisfactory reliability over both the childhood and adolescent periods, provided that it was administered by experienced child psychiatrists. In summary, Kolvin et al. (1991) reported that the SPI can be employed, using concepts and definitions of disorders geared more usually to adults, allowing both a clinical diagnosis of depression and rating of severity of disorder. Thus, major depressive episodes can be identified that are relatively discrete and associated with a specified number of symptoms of the depressive syndrome.

However, the most commonly used and validated schedule in assessing depression in children is the Kiddie-SADS (Ryan et al., 1987), which has now been updated (Kaufman et al., 1997). It is essentially a modification of the Schedule for Affective Disorders and Schizophrenia (Spitzer et al., 1978), and has been employed with children between 6 and 17 years of age (Orvaschel et al., 1982; Chambers et al., 1985). This is a reliable instrument for measuring symptoms of depression and conduct disorders, although ratings of anxiety disorders have not been as consistent.

The schema devised by Weinberg et al. (1973) is one of the better-known of the earlier schemas: it offers a list of primary and secondary symptoms based on the criteria for diagnosis of depression in adulthood (Feighner et al., 1972). To be diagnosed as depressed, children need to display primary symptoms of dysphoric mood and self-deprecation, plus two of a further eight symptoms. In the original version there was no guideline as to duration or severity of symptomatology; this gave rise to problems of broadness of the inclusion criteria and hence to high rates of depression in the populations in which it was used.

One of the newer instruments is the Newcastle Depression Inventory (Kolvin et al., 1984, 1989, 1991, 1992), which has been upgraded and modified.

The inventory has themes borrowed from the Kiddie-SADS but with the ratings of symptoms reorganized so that they are scored on an ordinal scale to reflect severity (1, 2, 3 and 4), with subsequent recoding on a binary scale (0, 0, 1, 1). The technique allows either categorical rating of depression based on a clinical algorithm, or a dimension of severity of depression, based on the summation of the satisfied criteria. Alternatively, it can be used for diagnosis, primarily being guided by *DSM-III* diagnostic categories.

Kolvin et al. (1991) have reported that, once the severity of diagnostic criteria had been taken into account, substantial agreement was found between such different schemas as the Weinberg and the Newcastle, each being equally valid in relation to an independent clinical assessment. Further, as all the diagnostic criteria are rated on ordinal scales, summation allows the emergence of quantitative variations within qualitatively distinct disorders (Rutter, 1986; Kolvin et al., 1991).

Diagnostic algorithms

The distinction between symptoms and syndromes of depression in adulthood has been complemented by the specification of diagnostic criteria for depressive disorders by Feighner et al. (1972) and Spitzer et al. (1978). In a similar way, over the last decade, clinicians in the field of child and adolescent psychiatry have explored the distinction between symptoms and syndromes, and such work has facilitated the development of diagnostic interviews or checklists. One such checklist that has emerged is that of Kolvin et al. (1992); its utility is that not only does it allow a discrimination between depressed and nondepressed children attending a consulting child psychiatry clinic, but also it includes features of the two subtypes of childhood depression – endogenous and negative cognitions. The latter work focused on a brief inventory that had been developed previously in relation to distinction between those children with school phobias who were depressed or not depressed (Kolvin et al., 1984). It has been used as a research instrument and was intended to provide a reasonably rapid assessment of the presence of depression with a satisfactory degree of reliability and validity.

The questionnaire was intended primarily as a clinical interview instrument and the updated version also provides an algorithm for diagnosis of depressive syndromes of varying severity. These authors (Kolvin et al., 1992) have provided evidence that dysphoria is not a mandatory criterion for childhood depression; this supports the view, previously mentioned, that although dysphoria is commonly viewed as a necessary characteristic of depression, it is not a sufficient criterion in itself (Hamilton, 1982; Rutter, 1988).

The extended questionnaire consists of 13 items and, although only slightly longer than the original, has many advantages. First, the constituent items offer a better representation of the different factors or clusters than the original scale; this is especially true of those reflecting depressive cognitions on the one hand and endogenous depression on the other. Second, there is good evidence of validity, although it could be argued that the validation levels may have been inflated by the methods used to select items. The items that have been identified and selected are as follows: dysphoric mood; anhedonia; feeling unloved; weeping; loss of energy; loss of interest; loss of appetite; lack of concentration; sense of emptiness; depersonalization; suicidal ideation; depressive thoughts; sense of hopelessness.

This brief scale is likely to make a useful contribution to symptomatic diagnosis of either marked or moderate depression, utilizing a diagnostic algorithm, especially when used by a less-experienced clinician. In the circumstances, the inventory is used with a cut-off of 5 on a binary scale, for symptomatic diagnosis of marked depression, or with a cut-off of 4, for moderate depression, including endogenous depression.

The use of binary and ordinal scales in diagnosing depression merits further comment. It is essential that the clinician bears in mind the distinction between substantial and marginal symptomatology, to avoid giving equal importance to a large number of symptoms, some of which may have little diagnostic significance. For instance, when using a four-point ordinal scale, a subject scoring 2 on each of the 13 items would score 26 but is unlikely to be depressed, whereas a subject scoring 4 on 4 items and only 1 on each of the other nine items will have a total of 25 points, and could well be depressed. Thus, the simple summation of scores when using an ordinal scale provides a good representation of overall severity, but could be misleading diagnostically; hence, a binary system of recoding is recommended as an essential supplement to the use of an ordinal scale, as it is likely to contribute to the valid discrimination of depression.

A fundamental drawback of the algorithm approach (and this is true for self-rating scales also) is the inability to incorporate criteria of impairment or of psychosocial or behavioural handicap. Such features may contribute to improving the reliability and validity of diagnosis (Weissmann, 1990).

Summary and conclusions

The advent of reliable and valid measures of present mental state in children and adolescents has greatly advanced our understanding of the phenomenology of major (unipolar) depression. School-aged children (and perhaps even younger) are capable of reporting their feelings and thoughts. In some cases of depression, the parents are not fully aware of their child's symptoms. Direct interviewing of the child provides a more accurate assessment of certain aspects of the child's mental state than interviewing of a parent, but complementary interviewing of the parents is well advised (Barrett et al., 1991). Parental information may be informative, especially for the less subjective and more externalizing symptoms, and for chronology of onset, history of duration and stressors.

The features of depression in school-aged children and adolescents are similar to those found in adults. There are, however, important developmental variations. Further research is required into the mechanisms of these developmental influences on the expression of depressive syndromes.

There are some final points. First, much more needs to be discovered about the natural history and outcome of different types of childhood depression right into adulthood. So far, longitudinal research has revealed evidence of psychopathological progression and shifts. The most prominent shift is where an MDD becomes superimposed on a DD, giving rise to a double depressive disorder. A progression is exemplified by anxiety disorder moving into an MDD and enhancing the severity of the latter. Further, a DD has a high risk of spawning an externalizing disorder which may persist after the depression remits. Depression may not only be followed by suicidal behaviour but, on occasions, may be secondary to it. Second, the notion of gateway (Kovacs et al., 1994) to major depression needs to be widened to incorporate not only dysthymic but also anxiety disorder. Third, the social and self-esteem consequences of different types of comorbidity need further exploration.

What has not yet emerged is a clear idea of the proportions of the prior disorders which shift into major depression, and the proportion of MDDs that remain 'uncontaminated' by comorbidity. Lastly, the endogenous and the negative cognition subcategories of major depression in childhood and dysthymia have not yet been elucidated (Ryan et al., 1987; Kolvin et al., 1991). Further studies are required into whether these are two distinct subgroups with regard to their biological bases, genetic loading for MDD and in their response to different forms of therapy (cognitive behavioural, psychodynamic and psychopharmacological).

REFERENCES

Aldenderfer, M. S. & Blashfield, R. K. (1984). *Cluster Analysis*. London: Sage Publications.

American Psychiatric Association (1994). *Diagnostic and Statistical Manual of Mental Disorders*, (DSM-IV) 4th edn. Washington, DC: American Psychiatric Association.

Angold, A. & Costello, E. J. (1993). Depressive comorbidity in children and adolescents: empirical, theoretical, and methodological issues. *American Journal of Psychiatry*, **150**, 1779–1.

Angold, A., Costello, E. J. & Erkanli, A. (1999). Comorbidity. *Journal of Child Psychology and Psychiatry*, **40**, 57–87.

Asarnow, J. R. & Ben-Meir, S. (1988). Children with schizophrenia spectrum of depressive disorders: a comparative study of premorbid adjustment, onset pattern and severity of impairment. *Journal of Child Psychology and Psychiatry*, **29**, 477–88.

Barrett, L. M., Berney, T. P., Bhate, S. et al. (1991). Diagnosing childhood depression: who should be interviewed – parent or child? *British Journal of Psychiatry*, **159** (Suppl. 11), 22–7.

Bernstein, G. A., Borchardt, C. M. & Perwein, A. R. (1996). Anxiety disorders of childhood and adolescence; a review of the past ten years. *Journal of the American Academy of Child and Adolescent Psychiatry*, **35**, 1110–19.

Biederman, J., Rosenbaum, J. F., Bolduc-Murphy, E. A. et al. (1993). A three-year follow-up of children with and without behavioural inhibition. *Journal of the American Academy of Child and Adolescent Psychiatry*, **32**, 814–21.

Biederman, J., Faraone, S., Mick, E. & Lelon, E. (1995). Psychiatric comorbidity among referred juveniles with major depression: fact or artifact? *Journal of the American Academy of Child and Adolescent Psychiatry*, **34**, 579–90.

Birmaher, B., Ryan, N. D., Williamson, D. E. et al. (1996). Childhood and adolescent depression: a review of the past 10 years. Part I. *Journal of the American Academy of Child and Adolescent Psychiatry*, **35**, 1427–39.

Brent, D. A., Kolko, D. J., Allan, M. J. & Brown, R. V. (1990). Suicidality in affectively disordered adolescent inpatients. *Journal of the American Academy of Child and Adolescent Psychiatry*, **29**, 586–93.

Carlson, G. A. & Cantwell, D. P. (1980a). Unmasking masked depression in children and adolescents. *American Journal of Psychiatry*, **137**, 44–9.

Carlson, G. A. & Cantwell, D. P. (1980b). A survey of depressive symptoms and disorder in a child psychiatric population. *Journal of Child Psychology and Psychiatry*, **21**, 19–25.

Carlson G. A. & Kashani, J. H. (1988). Phenomenology of major depressive disorder from childhood through adulthood. Analysis of three studies. *American Journal of Psychiatry*, **145**, 1222–5.

Carney, M. W. P., Roth, M. & Garside, R. F. (1965). The diagnosis of depressive syndromes and prediction of ECT response. *British Journal of Psychiatry*, **111**, 659–74.

Chambers, W. J., Puig-Antich, J., Hires, M. et al. (1985). The assessment of affective disorders in children and adolescents by semi-structured interview. *Archives of General Psychiatry*, **42**, 696–702.

Cole, D. A., Peeke, L. G., Martin, J. M., Truglio, R. & Seroczynski, A. D. (1998). A longitudinal look at the relation between depression and anxiety in children and adolescents. *Journal of Consulting and Clinical Psychology*, **66**, 451–60.

Compas, B. E., Sydney, E. & Grant, K. E. (1993). Taxonomy, assessment, and diagnosis of depression during adolescence. *Psychological Bulletin*, **114**, 323–44.

Cooper, P. J. & Goodyer, I. (1993). A community study of depression in adolescent girls. I:

Estimates of symptom and syndrome prevalence. *British Journal of Psychiatry*, **163**, 369–74.

Cytryn, L. & McKnew, D. H. (1972). Proposed classification of childhood depression. *American Journal of Psychiatry*, **129**, 149–55.

Cytryn, L., McKnew, D. H. & Bunney, W. E. (1980). Diagnosis of depression in children: a reassessment. *American Journal of Psychiatry*, **137**, 22–5.

Feighner, J. P., Robins, E., Guze, S. B. et al. (1972). Diagnostic criteria for use in psychiatric research. *Archives of General Psychiatry*, **26**, 57–63.

Ferro, T., Carlson, G. A., Grayson, P. & Klein, D. N. (1994). Depressive disorders: distinctions in children. *Journal of the American Academy of Child and Adolescent Psychiatry*, **33**, 664–70.

Finch, A., Saylor, C. & Edwards, G. (1985). Children's depression inventory: sex and grade norms for normal children. *Journal of Consulting and Clinical Psychology*, **53**, 424–5.

Flisher, A. J. (1999). Annotation. Mood disorder in suicidal children and adolescents: recent developments. *Journal of Child Psychology and Psychiatry*, **40**, 315–24.

Flisher, A. J. & Schaffer, D. (1997). Relations entre suicide et depression dans l'enfance et l'adolescence. In *Les Depressions chez l'enfant et l'adolescent. Faits et questions*, ed. M. C. Mouren-Simeoni & R. G. Klein. Paris: Expansion Scientifique Publishers.

Glaser, K. (1968). Masked depression in children and adolescents. *Annual Progress in Child Psychiatry and Child Development*, **1**, 345–55.

Goldberg, D. P., Cooper, B., Eastwood, M. R. et al. (1970). A standardised psychiatric interview suitable for use in community surveys. *British Journal of Preventative Social Medicine*, **24**, 18–27.

Goodyer, I. & Cooper, P. J. (1993). A community study of depression in adolescent girls. II: The clinical features of identified disorder. *British Journal of Psychiatry*, **163**, 374–80.

Goodyer, I., Wright, C. & Altham, P. (1989). Recent friendships in anxious and depressed school age children. *Psychological Medicine*, **19**, 165–74.

Goodyer, I. M., Herbert, J., Secher, S. M. & Pearson, J. (1997). Short-term outcome of major depression: I. Comorbidity and severity at presentation as predictors of persistent disorder. *Journal of the American Academy of Child and Adolescent Psychiatry*, **36**, 179–87.

Hamilton, M. (1982). Symptoms and assessment of depression. In *Handbook of Affective Disorders*, ed. E. S. Paykel, pp. 3–11. Edinburgh: Churchill-Livingstone.

Kashani, J. H. & Carlson, G. A. (1985). Major depressive disorder in a preschooler. *Journal of the American Academy of Child and Adolescent Psychiatry*, **24**, 490–4.

Kashani, J. H. & Carlson, G. A. (1987). Seriously depressed preschoolers. *American Journal of Psychiatry*, **144**, 348–50.

Kashani, J. H., Ray, J. S. & Carlson, G. A. (1984). Depression and depressive-like states in preschool-age children in a child development unit. *American Journal of Psychiatry*, **141**, 1397–402.

Kashani, J. H., Carlson, G. A., Beck, N. C. et al. (1987). Depression, depressive symptoms, and depressed mood among a community sample of adolescents. *American Journal of Psychiatry*, **144**, 931–4.

Kashani, J. H., Wesley, D. A., Beck, N. C., Bledsoe, Y. & Reid, J. (1997). Dysthymic disorder in clinically referred preschool children. *Journal of the American Academy of Child and Adolescent Psychiatry*, **36**, 1426–33.

Kaufman, J., Birmaher, B., Brent, D. et al. (1997). Schedule for Affective Disorders and Schizophrenia for School-age children – Present and Lifetime version (K-SADS-PL). *Journal of the American Academy of Child and Adolescent Psychiatry*, **36**, 980–8.

Keller, M. B. & Shapiro, R. W. (1982). 'Double depression': superimposition of acute depressive episodes on chronic depressive disorders. *American Journal of Psychiatry*, **139**, 438–42.

Keller, M. B. & Lavori, P. W., Endicott, J., Coryell, W. & Klerman, G. L. (1983). 'Double depression': two year follow-up. *American Psychiatry*, **140**, 689–94.

Kendell, R. E. (1968). *The Classification of Depressive Illnesses*. London: Oxford University Press.

Kendell, R. E. (1975). *The Role of Diagnosis in Psychiatry*. Philadelphia, PA: J. B. Lippincott.

Kiloh, L. & Garside, R. F. (1963). The independence of neurotic depression and endogenous depression. *British Journal of Psychiatry*, **109**, 451–63.

Kolvin, I., Berney, T. P. & Bhate, S. (1984). Classification and diagnosis of depression in school phobia. *British Journal of Psychiatry*, **145**, 347–57.

Kolvin, I., Barrett, L., Berney, T. P. et al. (1989). The Newcastle child depression project: studies in the diagnosis and classification of childhood depression. In *Contemporary Themes in Psychiatry, A tribute to Sir Martin Roth*, ed. K. Davison & A. Kerr, pp. 149–55. London: Gaskell.

Kolvin, I., Barrett, L. M., Bhate, S. R. et al. (1991). Issues in the diagnosis and classification of childhood depression. *British Journal of Psychiatry*, **159** (Suppl. 11), 9–11.

Kolvin, I., Berney, T. P., Barrett, L. M. & Bhate, S. (1992). Development and evaluation of a diagnostic algorithm for depression in childhood. *European Child and Adolescent Psychiatry*, **1**, 1–13.

Kovacs, M. (1986). A developmental perspective on methods and measures in the assessment of depressive disorders: the clinical interview. In *Depression in Young People. Developmental and clinical perspectives*, ed. M. Rutter, C. Izard & P. Read, pp. 435–65. New York: Guilford Press.

Kovacs, M. & Devlin, B. (1998). Internalizing disorders in childhood. *Journal of Child Psychology and Psychiatry*, **39**, 47–63.

Kovacs, M., Feinberg, T. L., Crouse-Novak, M. A. et al. (1984a). Depressive disorders in childhood. I. A longitudinal prospective study of characteristics and recovery. *Archives of General Psychiatry*, **41**, 229–37.

Kovacs, M., Feinberg, T. L., Crouse-Novak, M. A. et al. (1984b). Depressive disorders in childhood. II. A longitudinal study of the risk of subsequent major depression. *Archives of General Psychiatry*, **41**, 643–9.

Kovacs, M., Gatsonis, C., Paulauskas, S. L. & Richards, C. (1989). Depressive disorders in childhood IV. A longitudinal study of comorbidity with and risk for anxiety disorders. *Archives of General Psychiatry*, **46**, 776–82.

Kovacs, M., Goldston, D. & Gatsonis, C. (1993). Suicidal behaviours and childhood-onset depressive disorders: a longitudinal investigation. *Journal of the American Academy of Child and Adolescent Psychiatry*, **32**, 8–20.

Kovacs, M., Akiskal, H. S., Gatsonis, C. & Parrone, P.L. (1994). Childhood-onset dysthymic disorder. *Archives of General Psychiatry*, **51**, 365–74.

Kovacs, M., Obrosky, S., Gatsonis, C. & Richards, C. (1997). First-episode major depressive and dysthymic disorder in childhood: clinical and sociodemographic factors in recovery. *Journal of* the *American Academy of Child and Adolescent Psychiatry*, **36**, 777–84.

Lewinsohn, P. M., Rohde, P., Seeley, J. R. & Hops, H. (1991). Comorbidity of unipolar depression: I. Major depression with dysthymia. *Journal of Abnormal Psychology*, **100**, 205–13.

McCauley, E., Myers, K., Mitchell, J. et al. (1993). Depression in young people: initial presentation and clinical course. *Journal of the American Academy of Child and Adolescent Psychiatry*, **32**, 714–22.

McConville, B. J., Boag. L. C. & Purohit, A. (1973). Three types of childhood depression. *Canadian Psychiatric Association Journal*, **18**, 133–8.

McGee, R., Feehan, M., Williams, S. & Anderson, J. (1992). DSM-III disorders from age 11 to 15 years. *Journal of the American Academy of Child and Adolescent Psychiatry*, **31**, 51–9.

McLeer, S., Callaghan, M., Henry, D. & Wallen, J. (1994). Psychiatric disorders in sexually abused children. *Journal of the American Academy of Child and Adolescent Psychiatry*, **33**, 313–19.

Maxwell, A. E. (1977). *Multivariate Analysis in Behavioural Research*. London: Chapman & Hall.

Mitchell, J., McCauley, E., Burke, P. M. & Moss, S. J. (1988). Phenomenology of depression in children and adolescents. *Journal of the American Academy of Child and Adolescent Psychiatry*, **27**, 12–20.

Nurcombe, B., Seifer, R., Scioll, A. et al. (1989). Is major depressive disorder in adolescence a distinct diagnostic entity? *Journal of the American Academy of Child and Adolescent Psychiatry*, **22**, 333–42.

Orvaschel, H., Thompson, W. D., Belanger, A. et al. (1982). Comparison of the 'family history' method to direct interview. *Journal of Affective Disorders*, **4**, 49–59.

Orvaschel, H., Lewinsohn, P. M. & Seeley, J. R. (1995). Continuity of psychopathology in a community sample of adolescents. *Journal of the American Academy of Child and Adolescent Psychiatry*, **35**, 1525–35.

Paykel, E. S. & Priest, R. G. (1992). Recognition and management of expression in general practice: consensus statement. *British Medical Journal*, **305**, 1192–202.

Puig-Antich, J. & Chambers, W. (1978). *The Schedule for Affective Disorders and Schizophrenia for School-aged Children*. New York: New York State Psychiatric Institute.

Ramana, R. & Paykel, E. S. (1992). Classification of affective disorders. *British Journal of Hospital Medicine*, **47**, 831–5.

Reinherz, H. Z., Giaconia, R. M., Pakis, B. et al. (1993). Psychosocial risks of major depression in late adolescence: a longitudinal community study. *Journal of American Academy of Child and Adolescent Psychiatry*, **32**, 1155–63.

Renouf, A. G., Kovacs, M. & Mukerji, P. (1997). Relationship of depressive, conduct, and comorbid disorders and social functioning in childhood. *Journal of the American Academy of Child and Adolescent Psychiatry*, **36**, 998–1004.

Rutter, M. (1986). The developmental psychopathology of depression: issues and perspectives. In *Depression in Young People: developmental and clinical perspectives*, ed. M. Rutter, C. E. Izard & P. V. Read, pp. 3–30. New York: Guilford Press.

Rutter, M. (1988). Epidemiological approaches to developmental psychopathology. *Archives of General Psychiatry*, **45**, 486–95.

Ryan, N. D., Puig-Antich, J., Ambrosini, P. et al. (1987). The clinical picture of major depression in children and adolescents. *Archives of General Psychiatry*, **44**, 854–61.

Sanford, M., Szatmari, P., Spinner, M. et al. (1995). Predicting the one-year course of adolescent major depression. *Journal of the American Academy of Child and Adolescent Psychiatry*, **34**, 1618–28.

Spitzer, T., Endicott, J. & Robins, E. (1978). Research diagnostic criteria rationale and reliability. *Archives of General Psychiatry*, **35**, 773–82.

Taylor, C. C. (1979). Principal component analysis and factor analysis of survey data. In *The Analysis of Survey Data*, vol. 1. *Exploring data structures*, eds. C. A. O'Muirchaertaigh & C. Payne. London: Wiley.

Trowell, J., Ugarte, B., Kolvin, I., Berelowitz, M., Sadowski, H. & LeCouteur, A. (1999). Behavioural psychopathology of child sexual abuse in schoolgirls referred to a tertiary centre. *European Child and Adolescent Psychiatry*, **8**, 107–16.

Verhulst, F. C. (1989). Childhood depression: problems of definition. *Israel Journal of Psychiatry and Related Sciences*, **26**, 3–11.

Verhulst, F. C., Akkerhuis, G. W. & Althaus, M. (1985). Mental health in Dutch children: (1) a cross-cultural comparison. *Acta Psychiatrica Scandinavica*, **72** (Suppl. 323), 1–108.

Weinberg, W. A., Rutman, J., Sullivan, L. et al. (1973). Depression in children referred to an educational diagnostic centre: diagnosis and treatment. Preliminary report. *Journal of Pediatrics*, **83**, 1065–72.

Weissmann, M. M. (1990). Applying impairment criteria to children's psychiatric diagnosis. *Journal of the American Academy of Child and Adolescent Psychiatry*, **29**, 789–95.

World Health Organization (1992). *The ICD-10 Classification of Mental and Behavioural Disorders*. Geneva: WHO.

Zeitlin, H. (1986). *The Natural History of Psychiatric Disorder in Children*. Institute of Psychiatry, Maudsley monograph no. 29. London: Oxford University Press.

6

The epidemiology of depression in children and adolescents

Adrian Angold and Elizabeth J. Costello

Many important questions about depression in young people can only be answered from general population studies (as opposed to studies of clinical samples). First, given that only a small minority of disturbed children are ever referred for psychiatric treatment (Costello et al., 1993), estimates of the rates of depression in children and adolescents cannot be determined from clinical data. Second, although clinical studies have often provided important leads to be followed up in epidemiological studies, the undeniable presence of referral biases (Berkson, 1946; Costello & Janiszewski, 1990; Cohen & Hesselbart, 1992; Cohen & Hesselbart, 1993; Goodman et al., 1997; Angold et al., 1998b) vitiates their use in describing patterns of diagnostic comorbidity or the sizes of impact of risk factors, or the level of need for services. Epidemiological studies are, therefore, important from both the administrative point of view (in determining needs for service provision or preventive interventions) and from the perspective of aetiological research.

Prevalence of depressive disorders in children and adolescents

Unipolar disorders

Table 6.1 presents prevalence estimates for unipolar depression from a number of general population studies that used the *DSM* diagnostic system (American Psychiatric Association, 1980, 1987, 1994). We have not included studies that used the *ICD* system because the existence of the categories of mixed disorders of conduct and emotions and depressive conduct disorder means that overall rates of depressive disorders are not usually ascertainable from reports from such studies. Where data are available from multiple waves of a longitudinal study, figures are reported for each wave separately.

It is immediately apparent that these estimates vary considerably from study to study. As Fleming & Offord (1990) pointed out in a trenchant review some years ago, much of this variation probably arises because there is no single

Table 6.1. Rates of unipolar depression from community studies (major depression and/or dysthymia)

Study	n	Age (years)	Time frame	Population rate of depression (%)
Kashani & Simonds, 1979 (*DSM-III*)	103	7–12		1.9
Dunedin Longitudinal Study				
Kashani et al., 1983 (*DSM-III*)	641	9	Current	1.8 major, 2.5 minor
Anderson et al., 1987 (*DSM-III*)	792	11	1 year	1.8
Frost et al., 1989 (*DSM-III*)	850	13	1 year	2.2
McGee et al., 1990 (*DSM-III*)	943	15	1 year	4.2
Deykin et al., 1987	424	16–19	Lifetime	6.8
Kashani et al., 1987 (*DSM-III*)	150	14–16	Lifetime	8.0
Pittsburgh Pediatric Study				
Costello et al., 1988 (*DSM-III*)	278	7–11	1 year	1.6
Costello, unpublished diagnoses from a 5-year follow-up of study 5 (*DSM-III-R*)	278	12–18	6 months	4.2
New York Longitudinal Study				
Velez et al., 1989 (*DSM-III-R*)	776	9–18	1 year	3.4
Velez et al., 1989 (*DSM-III-R*)	776	11–20	1 year	2.8
Ontario Child Health Study				
Fleming et al., 1989 ('*DSM-III-like*')	1153	6–11	6 months	0.6 high certainty, 2.7 medium certainty, 17.5 low certainty
Fleming et al., 1989 ('*DSM-III-like*')	1215	12–16	6 months	1.8 high certainty, 7.8 medium certainty, 43.9 low certainty

Study	N	Age	Time	Prevalence (%)
Oregon Adolescent Depression Project				
Rhode et al., 1991 (*DSM-III-R*)	1710	14–18	Current	2.9
Lewinsohn et al., 1993 (*DSM-III-R*)	1170	15–18	Lifetime	20.4
Cooper & Goodyer, 1993	368 (girls)	11–16		8.9
Bird et al., 1993 (*DSM-III*)	222	9–16	6 months	8.0
Fergusson et al., 1993 (*DSM-III-R*)	986	15	6 months	6.6
Reinherz et al., 1993b	386	18	6 months	6.0
Shaffer et al., 1996 (*DSM-III-R*)	1285	9–17	6 months	6.2 mild; 4.5 moderate; 2.5 severe
Great Smoky Mountains Study				
Costello et al., 1996 (*DSM-III-R*)	1015	9–13	3 months	1.5
Angold et al., 1998a (*DSM-IV*)	970	10–14	3 months	3.1
Angold et al., 1998a (*DSM-IV*)	928	11–15	3 months	3.2
Angold et al., 1998a (*DSM-IV*)	820	12–16	3 months	2.7
American Indian Study				
Costello et al., 1997 (*DSM-III-R*)	323	9–13	3 months	0.31
Costello et al., 1997 (*DSM-IV*)	317	10–14	3 months	1.6
Costello et al., 1997 (*DSM-IV*)	304	11–15	3 months	4.3
Costello et al., 1997 (*DSM-IV*)	289	12–16	3 months	1.7
Simonoff et al., 1997 (*DSM-III-R*)	2762	8–16	3 months	1.2
Angold et al., 2000a	921	9–17	3 months	1.3 major depressive disorder dysthymia, 2.7 minor

agreed-upon method for determining whether depression is present or not. Indeed, it can be seen that even the length of time over which depression is assessed varies dramatically from study to study. However, there is perhaps less disagreement here than it seems at first. If we ignore estimates of lifetime prevalence and consider only studies involving those under 18, the range is from 1.6–8.9%. Consider, however, the three values given from the Methods for the Epidemiology of Child and Adolescent (MECA) mental disorders study (Shaffer et al., 1996). Depending on the level of psychosocial impairment considered necessary for diagnosis, the prevalence estimate varied from 2.5% (for severe depression) to 6.2% (for mild to severe depression). In the Caring for Children in the Community Study (CCCS), similarly, the addition of *DSM-IV* minor depression moved the estimate from that study from 1.3% to 4.0% (Angold et al., 1998a). In the Ontario Child Health Study, high-certainty depressive diagnoses occurred in 1–2%, while medium-certainty diagnoses were observed in 3–8%.

Determining the prevalence of any disorder always involves some arbitrary decisions concerning where to place the cut points between sick and well. Consider the changing definitions of AIDS, for example. In addition, the implementation of any set of criteria for psychiatric disorder always involves arbitrary decisions about where to place cut points for symptom and impairment criteria. It is, therefore, not surprising that very disparate rates for disorders arise from different decision rules. Ignoring however the terminological differences between mild, minor and medium-certainty depression, it seems reasonable to interpret Table 6.1 as suggesting that around 2% of school-age children and adolescents have a severe unipolar depressive disturbance, and that around another 4% has a mild to moderate unipolar depressive disturbance. The estimate of 8.9% is for a sample of adolescent girls only (all the other studies included boys): a group that we will see below is expected to have higher rates of depression than others.

We also know that most of those with either disturbance are not receiving treatment. For instance, in the Great Smoky Mountains Study (GSMS) only 23% of those with a depressive disorder had seen a mental health professional in the 3 months preceding their interview. So, from a public health point of view, we have reasonable estimates that we need to identify and treat five times as many juveniles with depression as at present.

Bipolar disorders

Much less attention has been paid to bipolar disorders (BPDs) in the child and adolescent epidemiological literature. This is not surprising because BPDs are uncommon, and none of the existing epidemiological studies is large enough to include substantial samples of bipolar individuals. The Oregon Adolescent Depression Project reported that the lifetime prevalence of BPDs by age 14–18 was 0.94%, with point prevalences of 0.29% and 0.20% at two assessments 1 year apart (Lewinsohn et al., 1993, 1995b). The GSMS found a similarly low rate of BPDs (3-month prevalence 0.41%: Angold et al., 1999).

It has recently been suggested (Faraone et al., 1997) that the co-occurrence of attention deficit hyperactivity disorder (ADHD) and BPD is not a rare event. Clinical studies of children and adolescents show that rates of ADHD range from 57% to 98% in bipolar patients (Borchardt & Bernstein, 1995; Geller et al., 1995; West et al., 1995, 1996; Wozniak et al., 1995) and rates of BPD range from 11% to 22% in ADHD patients (Butler et al., 1995; Biederman et al., 1996). However, the epidemiological data show that rates of comorbidity between ADHD and BPD are much lower than suggested by these clinical studies. In the Oregon Adolescent Depression Project only 11% of bipolar adolescents also had ADHD (Lewinsohn et al., 1995b). In the GSMS (Costello et al., 1996), only six children or adolescents out of 1420 were observed to have been in a manic or hypomanic episode during the 3 months preceding any one of four annual interviews (a weighted population prevalence rate of 0.41%), while 92 (weighted 3.4%) met criteria for ADHD at at least one wave. Only one subject had both a manic episode and met criteria for ADHD, giving weighted population estimates of 0.9% for the rate of mania in those with ADHD (vs. 0.39% in those without ADHD), and a rate of 7% for ADHD in those with mania (vs. 3% in those without mania).

Neither of these studies proves that there is no association between ADHD and BPD, but they seriously challenge the notion that co-occurrence of ADHD and BPD is not a rare event. Both studies indicate that the co-occurrence of these disorders in the general population is a very rare event. On the other hand, it is easy to see how their co-occurrence would be very likely to result in referral to specialist services at a major centre with a particular interest in such problems. The point here is not to condemn clinical studies of rates of comorbidity, but to sound a warning about their interpretation. In following up this question, Faraone and his colleagues (1997) have produced evidence from a family study that comorbid ADHD and BPD may indeed be familially distinct from other forms of ADHD. It may be rare, but at present it appears that it does exist.

Gender, age and the diagnosis of unipolar depression

In our chapter on the epidemiology of depression in the first edition of this book (written in 1993), we pointed out that the evidence that there were changes in rates of depression in adolescence was actually very weak. Happily, that situation has now changed substantially, although some questions remain about exactly what happens in boys.

Studies of adults from several countries have emphatically documented that women have 1.5–3 times more current and lifetime unipolar depression than do men (Weissman & Klerman, 1977; Bebbington et al., 1981; Canino et al., 1987; Lee et al., 1987; Bland et al., 1988a,b; Cheng, 1989; Hwu et al., 1989; Wells et al., 1989; Wittchen et al., 1992; Weissman et al., 1993; Kessler et al., 1993; Blazer et al., 1994). In later life (after age 55), the female excess of depressions diminishes, mostly because of falling rates in women. Indeed, there is growing evidence that depression may be more common in men after age 55 (Bebbington, 1996; Bebbington et al., 1998; Jorm, 1987).

Using retrospective data, studies of adults have pointed to adolescence as the time when the gender difference first appears. For example, the Epidemiological Catchment Area (ECA) studies (Burke et al., 1990) suggested that unipolar depression onset rates were equal in males and females until age 15–19, while the National Comorbidity Survey (NCS: Kessler et al., 1993) provided evidence for the emergence of an onset differential by age 10–14.

The child and adolescent epidemiological literature generally agrees that rates of unipolar depression in prepubertal girls are not higher than those in prepubertal boys (Rutter et al., 1976; Anderson et al., 1987; Cohen & Brooks, 1987; Kashani et al., 1987; Bird et al., 1988; McGee & Williams, 1988; Guyer et al., 1989; Velez et al., 1989; Fleming & Offord, 1990; McGee et al., 1990, 1992; Nolen-Hoeksema et al., 1991; Angold & Rutter, 1992; Cohen et al., 1993a,b; E. J. Costello et al., unpublished paper; Reinherz et al., 1993a; Lewinsohn et al., 1995a; Angold et al., 1998a, 1999; Hankin et al., 1998). Indeed, the opposite may be the case (see below).

Adolescence is associated with increasing prevalence of depression in girls

Since the Isle of Wight studies (Rutter et al., 1970, 1976), child and adolescent studies using diagnostic interviews have generally suggested that rates of depression rise in adolescent girls (Rutter et al., 1976; Anderson et al., 1987; Cohen & Brooks, 1987; Kashani et al., 1987, 1989; Bird et al., 1988; McGee & Williams, 1988; Guyer et al., 1989; Velez et al., 1989; Fleming & Offord, 1990; McGee et al., 1990; Nolen-Hoeksema et al., 1991; Angold & Rutter, 1992; E. J. Costello et al., unpublished paper; Reinherz et al., 1993a; Lewinsohn et al.,

1995a; Hankin et al., 1998). In earlier research, the small numbers of depressed individuals in each study precluded formal statistical testing of this conclusion, but more recent epidemiological studies have confirmed it statistically (Angold et al., 1998a, 1999; Angold & Rutter, 1992; Lewinsohn et al., 1993; Reinherz et al., 1993b; Hankin et al., 1998).

The four child and adolescent general population studies examining the effects of age on depression with sufficient extension at the lower end of the age range (the Dunedin Longitudinal Study, Cohen's New York Study, the GSMS and CCCS) all agree that this change only becomes apparent at or after age 13 (Velez et al., 1989; McGee et al., 1992; Angold et al., 1998a; Hankin et al., 1998). An important implication of this timing is that an effect occurring around age 13 cannot be attributed to adrenarche, which occurs in middle to late childhood.

In childhood depression may be more common in boys

It is usually said that depression is equally common in prepubertal boys and girls (American Psychiatric Association, 1994), but the weight of the evidence now suggests that this is not so. Until recently, no diagnostic studies of younger/immature children had sufficient power to detect anything but enormous differences in rates of depression between boys and girls. It is worth noting that, of the three older studies with sufficient extension at younger ages, two found that depressive disorders were nonsignificantly more common in boys under 12 than girls under 12 (Anderson et al., 1987; Costello et al., 1988). The exception was Bird and colleagues' Puerto Rican Study (reported in Angold & Costello, 1995). The Dunedin Longitudinal Study noted a 5:1 male excess of 'pure' (noncomorbid) depression at age 13 (no gender breakdown was given for those with comorbid disorders), which was replaced by an excess of females from age 15 on (McGee et al., 1990; Hankin et al., 1998). In a reanalysis of these data (Hankin et al., 1998), extended to age 21, that involved only the 653 participants in the Dunedin Longitudinal Study with data available for all of ages 11, 13, 15, 18 and 21, boys were found to have an almost significantly higher rate of depression at age 11 than girls. Two studies have also now found that depression was two to three times more common in boys than in girls before age 13 or Tanner stage III–IV (Angold et al., 1998a, 1999), and both of these findings were statistically significant (Figure 6.1).

Scale score studies of gender and age effects on depression

Whereas studies using diagnosis of a depressive disorder as the criterion have shown consistent results, the findings from studies using questionnaires and scale scores have been notably mixed, providing little support for the idea that

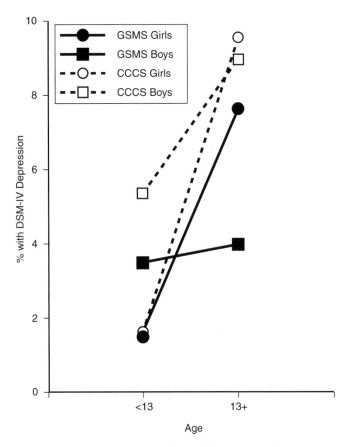

Figure 6.1. Age and 3-month prevalence of depression in the GSMS and CCCS.

mean depression scale scores are higher in adolescent girls than they are in adolescent boys or than they are in preadolescent girls (Kazdin et al., 1983; Kovacs, 1983; Helsel & Matson, 1984; Faust et al., 1985; Finch et al., 1985; Haley et al., 1985; Bartell & Reynolds, 1986; Smucker et al., 1986; Huntley et al., 1987; Doerfler et al., 1988; Gates et al., 1988; Reinherz et al., 1990; Petersen et al., 1991; Roberts & Chen, 1995; Compas et al., 1997; Wichstrøm, 1999). The failure to find sex differences in mean symptom scores of samples that are predominantly nondepressed extends into the college years (Hammen & Padesky, 1977; King & Buchwald, 1982).

However, several studies have now found that, in situations where there are few or no differences by age and gender in mean scores, the proportions of girls with relatively extreme high questionnaire scores increases significantly in adolescence (Teri, 1982; Roberts & Chen, 1995; Roberts et al., 1995; Compas et al., 1997; Angold et al., 1999).

Puberty and depression

It is hardly surprising that the changing age and gender distributions of depression from childhood to adolescence have led to examination of a variety of aspects of puberty in relation to depression. However, it is only recently that studies have moved beyond mean depression scale scores to examine depression diagnoses. As we saw above, mean scores do not well reflect the impact of adolescence on depression, so we need not be surprised that the earlier studies resulted in a confusing picture. An additional difficulty with this literature is that puberty is a complex developmental process, and there is no reason to assume that all aspects of that process will act in the same way in relation to depression. Indeed, a key objective from the aetiological point of view must be to try to determine which (if any) of the many different components of puberty are most centrally involved in generating increased rates of depression in adolescent girls.

Morphological stage and pubertal timing
Studies not using diagnostic measures

A number of studies of menarche or morphological development (secondary sex characteristics, usually measured by Tanner stages: Tanner, 1962) have suggested that the *timing* of these pubertal markers may be significantly related to mood or other disturbances as measured by a wide variety of scales (Susman et al., 1987b; Olweus et al., 1988; Brooks-Gunn & Warren, 1989; Paikoff et al., 1991; Angold & Rutter, 1992; Ge et al., 1996). Early puberty has been associated with problem behaviours in girls, but with good adjustment in boys (see Stattin & Magnusson, 1990 for an excellent review). Stattin & Magnusson (1990) argued from their influential longitudinal study that the negative effects of early development in girls were generated by the impact of early maturity on girls' social lives, and their early introduction to sexual life, for which they might be cognitively unready. However, these effects had largely disappeared by the time the girls were in mid-adolescence, whereas the female excess of depressive disorders continues throughout adulthood. In the Carolina Longitudinal Study, Cairns & Cairns (1994) did not find any effect of early puberty on behavioural deviance.

Overall, this literature contains many failures to replicate findings from study to study (Greif & Ulman, 1982; Stattin & Magnusson, 1990), and it is uncertain how much this is because different studies used different designs and different measures of psychopathology and puberty. However, it cannot be said, by any means, to have provided very solid support for the idea that early puberty is a major factor in the emergence of the female excess of depression.

Studies using diagnostic measures

Hayward and colleagues (1997) found that onsets of internalizing symptoms measured by various scales were associated with earlier puberty. However, the effect for depression scores alone was not significant. In a much smaller subset of girls followed into high school they also reported a nonsignificant association (odds ratio 1.7) between earlier pubertal timing and the development of interview-based diagnoses of internalizing disorders (any of depression, sub-clinical bulimia, social phobia, agoraphobia or panic disorder).

Graber and colleagues' study from the Oregon Adolescent Depression Project (Graber et al., 1997) produced contradictory results. Self-reported early maturers (the adolescents were asked whether they thought they were early, on time or late) had higher lifetime rates of depression than on-time maturers (30.2% vs. 22.1%), but late maturers had the highest lifetime rates of all (33.8%). Both of these effects were statistically significant. On the other hand, rates of current major depression were lowest in the early maturers (2.3%), intermediate in the on-time group (3.5%) and highest in the late maturers (3.9%). None of these differences was statistically significant.

Only two studies of depression diagnoses have attempted to separate out effects of different facets of puberty (Angold et al., 1998a, 1999). Both found that pubertal status (specifically, the achievement of Tanner stage III or IV) was associated with increased rates of depression in girls (odds ratios of 3–4), but that pubertal timing, recency of the transition to Tanner stage III and rate of transition through puberty were not.

So there are now two (three if one counts the mixture of diagnoses included in Hayward et al., 1997) studies that have failed to find an effect of pubertal timing on depression diagnoses observed at the time of interview. The only positive diagnostic study is that of Graber and colleagues (1997), which found a significant relationship between lifetime histories of depression (which could include prepubertal depressions) and self-ratings of the relative timing of puberty. At best, early puberty has been associated with apparently transient elevations in depression scale scores, and perhaps more strongly with other (nondepressive) forms of behavioural disturbance. Overall we would argue that there is no convincing evidence linking pubertal timing with the emergence of the adult gender ratio in depression, but evidence for substantial effects of pubertal status in two different samples. These findings argue against formulations that suggest that increased rates of depression occur in a subset of girls who mature early physically and then find themselves being subjected to relationship and behavioural pressures for which they are not yet cognitively fitted or socially adapted (Stattin & Magnusson, 1990).

Hormonal studies of puberty and psychopathology

The National Institute of Mental Health study of puberty and psychopathology (Nottelmann et al., 1987a,b; Susman et al., 1987a,b) found negative associations between testosterone : oestradiol ratio, sex hormone binding globulin, and androstenedione concentration and negative emotional tone in boys. These workers also reported an association of early maturation (measured by oestradiol and testosterone : oestradiol ratio) with reduced negative emotional tone in boys, but more negative emotional tone in girls. Adrenal androgen levels correlated with negative emotional tone in boys but not girls, while the opposite was the case for follicle-stimulating hormone (Nottelmann et al., 1990; Susman et al., 1985). Brooks-Gunn & Warren (1989) found that negative affect increased in 10–14-year-old girls during rapid oestrogen rise. A 1-year follow-up of 72 girls (Paikoff et al., 1991) found a significant linear relationship between oestradiol level at the first observation and depression 1 year later according to one depression scale, but no such effect in relation to two other depression scales.

None of these hormonal studies had sufficient power to tease apart the possible contributions of age itself, the indirect psychosocial impacts of morphological pubertal status and the more direct impact of the different groups of hormones that change at puberty. In addition, all of them used only depression scale scores, rather than interview-based diagnoses. The exception to these strictures is work from the GSMS. There, neither of the tropic hormones measured (follicle-stimulating hormone or luteinizing hormone) had any significant effect on depression over and above that of Tanner stage. However, both testosterone and oestradiol had very substantial effects that effaced those of Tanner stage. The adrenal androgens androstenedione and dehydroepiandrosterone sulphate could be shown to be correlated with depression status, but these effects disappeared when testosterone was included in the regression models. These findings, plus the timing of effects of age and pubertal status, suggest that adrenarche has little impact on depression status in girls, but that there are substantial effects of changes in levels of circulating testosterone and oestradiol that occur during mid to late puberty.

Further discussions of DHEA and other hormones and their relations with psychopathology are to be found in Chapters 4, 8 and 9.

Ethnicity and depression

Epidemiological studies of childhood and adolescent depression in minority adolescents are few and far between (Bird, 1996). *DSM-III* depression (American Psychiatric Association, 1980) was found in 5.9% of Puerto Rican children aged between 4 and 16 (Canino et al., 1987), and a score of over 30 on the Center for Epidemiologic Studies Depression (CES-D: Radloff, 1977) scale scores was reported in 18% of Mexican American youth aged 11–14, compared with 12.3% of Anglo youth (Roberts & Chen, 1995). Garrison's longitudinal study of depressive symptoms in adolescence included 812 African-American females at the screening stage, of whom 52 received a Kiddie-SADS (Schedule for Affective Disorders and Schizophrenia for School-age Children) diagnostic interview. However, data on the prevalence or incidence of depressive diagnoses were not given by sex and/or race (Garrison et al., 1997). In contrast to federal data, which show African-American females as the gender-by-ethnicity group at lowest risk for suicide (CDC, 1998), this study found that Black girls were more likely than white girls to report a suicide attempt requiring medical treatment. Among those who completed all three waves of this study, African-American girls ($n = 40$) had consistently higher mean CES-D depression scores, the highest scores on a scale of suicidal ideation (Garrison et al., 1991), and the highest correlation between scores over time, indicating greater persistence (Garrison et al., 1990). Angold et al. (2000b) found no significant differences in rates of depression between African-Americans and whites.

Ethnic differences in the adult ECA national prevalence studies of the 1980s are only available for the North Carolina site (Blazer et al., 1985). The 6-month prevalence of *DSM-III* major depression was 1.7%. The odds ratio associated with being nonwhite was 1.1. Data were not reported separately for the youngest nonwhite females. The NCS reported overall 1-month and lifetime rates of depression in adult Black and white females that did not differ much, with Blacks having slightly lower rates of depression overall. However, the disparity between Black and white females was greater for the youngest cohort (15–24 years): 4.5% vs. 8.6% 30-day, 9.2% vs. 23.1% lifetime. Hispanics had significantly higher rates than other ethnic groups in the NCS (Blazer et al., 1994) Overall, therefore, there is some evidence that there may be ethnic differences in rates of childhood and adolescent depression – particularly that rates of depression are higher in Hispanic Americans – but this is by no means certain.

Comorbidity

In a recent review and metaanalysis of epidemiological studies of comorbidity (Angold et al., 1999) we summarized the incontrovertible evidence that comorbidity between depression, conduct disorder or oppositional defiant disorder (ODD), anxiety, ADHD and substance abuse is much more common in the general population of children and adolescents than expected from the base rates of these disorders. We also addressed and rejected the possibility that comorbidity could be explained away as a result of a range of methodological problems. We concluded that comorbidity was not simply the result of: (1) Berkson's bias (Berkson, 1946); (2) referral bias; (3) interviewer expectancies (halo effects); (4) the use of multiple informants for diagnostic purposes; (5) multiple symptom codings resulting from single behaviours; and (6) the inclusion of nonspecific symptoms in the criterion sets for multiple diagnoses. Neither is it simply the result of the imposition of arbitrary groupings of symptoms into diagnoses, because factor analytically derived scale measures of psychopathology also find substantial correlations between different factors (McConaughy & Achenbach, 1994; Garnefski & Diekstra, 1997). In other words, comorbidity is a real characteristic of the phenomenology of child and adolescent depressive disorders. The metaanalytically derived average strengths of the associations of depressive disorders (major depressive disorder (MDD) and/or dysthymia) with anxiety disorders, ADHD and conduct disorder/ODD are shown in Figure 6.2. Comorbidity with substance abuse and dependence was not included in that metaanalysis, but there is no doubt that such comorbidity exists.

Homotypic vs. heterotypic comorbidity

Developmental psychopathologists are used to the concepts of homotypic and heterotypic continuity. The first refers to continuity of some phenomenon over time in a form that changes relatively little. For instance, the fact that depressed adolescents are more likely than nondepressed adolescents to be depressed in adulthood points to a degree of homotypic continuity in depression. Heterotypic continuity, on the other hand, refers to a continuous process that generates manifestations of different form over time. By analogy, studies of comorbidity may be seen as being of two types: first, those that examine comorbidity between disorders within a diagnostic grouping (such as the co-occurrence of major depression and dysthymia); and second, those that deal with comorbidity between disorders from different diagnostic groupings (such as depression and conduct disorder). We call the first studies of homotypic

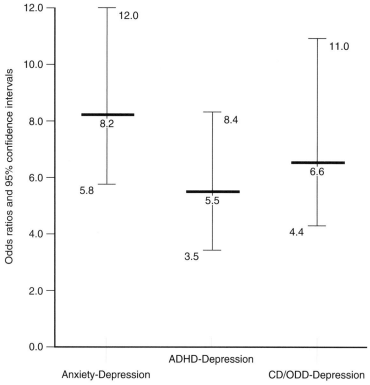

Figure 6.2. Strengths of comorbid associations between depression, anxiety, ADHD and CD/ODD.

comorbidity and the second studies of heterotypic comorbidity. We can make no *rigid* distinction between homotypic and heterotypic comorbidity. None the less, the distinction is useful because the implications of these two types of comorbidity tend to be rather different, and they are rarely addressed in the same paper.

Concurrent vs. successive comorbidity

One problem with the term 'comorbidity' is that it has been used to include a multitude of different temporal relationships amongst disorders. While some child and adolescent studies have considered disorders co-occurring over a relatively short span of time, others have reported rates of co-occurrence over 6 months, 1 year, 3 years or the individual's lifetime to date. Clearly such different time spans will allow very different types of temporal relationships between comorbid disorders. For instance, comorbidity between current disorders at the time of assessment means that both must be present at the same time. Although their times of onset and offset may not be coterminous, during some period they must have been present concurrently. We propose to label such co-occurrence concurrent comorbidity. The two disorders run together, perhaps not only in time but also in phenomenology.

When considering reports of lifetime comorbidity, the disorders in question may never have been present simultaneously, but may have occurred widely separated in time. When two disorders do not overlap in time, we suggest that the term successive comorbidity could be used. At least it would be helpful to know more about the degree to which comorbidity represents the occurrence of multiple disorders in succession as opposed to multiple disorders occurring at the same points in time. Data from the Oregon Adolescent Depression Project (Rhode et al., 1991) indicate that current (and, therefore, necessarily concurrent) and lifetime comorbidity rates can be very different. For instance, they found that the odds ratio for current comorbidity between unipolar depression and any other diagnosis was 9.6, while that for lifetime comorbidity was only 2.8. This implies that adolescents who had formerly been depressed but were not currently depressed, were unlikely also to have had other disorders. However, studies of rates of concurrent comorbidity in younger children do not support this implication. This suggests that lifetime recall probably underestimates comorbidity rates quite substantially. One obvious problem here is that estimates of lifetime comorbidity rely upon individuals remembering the symptoms of two separate disorders. The only way to avoid this apparent problem is to measure concurrent and successive comorbidity prospectively in longitudinal studies.

The meaning of comorbidity

As has been pointed out in numerous reviews (Achenbach, 1990; Caron & Rutter, 1991; Abikoff & Klein, 1992; Kendall et al., 1992; Angold & Costello, 1993; Hinshaw et al., 1993; Klein & Riso, 1993; Loeber & Keenan, 1994; Nottelmann & Jensen, 1995; Rutter, 1997; Angold et al., 1999), comorbidity has many implications for the study of psychopathology and its treatment, and there are many possible explanations for its occurrence. In what follows, we review results from studies that have moved beyond simply documenting the occurrence of comorbidity to attempting to understand how it arises.

Epiphenomenal comorbidity

The standard approach to quantifying comorbidity has been to look only at pairs of diagnoses. But when three conditions are all associated with one another, it is possible that one of the pairwise associations is nothing other than the mathematical product of the other two. We will refer to this possibility as epiphenomenal comorbidity (Angold et al., 2000a). The GSMS provided a large enough sample to test for this possibility, by controlling each pairwise comparison for the effects of other comorbidities. The results supported the epiphenomenal explanation for the relationship between depression and ADHD (via anxiety and conduct disorder), and for the relationship between conduct disorder and anxiety (via depression) and ODD and anxiety (via ADHD). For instance, the odds ratio for the association between anxiety and ODD fell from 3.0 to a nonsignificant 0.56 when other comorbidities were controlled for. In other words, there was no independent relationship between ODD and anxiety disorders. On the other hand, there were independent associations of conduct disorder with ODD, conduct disorder and ODD with depression and ADHD, and ADHD and depression with anxiety. The apparent pairwise covariation of ADHD with depression, and conduct disorder and ODD with anxiety was explained by comorbidity between other pairs of disorders; it was an epiphenomenon of the relationships between other pairs of disorders. These results need to be replicated, but they do suggest that some simplification of the problem of comorbidity may be at hand – we may have to explain only a subset of the possible pairings of disorders. We should note that this does not mean that those who do have both depression and ADHD do not have 'real' depression or ADHD (Biederman et al., 1998). It simply means that, in the absence of comorbid anxiety, conduct disorder or ODD, depressed individuals are not more likely to have ADHD than psychiatrically well children.

Homotypic comorbidity between major depression and dysthymia – a marker of homotypic continuity?

Some adult studies have suggested that major depression, dysthymia and the simultaneous comorbidity of the two represent nothing more than separate phases or manifestations of the same disorder (Keller et al., 1982a,b, 1992; Klein, 1990) or points on a continuum of severity of depressive conditions (Angst & Dobler-Mikola, 1984; Angst et al., 1984). Several studies have identified differences between children with dysthymia, major depression and double depression in symptomatology, impairment, heterotypic comorbidity and rates of suicidality (Fine et al., 1985; Ryan et al., 1987; Shain et al., 1991; Asarnow &

Ben-Meir, 1994; Ferro et al., 1994), but even these can be interpreted as indicating that 'major depression may be the driving force behind the expression of depressive symptomatology, regardless of whether the child is acutely or chronically depressed' (Ferro et al., 1994).

Longitudinal studies of children have, on the whole, given a similar impression (Kovacs et al., 1984), but Kovacs' 12-year clinical follow-up of children with major depressive episodes and dysthymia resulted in a rather more differentiated conclusion. By the 12-year follow-up (Kovacs, 1996), 76% of children whose first depression was dysthymic disorder had a subsequent major depressive disorder and 13% had a bipolar disorder. Of those whose first episode was a major depressive episode, 48% later met criteria for dysthymia and 15% had bipolar disorders. These writers go on to emphasize that childhood dysthymia in their sample did not persist into adulthood itself, but exerted its influence on later risk for affective disorder through major depressive episodes. They now regard childhood-onset dysthymic disorder as an 'early marker of recurrent affective illness'. However, Kovacs and colleagues suggest that we should maintain the distinction between early-onset dysthymic disorder (with somewhat modified diagnostic criteria) and major depressive disorder, because the former had an earlier age of onset (Ferro et al., 1994). In addition, a subset of early dysthymics did not develop MDD, dysthymia was associated with shorter disorder-free periods than MDD without dysthymia, and first-episode dysthymia and MDD carried different levels of risk for later affective and substance use disorders. There are interesting parallels here with Lewinsohn and colleagues' work on older adolescents (1991). They found that lifetime comorbidity between MDD and dysthymia was twice as high in their adolescent general population sample as in an adult sample, and that dysthymia nearly always preceded MDD when both occurred. However, MDD was vastly more common than dysthymia in adolescents.

Heterotypic comorbidity as a marker of severity

Comorbidity has often been associated with increased levels of symptomatology within each of the disorders making up the comorbid group, and with increased levels of impairment in functioning. Individuals with more than one diagnosis also tend to have suffered from higher levels of psychosocial adversity. For instance, individuals with comorbid ADHD and depression or anxiety disorders have been reported to have more severe disorders than those with ADHD alone (Jensen et al., 1993). Other data suggest that comorbidity between ADHD and internalizing disorders may not necessarily be indicative of more severe ADHD (Pliszka, 1992; August et al., 1996). Depression seems to have little effect on the course of conduct disorder (Capaldi, 1992; Zoccolillo, 1992), though the latter may be associated with more severe concurrent depressions (Marriage et al., 1986; Noam et al., 1994; Rudolph et al., 1994), but perhaps with less risk that depression will continue into adulthood (Harrington et al., 1991). Comorbidity between conduct disorder and depression is however strongly associated with suicide, especially when combined with alcohol use (Shaffer & Fisher, 1981; Brent et al., 1988; Martunnen et al., 1991; Rhode et al., 1991; Andrews & Lewinsohn, 1992; Shaffer, 1993; Lewinsohn et al., 1994b). Both anxiety and depression may also be more severe when they occur together (Last et al., 1996).

It is difficult to draw any hard-and-fast conclusions from this confusing literature, but it cannot be said to indicate that comorbidity is just a marker for overall severity of the component disorders. Rather, it points to complex relationships among disorders over time, and in the case of suicide, to the particularly negative effects of depression and conduct disorder.

Comorbidity between conduct disorders and depressive disorders

Zoccolillo's (1992) helpful review of the relationships between conduct disorder and depressive and emotional disorders concluded that separate disorders should be diagnosed when conditions comorbid with conduct disorder are observed, and rejected the *ICD-10* category of depressive conduct disorder (World Health Organization, 1993). In considering the very limited evidence on a variety of explanations for conduct disorder comorbidity, he concluded that the best solution might be to regard conduct disorder as a 'disorder of multiple dysfunction', with depression or anxiety representing dysfunctions in affect. Given the evidence cited, it seems that this conclusion is only meant to apply to life course persistent conduct problems. His key lines of evidence were: (1) the more severe the antisocial behaviour, the greater the likelihood of comorbidity with nonantisocial disorders; (2) conduct disorder only predicts adult affective disturbance in individuals who have persistent antisocial behaviour in adulthood; and (3) conduct disorder is associated with earlier onset of affective disturbances, at around the same time as the first conduct disorder symptoms appear. A good deal of additional work is needed to provide convincing evidence on each of these topics, but they also admit of an alternative explanation – that conduct disorder causes affective disorders. Aggressive and conduct disorder children often interpret the social actions of others as being hostile (Quiggle et al., 1992), have problems in all sorts of social relationships, do poorly at school, get into serious trouble with the authorities, and are often told that they are bad. The literatures on life events, chronic difficulties and hassles, and cognitive styles in depression suggest that these correlates of conduct disorder could cause depression (see Capaldi, 1992 for a version of this model). This suggests the hypothesis that individuals with conduct disorder who had lower rates of difficulties arising from their conduct disorder behaviour would manifest less depression. If specific predictors of the appearance of depression in conduct disorder (other than just the severity of conduct disorder itself) could be identified, and some or all of those predictors were effects of conduct disorder, then it would be reasonable to regard conduct disorder as causing depression. If depression were simply a manifestation of the diathesis underlying conduct disorder, no such specific risk factors should be identified because conduct disorder itself is the risk.

An alternative approach was employed by Fergusson and colleagues (1996). They fit structural equation models to their general population data to test the contrasting hypotheses that the relationship between conduct disorder and depression was the result of correlations among the risk factors for the two disorders or the result of reciprocal causation. They found no support for the idea that either disorder caused the other, but noted that a substantial amount of the covariation between them could be explained by their having common or correlated risk factors. This elegant study underscores the usefulness of having measures of comorbidity on individuals at more than one point in time, and suggests an analytic approach that could be replicated with data from several of the general population studies listed in Table 6.1.

The work of Cohen and colleagues (1990) illustrates another approach involving direct statistical comparisons among the relationships of risk factors measured in childhood with internalizing, externalizing and substance abuse problems measured 8 years later. This study found that certain risk factors were common to more than one problem outcome. For instance, parental mental illness and remarriage were associated with both internalizing and externalizing problems. Other factors appeared to be relatively specific to only one sort of problem. For instance, residential instability was protective against substance abuse, but had no significant effect on either internalizing or externalizing problems. Family social isolation was related only to internalizing problems. The key strengths of this study are that it involves simultaneous examination of the effects of multiple risk factors on multiple outcomes measured at multiple points in time. Using a similar approach, Lewinsohn et al. (1995) compared risk factors associated with depression and substance abuse. They found that life events, physical problems and previous episodes of depression, anxiety or suicidal behaviour were specifically associated with depression, while previous internalizing and externalizing symptom scores, poor coping skills, interpersonal conflicts with parents and dissatisfaction with grades were associated with both depression and substance abuse. Many statistical approaches to complex longitudinal data are now available and, although it is often difficult to decide exactly how to implement the effects of comorbidity in such models, this general approach is one that deserves to be much more widely employed.

The genetic epidemiology of unipolar depression

Comorbidity occurs not only within individuals – it also occurs within families. The children of depressed parents clearly have elevated rates of depression compared to the children of the nondepressed, but they are also at higher risk of having anxiety and disruptive behaviour disorders (Morrison & Stewart 1971; Welner et al., 1977; Decina et al., 1983; Gershon et al., 1985; Klein & Depue, 1985; Hammen et al., 1987; Last et al., 1987; Turner et al., 1987; Merikangas et al., 1988; Nurnberger et al., 1988; Orvaschel et al., 1988; Sylvester et al., 1988; McClellan et al., 1990; Moreau et al., 1990; Orvaschel, 1990; Grigoroiu-Serbanescu et al., 1991a,b; Hammen, 1992; Weissman et al., 1992; Lewinsohn et al., 1993; Warner et al., 1995; Beardslee et al., 1996; Beidel & Turner, 1997). While children of parents with 'pure' anxiety disorders have been found to have little but anxiety disorders, those with depressed or mixed anxious depressed parents have a much wider range of disorders (Beidel & Turner, 1997). Relatives of children with ADHD have higher rates of depression as well as antisocial personality disorder, hysteria, alcoholism and substance dependence (Cantwell, 1972; Morrison, 1980; Biederman et al., 1990, 1992; McCormick, 1995).

Twin studies have so far addressed only depression scale scores. In the Virginia Twin Study of Adolescent Behavioral Development, parent-based measures indicated the presence of a substantial additive genetic component (over 50%), but child self-report measures showed a much smaller genetic effect (less then 20%). However, Thapar & McGuffin (1994) found no such difference between parent and adolescent reports. Eley (1997) and Rende et al. (1993) found heritabilities for depression scores of 42% and 34% respectively. These studies disagree, however, on the importance of shared and nonshared environmental components, but that may be because there is a change from childhood to adolescence, with shared environment being more important before adolescence (Thapar & McGuffin, 1994). There is growing evidence that genetic risk for depression increases (particularly in girls) in adolescence, and that what is inherited involves not just a tendency to become depressed, but a tendency to have more life events (Harrington et al., 1990; Thapar & McGuffin, 1994; Thapar et al., 1998; Silberg et al., 1999). In other words, there is evidence for significant gene–environment correlation in the aetiology of depression. This perhaps explains the apparent absence of evidence for any genetic effect on depression from Eley et al.'s (1998) adoption study.

Environmental risk factors for depression

A number of epidemiological studies from the UK, the USA, New Zealand and Canada have reported on associations between a number of putative risk factors for depression and the presence of *DSM-III* (or similar) diagnoses of depression in children and adolescents. In summary (Costello, 1989; Lewinsohn et al., 1994a, 1996; Nolen-Hoeksema & Girgus, 1994), these studies found that low socioeconomic status (SES), high life stress, sexual abuse, physical illness, low academic achievement, depressive cognitions, low self-esteem and various measures of family disruption, disharmony and disorder are associated with the presence of psychiatric disorders in general, with each study finding slightly different patterns of effect. However, no pattern of risk factors has yet appeared that is specifically associated with depression except for the changes associated with puberty. The nonspecificity of risk factors may result, in part, from the crudity of most of our measures of them. For instance, family dysfunction comes in many forms and an overall measure of this potential risk factor may be lumping together apples and oranges. Thus a family with an alcoholic father may have all sorts of problems (Earls et al., 1988; Reich et al., 1988), as may a family with a depressed mother, and two such families might score equally highly on a questionnaire about family dysfunction. However, the nature of the difficulties experienced by children in each of these families might be quite different, and associated with substantially different psychiatric outcomes. This suggests that there would be value in looking at risk factors like family dysfunction in a more molecular fashion.

Little attention has been paid to the various possible actions of risk factors, or the important point that, in a developing organism, patterns of risk cannot be expected to be static (Costello & Angold, 1995). The task now is to investigate the processes by which risk factors interact to produce the end-point of an identifiable depressive disorder. As Rutter (1997) has noted:

the research issues [for developmental psychopathology] have been formulated in ways that depart in some respects from those that have been traditional in epidemiology. Most crucially, there is a focus on continuities and discontinuities rather than on rates of disorder as such. The developmental perspective is concerned with continuities and discontinuities over time, and the psychopathologic perspective with continuities and discontinuities over the span of behavioral variation. In both cases the findings are used to examine mechanisms and processes. In other words, the aim is to go beyond the identification of risk factors to the delineation of the chain of operations by which such factors lead to disorder.

Research on life events has begun to address some of these issues. First, it is clear that life events that carry a moderate to severe degree of personal negative impact for the child, are associated with depression (see Chapter 8) but, as we have seen above, the occurrence of life events is also heritable, along with depression. So, life events are not just random environmental occurrences, rather they appear to be part of a partially familial nexus of risk factors associated with depression. Goodyer et al. (1993) found that the presence of a maternal history of psychiatric disorder and the occurrence of a recent life event that carried a severe negative impact for the child, taking into account its developmental status, had additive effects on the likelihood of depression in 11–16-year-old girls.

However, the situation is also probably more complex than this, because one has also to consider the possibility that there are developmental changes in sensitivity to the depressogenic effects of life events, with the changes of puberty leading to greater likelihood of depression in the face of life stress in adolescent girls than in younger girls or adolescent boys (Simmons & Blyth, 1987; Simmons et al., 1987; Petersen et al., 1991). Furthermore, it is necessary to consider not just the event itself, but its meaning for the individual (Rutter & Sandberg, 1992). In other words, the role of life events in depression is neither simple nor developmentally invariant. There is every reason to suppose that the same will be true of other risk factors for depression. This means that the focus will need to be on the interactions among risk factors, with the result that much larger epidemiological studies will be needed than we have had so far. (For a more detailed discussion of how the salience of life experience for individuals has been incorporated into measures of life events and difficulties for children and adolescents over the past two decades, see Chapter 8.)

Where should we go from here?

Comparisons between this chapter in the first edition of this book and the new edition lead to the welcome conclusion that we have come a long way over the last 7 years. Now, the key unanswered questions concern the aetiology of depression and how it comes to be associated with so many other comorbid disorders. This sort of research calls for relatively large epidemiological studies that involve assessments of physiological and family / genetic status, and a wide range of risk factors. Clearly, everything cannot be studied at once, but we have to face the fact that bivariate analyses will not suffice to advance our understanding of the aetiology of depression. It is already clear that depression results from the interplay of numerous factors, and that these factors are not the same at all points in development. We already know that much of the action is in the interaction terms in our models, and we will not make much progress without studies with adequate power to test complex interaction models.

REFERENCES

Abikoff, H. & Klein, R. G. (1992). Attention-deficit hyperactivity and conduct disorder: comorbidity and implications for treatment. *Journal of Consulting and Clinical Psychology*, **60**, 881–92.

Achenbach, T. M. (1990). 'Comorbidity' in child and adolescent psychiatry: categorical and quantitative perspectives. *Journal of Child and Adolescent Psychopharmacology*, **1**, 271–8.

Achenbach, T. M. (1995). Diagnosis, assessment, and comorbidity in psychosocial treatment research. *Journal of Abnormal Child Psychology*, **23**, 45–65.

American Psychiatric Association (1980). *Diagnostic and Statistical Manual of Mental Disorders (DSM-III)*, 3rd edn. Washington, DC: American Psychiatric Press.

American Psychiatric Association (1987). *Diagnostic and Statistical Manual of Mental Disorders (DSM-IIIR)*, 3rd edn. Washington, DC: American Psychiatric Press.

American Psychiatric Association (1994). *Diagnostic and Statistical Manual of Mental Disorders (DSM-IV)*, 4th edn. Washington, DC: American Psychiatric Press.

Anderson, J. C., Williams, S., McGee, R. & Silva, P. A. (1987). DSM-III disorders in preadolescent children: prevalence in a large sample from the general population. *Archives of General Psychiatry*, **44**, 69–77.

Andrews, J. A. & Lewinsohn, P. M. (1992). Suicidal attempts among older adolescents: prevalence and co-occurrence with psychiatric disorders. *Journal of the American Academy of Child and Adolescent Psychiatry*, **31**, 655–62.

Angold, A. & Costello, E. J. (1993). Depressive comorbidity in children and adolescents: empirical, theoretical, and methodological issues. *American Journal of Psychiatry*, **150**, 1779–91.

Angold, A. & Costello, E. J. (1995). The epidemiology of depression in children and adolescents. In *The Depressed Child and Adolescent: Developmental and Clinical Perspectives*, ed. I. M. Goodyer, pp. 127–47. Cambridge: Cambridge University Press.

Angold, A. & Rutter, M. (1992). The effects of age and pubertal status on depression in a large clinical sample. *Development and Psychopathology*, **4**, 5–28.

Angold, A., Costello, E. J. & Worthman, C. M. (1998a). Puberty and depression: the roles of age, pubertal status, and pubertal timing. *Psychological Medicine*, **28**, 51–61.

Angold, A., Messer, S. C., Stangl, D. et al. (1998b). Perceived parental burden and service use for child and adolescent psychiatric disorders. *American Journal of Public Health*, **88**, 75–80.

Angold, A., Costello, E. J. & Erkanli, A. (1999). Comorbidity. *Journal of Child Psychology and Psychiatry*, **40**, 57–87.

Angold, A., Costello, E. J. & Worthman, C. M. (1999). Pubertal changes in hormone levels and depression in girls. *Psychological Medicine*, **29**, 1043–53.

Angold, A., Erkanli, A., Egger, H. M. & Costello, E. J. (2000a). Comorbidity real and 'epiphenomenal' in the Great Smoky Mountains Study (in press).

Angold, A., Erkanli, A., Farmer, E. M. Z. et al. (2000b). Caring for children in the community. A study of psychiatric disorder, impairment and service use in rural African American and white youth. *Archives of General Psychiatry* (in press).

Angst, J. & Dobler-Mikola, A. (1984). The Zurich Study: II. The continuum from normal to pathological depressive mood swings. *European Archives of Psychiatry and Neurological Sciences*, **234**, 21–9.

Angst, J., Dobler-Mikola, A. & Binder, J. (1984). The Zurich study – a prospective epidemiological study of depressive, neurotic and psychosomatic syndromes. I. Problem, methodology. *European Archives of Psychiatry and Neurological Sciences*, **234**, 13–20.

Asarnow, J. R. & Ben-Meir, S. (1994). Children with schizophrenia spectrum and depressive disorders: a comparative study of premorbid adjustment, onset pattern and severity of impairment. *Journal of Child Psychology and Psychiatry*, **29**, 477–88.

August, G. J., Realmuto, G. M., MacDonaldI, A. W., Nugent, S. M. & Crosby, R. (1996). Prevalence of ADHD and comorbid disorders among elementary school children screened for disruptive behavior. *Journal of Abnormal Child Psychology*, **24**, 571–95.

Bartell, N. P. & Reynolds, W. M. (1986). Depression and self-esteem in academically gifted and nongifted children: a comparison study. *Journal of School Psychology*, **24**, 55–61.

Beardslee, W. R., Keller, M. B., Seifer, R. et al. (1996). Prediction of adolescent affective disorder: effects of prior parental affective disorders and child psychopathology. *Journal of the American Academy of Child and Adolescent Psychiatry*, **35**, 279–88.

Bebbington, P. (1996). The origins of sex differences in depressive disorder: bridging the gap. *International Review of Psychiatry*, **8**, 295–332.

Bebbington, P. E., Hurry, J., Tennant, C., Sturt, E. & Wing, J. K. (1981). Epidemiology of mental disorders in Camberwell. *Psychological Medicine*, **11**, 561–79.

Bebbington, P. E., Dunn, G., Jenkins, R. et al. (1998). The influence of age and sex on the prevalence of depressive conditions: report from the National Survey of Psychiatric Morbidity. *Psychological Medicine*, **28**, 9–10.

Beidel, D. & Turner, S. M. (1997). At risk for anxiety: I. Psychopathology in the offspring of anxious parents. *Journal of the American Academy of Child and Adolescent Psychiatry*, **36**, 918–24.

Berkson, J. (1946). Limitations of the application of fourfold table analysis to hospital data. *Biometrics Bulletin*, **2**, 47–52.

Biederman, J., Faraone, S. V., Keenan, K., Knee, D. & Tsuang, M. T. (1990). Family-genetic and psychosocial risk factors in DSM-III attention deficit disorder. *Journal of the American Academy of Child and Adolescent Psychiatry*, **29**, 526–33.

Biederman, J., Faraone, S. V., Keenan, K. et al. (1992). Further evidence for family-genetic risk factors in attention deficit hyperactivity disorder: patterns of comorbidity in probands and relatives in psychiatrically and pediatrically referred samples. *Archives of General Psychiatry*, **49**, 728–38.

Biederman, J., Faraone, S. V. & Mick, E. (1996). Attention deficit hyperactivity disorder and juvenile mania: an overlooked comorbidity? *Journal of the American Academy of Child and Adolescent Psychiatry*, **35**, 997–1008.

Biederman, J., Mick, E. & Faraone, S. V. (1998). Depression in attention deficit hyperactivity disorder (ADHD) children: 'true' depression or demoralization? *Journal of Affective Disorders*, **47**, 113–22.

Bird, H. R. (1996). Epidemiology of childhood disorders in a cross-cultural context. *Journal of Psychology and Psychiatry*, **37**, 35–49.

Bird, H. R., Canino, G., Rubio-Stipec, M. et al. (1988). Estimates of the prevalence of childhood maladjustment in a community survey in Puerto Rico: the use of combined measures. *Archives of General Psychiatry*, **45**, 1120–6.

Bird, H. R., Gould, M. S. & Staghezza, B. M. (1993). Patterns of diagnostic comorbidity in a community sample of children aged 9 through 16 years. *Journal of the American Academy of Child and Adolescent Psychiatry*, **32**, 361–8.

Bland, R. C., Newman, S. C. & Orn, H. (1988a). Lifetime prevalence of psychiatric disorders in Edmonton. *Acta Psychiatrica Scandinavica*, **77**, 24–32.

Bland, R. C., Newman, S. C. & Orn, H. (1988b). Period prevalence of psychiatric disorders in Edmonton. *Acta Psychiatrica Scandinavica*, **77**, 33–42.

Blazer, D. G., George, L. K., Landerman, R. et al. (1985). Psychiatric disorders: a rural/urban comparison. *Archives of General Psychiatry*, **42**, 651–6.

Blazer, D. G., Kessler, R. C., McGonagle, K. A. & Swartz, M. S. (1994). The prevalence and distribution of major depression in a national community sample: the national comorbidity survey. *American Journal of Psychiatry*, **151**, 979–86.

Borchardt, C. M. & Bernstein, G. A. (1995). Comorbid disorders in hospitalized bipolar adolescents compared with unipolar depressed adolescents. *Child Psychiatry and Human Development*, **26**, 11–18.

Brent, D. A., Perper, J. A., Goldstein, C. E. et al. (1988). Risk factors for adolescent suicide: a comparison of adolescent suicide victims with suicidal inpatients. *Archives of General Psychiatry*, **45**, 581–8.

Brent, D. A., Kolko, D. J., Allan, M. J. & Brown, R. V. (1990). Suicidality in affectively disordered adolescent inpatients. *Journal of the American Academy of Child and Adolescent Psychiatry*, **29**, 586–93.

Brent, D. A., Kolko, D. J., Wartella, M. E. et al. (1993a). Adolescent psychiatric inpatients' risk of suicide attempt at 6-month follow-up. *Journal of the American Academy of Child and Adolescent Psychiatry*, **32**, 95–105.

Brent, D. A., Perper, J. A., Moritz, G. et al. (1993b). Psychiatric risk factors for adolescent suicide: a case-control study. *Journal of the American Academy of Child and Adolescent Psychiatry*, **32**, 521–9.

Brooks-Gunn, J. & Warren, M. P. (1989). Biological and social contributions to negative affect in young adolescent girls. *Child Development*, **60**, 40–55.

Burke, K. C., Burke, J. D., Regier, D. A. & Rae, D. S. (1990). Age at onset of selected mental disorders in five community populations. *Archives of General Psychiatry*, **47**, 511–18.

Butler, S. F., Arredondo, D. E. & McCloskey, V. (1995). Affective comorbidity in children and adolescents with attention deficit hyperactivity disorder. *Annals of Clinical Psychiatry*, **7**, 51–5.

Cairns, R. B. & Cairns, B. D. (1994). *Lifelines and Risks: pathways of youth in our time*. New York, NY: Cambridge University Press.

Canino, G. J., Bird, H. R., Shrout, P. E. et al. (1987). The prevalence of specific psychiatric disorders in Puerto Rico. *Archives of General Psychiatry*, **44**, 727–35.

Cantwell, D. P. (1972). Psychiatric illness in the families of hyperactive children. *Archives of General Psychiatry*, **27**, 414–23.

Capaldi, D. M. (1992). Co-occurrence of conduct problems and depressive symptoms in early adolescent boys: II. A 2-year follow-up at grade 8. *Development and Psychopathology*, **4**, 125–44.

Caron, C. & Rutter, M. (1991). Comorbidity in child psychopathology: concepts, issues and research strategies. *Journal of Child Psychology and Psychiatry*, **32**, 1063–80.

CDC (1998). Suicide among black youths – United States, 1980–1995. *CDC MMWR Weekly*, **47**, 193–6.

Cheng, T. A. (1989). Sex difference in the prevalence of minor psychiatric morbidity: a social epidemiological study in Taiwan. *Acta Psychiatrica Scandinavica*, **80**, 395–407.

Cohen, P. & Brooks, J. S. (1987). Family factors related to the persistence of psychopathology in childhood and adolescence. *Psychiatry*, **50**, 332–45.

Cohen, P. & Hesselbart, C. S. (1992). Demographic factors in the use of children's mental health services. *American Journal of Public Health*, **83**, 49–52.

Cohen, P. & Hesselbart, C. S. (1993). Demographic factors in the use of children's mental health services. *American Journal of Public Health*, **83**, 49–52.

Cohen, P., Brook, J. S., Cohen, J., Velez, N. & Garcia, M. (1990). Common and uncommon pathways to adolescent psychopathology and problem behavior. In *Straight and Devious Pathways from Childhood to Adulthood*, ed. L. N. Robins, pp. 242–58. New York: Cambridge University Press.

Cohen, P., Cohen, J. & Brook, J. (1993a). An epidemiological study of disorders in late childhood and adolescence: 2. Persistence of disorders. *Journal of Child Psychology and Psychiatry*, **34**, 869–77.

Cohen, P., Cohen, J., Kasen, S. et al. (1993b). An epidemiological study of disorders in late childhood and adolescence: 1. Age- and gender-specific prevalence. *Journal of Child Psychology and Psychiatry and Allied Disciplines*, **34**, 851–67.

Compas, B. E., Oppedisano, G., Connor, J. K. et al. (1997). Gender differences in depressive symptoms in adolescence: comparison of national samples of clinically referred and nonreferred youths. *Journal of Consulting and Clinical Psychology*, **65**, 617–26.

Cooper, P. J. & Goodyer, I. (1993). A community study of depression in adolescent girls: I. Estimates of symptom and syndrome prevalence. *British Journal of Psychiatry*, **163**, 367–74.

Costello, E. J. (1989). The status of epidemiologic research into psychiatric disorders of childhood and adolescence. In *Children's Mental Health Services and Policy: building a research base*, ed. R. C. Friedman, pp. 304–16. Tampa, FL: Florida Mental Health Institute, University of South

Florida.

Costello, E. J. & Angold, A. (1995). Developmental epidemiology. In *Developmental Psychopathology*, ed. D. Cicchetti & D. Cohen, pp. 23–56. New York, NY: John Wiley.

Costello, E. J. & Janiszewski, S. (1990). Who gets treated? Factors associated with referral in children with psychiatric disorders. *Acta Psychiatrica Scandinavica*, **81**, 523–9.

Costello, E. J., Costello, A. J., Edelbrock, C. et al. (1988). Psychiatric disorders in pediatric primary care: prevalence and risk factors. *Archives of General Psychiatry*, **45**, 1107–16.

Costello, E. J., Burns, B. J., Angold, A. & Leaf, P. J. (1993). How can epidemiology improve mental health services for children and adolescents? *Journal of the American Academy of Child and Adolescent Psychiatry*, **32**, 1106–13.

Costello, E. J., Angold, A., Burns, B. J. et al. (1996). The Great Smoky Mountains study of youth: goals, designs, methods, and the prevalence of DSM-III-R disorders. *Archives of General Psychiatry*, **53**, 1129–36.

Costello, E., Farmer, E., Angold, A., Burns, B. & Erkanli, A. (1997). Psychiatric disorders among American Indian and white youth in Appalachia: the Great Smoky Mountains study. *American Journal of Public Health*, **87**, 827–32.

Decina, P., Kestenbaum, C., Farber, S. et al. (1983). Clinical and psychological assessment of children of bipolar probands. *American Journal of Psychiatry*, **140**, 548–53.

Deykin, E. Y., Levy, J. C. & Wells, V. (1987). Adolescent depression, alcohol and drug abuse. *American Journal of Public Health*, **77**, 178–81.

Doerfler, L. A., Felner, R. D., Rowlison, R. T., Raley, P. A. & Evans, E. (1988). Depression in children and adolescents: a comparative analysis of the utility and construct validity of two assessment measures. *Journal of Consulting and Clinical Psychology*, **56**, 769–72.

Earls, F., Reich, W., Jung, K. G. & Cloninger, C. R. (1988). Psychopathology in children of alcoholic and antisocial parents. *Alcoholism: Clinical and Experimental Research*, **12**, 481–7.

Eley, T. C. (1997). Depressive symptoms in children and adults: etiological links between normality and abnormality: a research note. *Journal of Child Psychology and Psychiatry*, **38**, 861–5.

Eley, T. C., Deater-Deckard, K., Fombonne, E., Fulker, D. W. & Plomin, R. (1998). An adoption study of depressive symptoms in middle childhood. *Journal of Child Psychology and Psychiatry*, **39**, 337–45.

Faraone, S. V., Biederman, J., Mennin, D., Wozniak, J. & Spencer, T. (1997). Attention-deficit hyperactivity disorder with bipolar disorder: a familial subtype? *Journal of the American Academy of Child and Adolescent Psychiatry*, **36**, 1378–87.

Faust, J., Baum, C. G. & Forehand, R. (1985). An examination of the association between social relationships and depression in early adolescence. *Journal of Applied Developmental Psychology*, **6**, 291–7.

Fergusson, D. M., Horwood, L. J. & Lynskey, M. T. (1993). Prevalence and comorbidity of DSM-III-R diagnoses in a birth cohort of 15 year olds. *Journal of the American Academy of Child and Adolescent Psychiatry*, **32**, 1127–34.

Fergusson, D. M., Lynskey, M. T. & Horwood, L. J. (1996). Origins of comorbidity between conduct and affective disorders. *Journal of the American Academy of Child and Adolescent*

Psychiatry, **35**, 451–60.

Ferro, T., Carlson, G. A., Grayson, P. & Klein, D. N. (1994). Depressive disorders: distinctions in children. *Journal of the American Academy of Child and Adolescent Psychiatry*, **33**, 664–70.

Finch, A. J., Saylor, C. F. & Edwards, G. L. (1985). Children's depression inventory: sex and grade norms for normal children. *Journal of Consulting and Clinical Psychology*, **53**, 424–5.

Fine, S., Moretti, M., Haley, G. & Marriage, K. (1985). Affective disorders in children and adolescents: the dysthymic disorder dilemma. *Canadian Journal of Psychiatry*, **30**, 173–7.

Fleming, J. E. & Offord, D. R. (1990). Epidemiology of childhood depressive disorders: a critical review. *Journal of the American Academy of Child and Adolescent Psychiatry*, **29**, 571–80.

Fleming, J. E., Offord, D. R. & Boyle, M. H. (1989). Prevalence of childhood and adolescent depression in the Community: Ontario child health study. *British Journal of Psychiatry*, **155**, 647–54.

Frost, L. A., Moffitt, T. E. & McGee, R. (1989). Neuropsychological correlates of psychopathology in an unselected cohort of young adolescents. *Journal of Abnormal Psychology*, **98**, 307–13.

Garnefski, N. & Diekstra, R. F. W. (1997). 'Comorbidity' of behavioral, emotional, and cognitive problems in adolescence. *Journal of Youth and Adolescence*, **26**, 321–38.

Garrison, C. Z., Jackson, K. L., Marsteller, F., McKeown, R. & Addy, C. (1990). A longitudinal study of depressive symptomatology in young adolescents. *Journal of the American Academy of Child and Adolescent Psychiatry*, **29**, 581–5.

Garrison, C. Z., Addy, C. L., Jackson, K. L., McKeown, R. E. & Waller, J. L. (1991). A longitudinal study of suicidal ideation in young adolescents. *Journal of the American Academy of Child and Adolescent Psychiatry*, **30**, 597–603.

Garrison, C. Z., Waller, J. L., Cuffe, S. P. et al. (1997). Incidence of major depressive disorder and dysthymia in young adolescents. *Journal of the American Academy of Child and Adolescent Psychiatry*, **36**, 458–65.

Gates, L., Lineberger, M. R., Crockett, J. & Hubbard, J. (1988). Birth order and its relationship to depression, anxiety, and self-concept test scores in children. *Journal of Genetic Psychology*, **149**, 29–34.

Ge, X., Conger, R. D. & Elder, G. H. (1996). Coming of age too early: pubertal influences on girls' vulnerability to psychological distress. *Child Development*, **67**, 3386–400.

Geller, B., Sun, K., Zimmerman, B., Frazier, J. & Williams, M. (1995). Complex and rapid-cycling in bipolar children and adolescents: a preliminary study. *Journal of Affective Disorders*, **34**, 259–68.

Gershon, E. S., McKnew, D., Cytryn, L. et al. (1985). Diagnoses in school-age children of bipolar affective disorder patients and normal controls. *Journal of Affective Disorders*, **8**, 283–91.

Goodman, S. H., Lahey, B. B., Fielding, B. et al. (1997). Representativeness of clinical samples of youths with mental disorders: a preliminary population-based study. *Journal of Abnormal Psychology*, **106**, 3–14.

Goodyer, I. M., Cooper, P. J., Vize, C. M. & Ashby, L. (1993). Depression in 11–16 year-old girls: the role of past parental psychopathology and exposure to recent life events. *Journal of Child Psychology and Psychiatry*, **34**, 1103–15.

Graber, J. A., Lewinsohn, P. M., Seeley, J. R. & Brooks-Gunn, J. (1997). Is psychopathology associated with the timing of pubertal development? *Journal of the American Academy of Child and Adolescent Psychiatry*, **36**, 1768–76.

Greif, E. B. & Ulman, K. J. (1982). The psychological impact of the menarche on early adolescent females: a review of the literature. *Child Development*, **53**, 1413–30.

Grigoroiu-Serbanescu, M., Christodorescu, D., Magureanu, S. et al. (1991a). Adolescent offspring of endogenous unipolar depressive parents and of normal parents. *Journal of Affective Disorders*, **21**, 185–98.

Grigoroiu-Serbanescu, M., Christodorescu, D., Totoescu, A. & Jipescu, I. (1991b). Depressive disorders and depressive personality traits in offspring aged 10–17 of bipolar and of normal parents. *Journal of Youth and Adolescence*, **20**, 135–48.

Guyer, B., Lescohier, I., Gallagher, S. S., Hausman, A. & Azzara, C. V. (1989). Intentional injuries among children and adolescents in Massachusetts. *New England Journal of Medicine*, **321**, 1584–9.

Haley, G. M., Fine, S., Marriage, K., Moretti, M. M. & Freeman, R. J. (1985). Cognitive bias and depression in psychiatrically disturbed children and adolescents. *Journal of Consulting and Clinical Psychology*, **53**, 535–7.

Hammen, C. (1992). The family–environmental context of depression: a perspective on children's risk. In *Developmental Perspectives on Depression – Rochester Symposium on Developmental Psychopathology*, ed. D. Cicchetti & S. L. Toth, pp. 251–81. Rochester: University of Rochester Press.

Hammen, C. L. & Padesky, C. A. (1977). Sex differences in the expression of depressive responses on the Beck Depression Inventory. *Journal of Abnormal Psychology*, **86**, 609–14.

Hammen, C., Gordon, D., Burge, D. et al. (1987). Maternal affective disorders, illness and stress: risk for children's psychopathology. *American Journal of Psychiatry*, **144**, 736–41.

Hankin, B. L., Abramson, L. Y., Moffitt, T. E. et al. (1998). Development of depression from preadolescence to young adulthood: Emerging gender differences in a 10-year longitudinal study. *Journal of Abnormal Psychology*, **107**, 128–40.

Harrington, R., Fudge, H., Rutter, M., Pickles, A. & Hill, J. (1990). Adult outcomes of childhood and adolescent depression. *Archives of General Psychiatry*, **47**, 465–73.

Harrington, R., Fudge, H., Rutter, M., Pickles, A. & Hill, J. (1991). Adult outcomes of childhood and adolescent depression: II. Links with antisocial disorders. *Journal of the American Academy of Child and Adolescent Psychiatry*, **30**, 434–9.

Hayward, C., Killen, J. D., Wilson, D. M. et al. (1997). Psychiatric risk associated with early puberty in adolescent girls. *Journal of the American Academy of Child and Adolescent Psychiatry*, **36**, 255–62.

Helsel, W. J. & Matson, J. L. (1984). The assessment of depression in children: the internal structure of the Child Depression Inventory (CDI). *Behavior Research and Therapy*, **22**, 289–98.

Hinshaw, S. P., Lahey, B. B. & Hart, E. L. (1993). Issues of taxonomy and comorbidity in the development of conduct disorder. Special issue: toward a developmental perspective on conduct disorder. *Development and Psychopathology*, **5**, 31–49.

Huntley, D. K., Phelps, R. E. & Rehm, L. P. (1987). Depression in children from single-parent families. *Journal of Divorce*, **10**, 153–61.

Hwu, H. G., Yeh, E. K. & Chang, L. Y. (1989). Prevalence of psychiatric disorders in Taiwan defined by the Chinese Diagnostic Interview Schedule. *Acta Psychiatrica Scandinavica*, **79**, 136–47.

Jensen, P. S., Shervette, R. E., Xenakis, S. N. & Richters, J. (1993). Anxiety and depressive disorders in attention deficit disorder with hyperactivity: new findings. *American Journal of Psychiatry*, **150**, 1203–9.

Jorm, A. F. (1987). Sex and age differences in depression: a quantitative synthesis of published research. *Australian and New Zealand Journal of Psychiatry*, **21**, 46–53.

Kashani, J. H. & Simonds, J. F. (1979). The incidence of depression in children. *American Journal of Psychiatry*, **136**, 1203–5.

Kashani, J. H., McGee, R. O., Clarkson, S. E. et al. (1983). Depression in a sample of 9-year-old children: prevalence and associated characteristics. *Archives of General Psychiatry*, **40**, 1217–23.

Kashani, J. H., Beck, N. C., Hoeper, E. W. et al. (1987). Psychiatric disorders in a community sample of adolescents. *American Journal of Psychiatry*, **144**, 584–9.

Kashani, J. H., Orvaschel, H., Rosenberg, M. A. & Reid, J. C. (1989). Psychopathology in a community sample of children and adolescents: a developmental perspective. *Journal of the American Academy of Child and Adolescent Psychiatry*, **28**, 701–6.

Kazdin, A. E., French, N. H. & Unis, A. S. (1983). Child, mother, and father evaluations of depression in psychiatric inpatient children. *Journal of Abnormal Child Psychology*, **11**, 167–80.

Keller, M. B., Shapiro, R. W., Lavori, P. W. & Wolfe, N. (1982a). Recovery in major depressive disorder analysis with the life table and regression models. *Archives of General Psychiatry*, **39**, 905–10.

Keller, M. B., Shapiro, R. W., Lavori, P. W. & Wolfe, N. (1982b). Relapse in major depressive disorder: analysis with the life table. *Archives of General Psychiatry*, **39**, 911–15.

Keller, M. B., Lavori, P. W., Mueller, T. I. et al. (1992). Time to recovery, chronicity, and levels of psychopathology in major depression: a 5-year prospective follow-up of 431 subjects. *Archives of General Psychiatry*, **49**, 809–16.

Kendall, P. C., Kortlander, E., Chansky, T. E. & Brady, E. U. (1992). Comorbidity of anxiety and depression in youth: treatment implications. *Journal of Consulting and Clinical Psychology*, **60**, 869–80.

Kessler, R. C., McGonagle, K. A., Swartz, M. S., Blazer, D. G. & Nelson, C. B. (1993). Sex and depression in the national comorbidity survey: I. Lifetime prevalence, chronicity and recurrence. *Journal of Affective Disorders*, **29**, 85–96.

Kessler, R. C., McGonagle, K. A., Nelson, C. B. et al. (1994). Sex and depression in the national comorbidity survey: II. Cohort effects. *Journal of Affective Disorders*, **30**, 15–26.

King, D. A. & Buchwald, A. M. (1982). Sex differences in subclinical depression: administration of the Beck Depression Inventory in public and private disclosure situations. *Journal of Personality and Social Psychology*, **42**, 963–9.

Klein, D. F. (1990). Symptom criteria and family history in major depression. *American Journal of Psychiatry*, **147**, 850–4.

Klein, D. W. & Depue, R. A. (1985). Obsessional personality traits and risk for bipolar affective disorder: an offspring study. *Journal of Abnormal Psychology*, **84**, 291–7.

Klein, D. N. & Riso, L. P. (1993). Psychiatric disorders: problems of boundaries and comorbidity. In *Basic Issues in Psychopathology*, ed. C. G. Costello, pp. 19–66. New York: Guilford Press.

Kovacs, M. (1983). *The Children's Depression Inventory: a self-rated depression scale for school-aged youngsters*. Pittsburgh, PA: University of Pittsburgh School of Medicine.

Kovacs, M. (1992). *Children's Depression Inventory (CDI) Manual*. North Tonawanda, NY: Multi-Health Systems.

Kovacs, M. (1996). Presentation and course of major depressive disorder during childhood and later years of the life span. *Journal of the American Academy of Child and Adolescent Psychiatry*, **35**, 705–15.

Kovacs, M., Feinberg, T. L., Crouse-Novak, M. A. et al. (1984). Depressive disorders in childhood: II. A longitudinal study of the risk for a subsequent major depression. *Archives of General Psychiatry*, **41**, 643–9.

Last, C. G., Hersen, M., Kazdin, A. E., Francis, G. & Grubb, H. J. (1987). Psychiatric illness in the mothers of anxious children. *American Journal of Psychiatry*, **144**, 1580–3.

Last, C. G., Perrin, S., Hersen, M. & Kazdin, A. E. (1996). A prospective study of childhood anxiety disorders. *Journal of the American Academy of Child and Adolescent Psychiatry*, **35**, 1502–10.

Lee, C. K., Han, J. H. & Choi, J. O. (1987). The epidemiological study of mental disorders in Korea (IX): alcoholism, anxiety, and depression. *Seoul Journal of Psychiatry*, **12**, 183–91.

Lewinsohn, P. M., Rohde, P., Seeley, J. R. & Hops, H. (1991). Comorbidity of unipolar depression: I. Major depression with dysthymia. *Journal of Abnormal Psychology*, **100**, 205–13.

Lewinsohn, P. M., Hops, H., Roberts, R. E., Seeley, J. R. & Andrews, J. A. (1993). Adolescent psychopathology: I. Prevalence and incidence of depression and other DSM-III-R disorders in high school students. *Journal of Abnormal Psychology*, **102**, 133–44.

Lewinsohn, P. M., Roberts, R. E., Seeley, J. R. et al. (1994a). Adolescent psychopathology: II. Psychosocial risk factors for depression. *Journal of Abnormal Psychology*, **103**, 302–15.

Lewinsohn, P. M., Rohde, P. & Seeley, J. R. (1994b). Psychosocial risk factors for future adolescent suicide attempts. *Journal of Consulting and Clinical Psychology*, **62**, 297–305.

Lewinsohn, P. M., Gotlib, I. H. & Seeley, J. R. (1995a). Adolescent psychopathology: IV. Specificity of psychosocial risk factors for depression and substance abuse in older adolescents. *Journal of the American Academy of Child and Adolescent Psychiatry*, **34**, 1221–9.

Lewinsohn, P. M., Klein, D. N. & Seeley, J. R. (1995b). Bipolar disorders in a community sample of older adolescents: prevalence, phenomenology, comorbidity, and course. *Journal of the American Academy of Child and Adolescent Psychiatry*, **34**, 454–63.

Lewinsohn, P. M., Seeley, J. R., Hibbard, J., Rohde, P. & Sack, W. H. (1996). Cross-sectional and prospective relationships between physical morbidity and depression in older adolescents. *Journal of the American Academy of Child and Adolescent Psychiatry*, **35**, 1120–9.

Loeber, R. & Keenan, K. (1994). Interaction between conduct disorder and its comorbid conditions: effects of age and gender. *Clinical Psychology Review*, **14**, 497–523.

Marriage, K., Fine, S., Moretti, M. & Haley, G. (1986). Relationship between depression and conduct disorder in children and adolescents. *Journal of the American Academy of Child Psychiatry*, **25**, 687–91.

Martunnen, M. J., Aro, H. M., Henriksson, M. M. & Lönnqvist, J. K. (1991). Mental disorders in adolescent suicide: DSM-III-R axes I and II diagnoses in suicides among 13 to 19 year-olds in Finland. *Archives of General Psychiatry*, **48**, 834–9.

McClellan, J. M., Rubert, M. P., Reichler, R. J. & Sylvester, C. E. (1990). Attention deficit disorder in children at risk for anxiety and depression. *Journal of the American Academy of Child and Adolescent Psychiatry*, **29**, 534–9.

McConaughy, S. H. & Achenbach, T. M. (1994). Comorbidity of empirically based syndromes in matched general population and clinical samples. *Journal of Child Psychology and Psychiatry*, **35**, 1141–57.

McCormick, L. H. (1995). Depression in mothers of children with attention deficit hyperactivity disorder. *Family Medicine*, **27**, 176–9.

McGee, R. & Williams, S. (1988). A longitudinal study of depression in nine-year-old children. *Journal of the American Academy of Child and Adolescent Psychiatry*, **27**, 342–8.

McGee, R., Feehan, M., Williams, S. et al. (1990). DSM-III disorders in a large sample of adolescents. *Journal of the American Academy of Child and Adolescent Psychiatry*, **29**, 611–19.

McGee, R., Feehan, M., Williams, S. & Anderson, J. (1992). DSM-III disorders from age 11 to age 15 years. *Journal of the American Academy of Child and Adolescent Psychiatry*, **31**, 51–9.

Merikangas, K. R., Prusoff, B. A. & Weissman, M. M. (1988). Parental concordance for affective disorders: psychopathology in offspring. *Journal of Affective Disorders*, **15**, 279–90.

Moreau, D. L., Weissman, M. & Warner, V. (1990). Panic disorder in children at high risk for depression. *Annual Progress in Child Psychiatry and Child Development*, **146**, 363–7.

Morrison, J. L. (1980). Adult psychiatric disorder in parents of hyperactive children. *American Journal of Psychiatry*, **137**, 825–7.

Morrison, J. L. & Stewart, M. A. (1971). A family study of the hyperactive child syndrome. *Biological Psychiatry*, **3**, 189–95.

Noam, G. G., Paget, K., Valiant, G., Borst, S. & Bartok, J. (1994). Conduct and affective disorders in developmental perspective: a systematic study of adolescent psychopathology. *Development and Psychopathology*, **6**, 519–32.

Nolen-Hoeksema, S. & Girgus, J. S. (1994). The emergence of gender differences in depression during adolescence. *Psychological Bulletin*, **115**, 424–41.

Nolen-Hoeksema, S., Girgus, J. S. & Seligman, M. E. P. (1991). Sex differences in depression and explanatory style in children. *Journal of Youth and Adolescence*, **20**, 233–45.

Nottelmann, E. D. & Jensen, P. S. (1995). Comorbidity of disorders in children and adolescents: developmental perspectives. In *Advances in Clinical Child Psychology*, ed. T. H. Ollendick & R. J. Prinz, pp. 109–55. New York: Plenum Press.

Nottelmann, E. D., Susman, E. F., Dorn, L. D. et al. (1987a). Developmental processes in early adolescence: relations among chronological age, pubertal stage, height, weight, and serum levels of gonadotropins, sex steroids, and adrenal androgens. *Journal of Adolescent Health Care*, **8**, 246–60.

Nottelmann, E. D., Susman, E. J., Inoff-Germain, G., Cutler, G. et al. (1987b). Developmental processes in early adolescence: relationships between adolescent adjustment problems and chronological age, pubertal stage, and puberty-related serum hormone levels. *Journal of Pediatrics*, **110**, 473–80.

Nottelmann, E. D., Inoff-Germain, G., Susman, E. J. & Chrousos, G. P. (1990). Hormones and behavior at puberty. In *Adolescence and Puberty*, ed. J. Bancroft & J. M. Reinisch, pp. 88–123. New York: Oxford Press.

Nurnberger, J. I., Hamovit, J., Hibbs, E. et al. (1988). A high-risk study of primary affective disorder: selection of subjects, initial assessment, and 1- to 2-year follow-up. In *Relatives at Risk for Mental Disorder*, ed. D. L. Dunner, E. S. Gershon & J. E. Barrett, pp. 161–77. New York: Raven Press.

Olweus, D., Mattsson, A., Schalling, D. & Low, H. (1988). Circulating testosterone levels and aggression in adolescent males: a causal analysis. *Psychosomatic Medicine*, **50**, 261–72.

Orvaschel, H. (1990). Early onset psychiatric disorder in high risk children and increased familial morbidity. *Journal of the American Academy of Child and Adolescent Psychiatry*, **29**, 184–8.

Orvaschel, H., Walsh-Allis, G., Ye, W. & Walsh, G. T. (1988). Psychopathology in children of parents with recurrent depression. *Journal of Abnormal Child Psychology*, **16**, 17–28.

Paikoff, R. L., Brooks-Gunn, J. & Warren, M. P. (1991). Effects of girls' hormonal status on depressive and aggressive symptoms over the course of one year. *Journal of Youth and Adolescence*, **20**, 191–215.

Petersen, A. C., Sarigiani, P. A. & Kennedy, R. E. (1991). Adolescent depression: why more girls? *Journal of Youth and Adolescence*, **20**, 247–71.

Pliszka, S. R. (1992). Comorbidity of attention-deficit hyperactivity disorder and overanxious disorder. *Journal of the American Academy of Child and Adolescent Psychiatry*, **31**, 197–203.

Quiggle, N. L., Garber, J., Panak, W. F. & Dodge, K. A. (1992). Social information processing in aggressive and depressed children. *Child Development*, **63**, 1305–20.

Radloff, L. (1977). The CES-D scale: a self-report depression scale for research in the general population. *Applied Psychological Measurement*, **3**, 385–401.

Reich, W., Earls, F. & Powell, J. (1988). A comparison of the home and social environments of children of alcoholic and non-alcoholic parents. *British Journal of Addiction*, **83**, 831–9.

Reinherz, H. Z., Frost, A. K., Stewart-Berghauer, G. et al. (1990). The many faces of correlates of depressive symptoms in adolescents. *Journal of Early Adolescence*, **10**, 455–71.

Reinherz, H. Z., Giaconia, R. M., Lefkowitz, E. S., Pakiz, B. & Frost, A. K. (1993a). Prevalence of psychiatric disorders in a community population of older adolescents. *Journal of the American Academy of Child and Adolescent Psychiatry*, **32**, 369–77.

Reinherz, H. Z., Giaconia, R. M., Pakiz, B. et al. (1993b). Psychosocial risks for major depression in late adolescence: a longitudinal community study. *Journal of the American Academy of Child and Adolescent Psychiatry*, **32**, 1155–63.

Rende, R. D., Plomin, R., Reiss, D. & Hetherington, E. M. (1993). Genetic and environmental influences on depressive symptomatology in adolescence: individual differences and extreme scores. *Journal of Child Psychology and Psychiatry*, **34**, 1387–98.

Rhode, P., Lewinsohn, P. M. & Seeley, J. R. (1991). Comorbidity of unipolar depression: II. Comorbidity with other mental disorders in adolescents and adults. *Journal of Abnormal Psychology*, **100**, 214–22.

Roberts, R. E. & Chen, Y.-W. (1995). Depressive symptoms and suicidal ideation among Mexican-origin and anglo adolescents. *Journal of the American Academy of Child and Adolescent*

Psychiatry, **34**, 81–90.

Roberts, R. E., Lewinsohn, P. M. & Seeley, J. R. (1995). Symptoms of DSM-III-R major depression in adolescence: evidence from an epidemiological survey. *Journal of the American Academy of Child and Adolescent Psychiatry*, **34**, 1608–17.

Rudolph, K. D., Hammen, C. & Burge, D. (1994). Interpersonal functioning and depressive symptoms in childhood: addressing the issues of specificity and comorbidity. *Journal of Abnormal Child Psychology*, **22**, 355–71.

Rutter, M. (1997). Comorbidity: concepts, claims and choices. *Criminal Behavior and Mental Health*, **7**, 265–85.

Rutter, M. & Sandberg, S. (1992). Psychosocial stressors: concepts, causes, and effects. *European Child and Adolescent Psychiatry*, **1**, 3–13.

Rutter, M., Tizard, J. & Whitmore, K. (1970). *Education, Health, and Behaviour*. London: Longman.

Rutter, M., Graham, P., Chadwick, O. F. D. & Yule, W. (1976). Adolescent turmoil: fact or fiction? *Journal of Child Psychology and Psychiatry*, **17**, 35–56.

Ryan, N., Puig-Antich, J., Ambrosini, P. J. et al. (1987). The clinical picture of major depression in children and adolescents. *Archives of General Psychiatry*, **44**, 854–61.

Shaffer, D. (1993). Suicide: risk factors and the public health. *American Journal of Public Health*, **83**, 171–2.

Shaffer, D. & Fisher, P. W. (1981). The epidemiology of suicide in children and young adolescents. *Journal of the American Academy of Child Psychiatry*, **20**, 545–65.

Shaffer, D., Fisher, P. W., Dulcan, M. et al. (1996). The NIMH diagnostic interview schedule for children (DISC 2.3): description, acceptability, prevalences, and performance in the MECA study. *Journal of the American Academy of Child and Adolescent Psychiatry*, **35**, 865–77.

Shain, B. N., King, C. A., Naylor, M. & Alessi, N. E. (1991). Chronic depression and hospital course in adolescents. *Journal of the American Academy of Child and Adolescent Psychiatry*, **30**, 428–33.

Silberg, J., Pickles, A., Rutter, M. et al. (1999). The influence of genetic factors and life stress on depression among adolescents girls. *Archives of General Psychiatry*, **56**, 225–32.

Simmons, R. G. & Blyth, D. A. (1987). *Moving into Adolescence: the impact of pubertal change and school context*. Hawthorne, NY: Aldine de Gruyter.

Simmons, R. G., Burgeson, R. & Carlton-Ford, S. (1987). The impact of cumulative change in early adolescence. *Child Development*, **58**, 1220–34.

Simonoff, E., Pickles, A., Meyer, J. M. et al. (1997). The Virginia twin study of adolescent behavioral development: influences of age, sex and impairment on rates of disorder. *Archives of General Psychiatry*, **54**, 801–8.

Smucker, M. R., Craighead, W. E., Craighead, L. W. & Green, B. J. (1986). Normative and reliability data for the children's depression inventory. *Journal of Abnormal Child Psychology*, **14**, 25–39.

Stattin, H. & Magnusson, D. (1990). *Paths through Life*, vol. 2. *Pubertal Maturation in Female Development*. Hillsdale, NJ: Lawrence Erlbaum.

Susman, E. J., Nottelmann, E. D., Inoff-Germain, G. E. et al. (1985). The relation of relative hormonal levels and physical development and social-emotional behavior in young adolescents. *Journal of Youth and Adolescence*, **14**, 245–64.

Susman, E. J., Inoff-Germain, G., Nottelmann, E. D. et al. (1987a). Hormones, emotional dispositions, and aggressive attributes in young adolescents. *Child Development*, **58**, 1114–34.

Susman, E. J., Nottelmann, E. D., Inoff-Germain, G., Dorn, L. D. & Chrousos, G. P. (1987b). Hormonal influences on aspects of psychological development during adolescence. *Journal of Adolescent Health Care*, **8**, 492–504.

Sylvester, C. E., Hyde, T. S. & Reichler, R. J. (1988). Clinical psychopathology among children of adults with panic disorder. In *Relatives at Risk for Mental Disorder*, ed. D. L. Dunner, E. S. Gershon & J. E. Barrett, pp. 87–99. New York: Raven Press.

Tanner, J. M. (1962). *Growth at Adolescence: with a general consideration of the effects of hereditary and environmental factors upon growth and maturation from birth to maturity*. Oxford: Blackwell Scientific Publications.

Teri, L. (1982). The use of the Beck Depression Inventory with adolescents. *Journal of Abnormal Child Psychology*, **10**, 277–84.

Thapar, A. & McGuffin, P. (1994). A twin study of depressive symptoms in childhood. *British Journal of Psychiatry*, **165**, 259–65.

Thapar, A., Harold, G. & McGuffin, P. (1998). Life events and depressive symptoms in childhood – shared genes or shared adversity? A research note. *Journal of Child Psychology and Psychiatry*, **39**, 1153–8.

Turner, S. M., Beidel, D. C. & Costello, A. (1987). Psychopathology in the offspring of anxiety disorders patients. *Journal of Consulting and Clinical Psychology*, **55**, 229–35.

Velez, C. N., Johnson, J. & Cohen, P. (1989). A longitudinal analysis of selected risk factors of childhood psychopathology. *Journal of the American Academy of Child and Adolescent Psychiatry*, **28**, 861–4.

Warner, V., Mufson, L. & Weissman, M. M. (1995). Offspring at high and low risk for depression and anxiety: mechanisms of psychiatric disorder. *Journal of the American Academy of Child and Adolescent Psychiatry*, **34**, 786–97.

Weissman, M. M. & Klerman, G. L. (1977). Sex differences and the epidemiology of depression. *Archives of General Psychiatry*, **34**, 98–111.

Weissman, M. M., Bland, R., Joyce, P. R. et al. (1993). Sex differences in rates of depression: cross-national perspectives. *Journal of Affective Disorders*, **29**, 77–84.

Weissman, M. M., Bland, R. C., Canino, G. J. et al. (1996). Cross-national epidemiology of major depression and bipolar disorder. *Journal of the American Medical Association*, **276**, 293–9.

Weissman, M. M., Fendrich, M., Warner, V. & Wickramaratne, P. (1992). Incidence of psychiatric disorder in offspring at high and low risk for depression. *Journal of the American Academy of Child and Adolescent Psychiatry*, **31**, 640–8.

Wells, J. E., Bushnell, J. A., Hornblow, A. R., Joyce, P. R. & Oakley-Browne, M. A. (1989). Christchurch psychiatric epidemiology study, part I: methodology and lifetime prevalence for specific psychiatric disorders. *Australian and New Zealand Journal of Psychiatry*, **23**, 315–26.

Welner, Z., Welner, A., McCrary, M. D. & Leonard, M. A. (1977). Psychopathology in children of inpatients with depression. *Journal of Nervous and Mental Disorders*, **164**, 408–13.

West, S. A., McElroy, S. L., Strakowski, S. M., Keck, P. E. & McConville, B. J. (1995). Attention deficit hyperactivity disorder in adolescent mania. *American Journal of Psychiatry*, **152**, 271–3.

West, S. A., Strakowski, S. M., Sax, K. W. et al. (1996). Phenomenology and comorbidity of adolescents hospitalized for the treatment of acute mania. *Biological Psychiatry*, **39**, 458–60.

Wichstrøm, L. (1999). The emergence of gender difference in depressed mood during adolescence: the role of intensified gender socialization. *Developmental Psychology*, **35**, 232–45.

Wittchen, H.-U., Essau, C. A., von Zerssen, D., Krieg, J. C. & Zaudig, M. (1992). Lifetime and six-month prevalence of mental disorders in the Munich follow-up study. *European Archives of Psychiatry and Clinical Neuroscience*, **241**, 247–58.

World Health Organization (1993). *The ICD-10 Classification of Mental and Behavioural Disorders: Diagnostic Criteria for Research*. Geneva: World Health Organization.

Wozniak, J., Biederman, J., Kiely, K. et al. (1995). Mania-like symptoms suggestive of childhood-onset bipolar disorder in clinically referred children. *Journal of the American Academy of Child and Adolescent Psychiatry*, **34**, 867–76.

Zoccolillo, M. (1992). Co-occurrence of conduct disorder and its adult outcomes with depressive and anxiety disorders: a review. *Journal of the American Academy of Child and Adolescent Psychiatry*, **31**, 547–56.

7

Family-genetic aspects of juvenile affective disorders

Michael Strober

Introduction

Important among the distinguishing features of juvenile mood disorders are significant social morbidity, protracted courses of recovery, possibly indicative of greater resistance to currently available treatment modalities, an unusually high propensity for manic switches, and episode recurrence (Birmaher et al., 1996; Strober, 1996). These sobering 'truths' are underlined further by epidemiological data showing that affective disorders are becoming increasingly prevalent in the juvenile population, suggesting earlier ages of onset in those at risk (Klerman & Weissman, 1989). Factors accounting for these temporal changes in rates of illness are little understood, although both genetic and environmental effects can be assumed. The validity of these conditions as diagnostic entities in young people remains an important area for further research.

Disturbances of mood in young people encompass a wide range of clinical phenomena and associated risk factors. Similarities in the syndromic expression of depression in juveniles and adults are well documented (Ryan et al., 1987), but homogeneity of phenotype does not mean there is a single common disorder across all age groups. For example, while prepubertal major depression seems to breed true over time and recur through adolescence (Kovacs et al., 1984; Hammen et al., 1990), one follow-up study focusing on the adult psychiatric status of children and adolescents with depression showed that prospective continuity with adult major depression was considerably stronger among postpubertal subjects (Harrington et al., 1990). A subsequent analysis of data from this cohort illustrates, as well, how immensely important it is to take account of nondepressive comorbid states in mapping developmental linkages in efforts to establish nosological validity. Specifically, when the cohort was stratified by the presence versus absence of coexisting conduct disorder, only the purely depressed subjects were strongly predisposed to adult depressions, whereas comorbidity of depression and conduct disorder during childhood was predictive of adult alcoholism and criminality. These differential patterns of continuity are in line with clinical studies (Nurcombe et al., 1989; Seifer et al., 1989) which suggest an increasing incidence of adult-like depressive states with onset of puberty.

An important empirical question, then, is how research methodologies may be usefully applied in child psychiatry in investigations of nosological validity and the search for specific susceptibility factors and mediators of symptom expression and course of illness. This chapter focuses on the relevance of family–genetic studies to these issues. Substantive findings will be highlighted, along with methodological and conceptual problems that arise when applying this perspective to the study of causal influences. Since critical appraisals of this literature have appeared elsewhere (Beardslee et al., 1983; Orvaschel, 1983; Weissman, 1988, 1990; Downey & Coyne, 1990; Hammen, 1991), the present chapter will be more selective in its focus on recent controlled studies, and on studies that shed light on possible mediators of juvenile age of onset.

Family data in juvenile depression: prospects and caveats

Evidence that unipolar and bipolar affective disorders are transmitted across generations is impressive (Tsuang & Faraone, 1990). This fact makes the family study a highly informative complement to other conventional methods in testing the diagnostic validity of juvenile affective conditions. The intuitive appeal and straightforward simplicity of the family study are important virtues. If depression in juveniles is a valid entity, then lifetime risk of affective disorders in their adult relatives will be significantly greater than in the general population. Likewise, psychiatric assessment of the school-age offspring of affectively ill parents, when combined with longitudinal, prospective follow-up designs, should not only demonstrate concordance between parent and child diagnostic status, but illuminate risk and protective factors, as well as developmental effects on phenotypic expression of underlying vulnerabilities. The informativeness of family study data concerning juvenile affective disorder is, however, offset by significant challenges to their interpretation. As noted by others (Downey & Coyne, 1990; Coyne et al., 1992), research on children of depressed parents has paid surprisingly little attention to the unrepresentativeness of these samples, methodological complexities and the potential impact of contextual factors on measures of psychopathological adjustment in such a group. For example, with rare exceptions, studies of this type have recruited ill parents through treatment centres; but since most affectively disturbed adults do not seek treatment, these families may not be truly representative of the larger population. Only scant data are available on the psychiatric status of offspring of depressed adults in the community (Beardslee et al., 1988) to allow some gauge of the generality of findings from treated samples.

Equally problematical is the assumption – usually inferred, if not made explicit in these studies – that parent–child concordance for diagnostic status is accounted for by simple intergenerational transmission of risk. Yet conventional approaches to matching and statistical control may be inadequate to the task of separating spurious from causal influences in the multifactorial pathways of psychiatric risk linking parent to child (Coyne et al., 1992). Moreover, given that genetic and environmental effects are perfectly confounded in studies of intact families, and that diagnostic criteria for major depression are likely to encompass multiple disorders with distinct heritable and developmental antecedents, it becomes apparent how daunting is the challenge of decomposing transmissible risk into genetic, psychological and situational components. It is likely the case that 'depressed' offspring of affectively ill adults are a mixed lot, including true forms of inherited illness along with phenocopies arising from a combination of sources: chronic strains and adversities that accompany parental psychiatric impairment; lowered self-concept and peer rejection; deviant parenting behaviours resulting from depression; the effects of psychopathology in co-parents; and marital conflict, to cite but a few.

Empirical data attesting to the power of these variables in mediating associations between parent and child maladjustment are substantial (Downey & Coyne, 1990; Hammen, 1991; Coyne et al., 1992). Since these dysphorogenic stresses often cluster in families but are not particular to any one psychiatric disorder, they may spuriously inflate estimates from family data of the magnitude and specificity of affective risk transmitted from parent to child. Such cautions do not imply that the family study is too confounded to have practical or heuristic value in child psychiatry. To the contrary; as descriptive data on juvenile depression rapidly accumulates and methods in psychiatric genetics become more refined, the study of genetic and environmental risk factors in juvenile-onset affective disorders becomes an even more promising and clinically important endeavour. At this juncture, however, any review of the family–genetic literature must give proper acknowledgement to these complexities.

The offspring of affectively ill parents

At least 11 studies have utilized modern case-control methods and principles in assessing parent–child resemblance for affective disorder. Klein et al. (1985) examined 37 offspring, 15–21 years of age, of 24 patients with bipolar illness and

22 offspring of adults with nonaffective psychiatric disorders. Index and control parents were recruited through inpatient and outpatient treatment programmes of several large urban hospitals. Diagnoses were based on a review of medical records and personal interviews using the Schedule for Affective Disorders and Schizophrenia (SADS; Endicott & Spitzer, 1978) and Research Diagnostic Criteria (RDC; Spitzer et al., 1978). Diagnoses in offspring, based on RDC and *DSM-III* criteria (American Psychiatric Association, 1987) were established through personal interviews using the lifetime version of the SADS conducted by assessors who were blind to parental diagnostic status. Final diagnoses were determined independently by two experienced clinicians.

Gershon et al. (1985) reported diagnoses by *DSM-III* criteria in 29 children, 6–17 years of age, of bipolar parents recruited through the affective disorders programme at the National Institute of Mental Health (NIMH), and 37 children of normal control families. History of psychopathology in the offspring was obtained from separate parent and child interviews using the Kiddie-SADS (Schedule for Affective Disorders and Schizophrenia for School-age Children; Orvaschel et al., 1981). Although interviews with offspring were often conducted with knowledge of the parent's diagnostic status, final diagnoses were decided by two child psychiatrists who blindly evaluated parent and child interview forms. Beardslee et al. (1987) evaluated 108 offspring, 11–19 years of age, of adults with affective disorder (mainly unipolar major depression), and 64 offspring from a randomly selected sample of community control families free of psychiatric illness. Index families were recruited, in part, from subjects at the Boston site of the NIMH Collaborative Study of the Psychobiology of Depression (Katz & Klerman, 1979). Lifetime psychopathology in the offspring was assessed using the Diagnostic Interview for Children and Adolescents (DICA; Herjanic & Reich, 1982), administered separately to parent and child by independent assessors who were blind to parental diagnostic status. *DSM-III* diagnoses were made by combining parent and child data using predetermined consensus rating procedures. Breslau et al. (1987) reported rates of major depression and anxiety disorders in 331 mother–child dyads obtained from a geographically based probability sample. Psychiatric history information on mother and child was obtained by personal interview using adult and child versions of the Diagnostic Interview Schedule (Robins et al., 1981; Costello et al., 1984). With rare exception, the same interviewer examined mother and child; however, final *DSM-III* diagnoses were derived by computer algorithms. Rates of disorder are reported separately for children 8–17 years of age, and 18–23 years of age. Mothers' diagnostic status was trichotomized into: (1) generalized anxiety only; (2) major depression, of whom 80% had concurrent generalized anxiety; and (3) neither major depression nor generalized anxiety.

The study by Weissman et al. (1987) compared rates of disorder in 125 children, 6–23 years of age, of 56 unipolar depressed adults and 95 children of 35 controls without any history of psychiatric illness. Depressed adults were probands involved in the Yale Family Study of affective disorders, recruited through treatment clinics at the Yale University Depression Research Unit. History of psychiatric disorder in the offspring was determined by independent Kiddie-SADS interviews of parent and child conducted blind to parental diagnosis. *DSM-III* diagnoses were determined by consensus using a best estimate procedure in which two clinicians independently and blindly examined all available sources of information.

The study by Hammen et al. (1987) included 19 offspring of 13 mothers with recurrent unipolar depression, 12 offspring of nine mothers with bipolar illness, 18 offspring of 14 mothers with chronic physical disease, and 35 offspring of 22 mothers free of psychiatric disorder. Offspring ranged in age from 8 to 16 years. Affectively ill mothers were recruited through both private and public treatment facilities. Medical controls were obtained through advertisement in newsletters of the American Diabetes Association and Arthritis Foundation, and through speciality medical practices. Normals were recruited from schools matched demographically to socioeconomic profiles of the affective probands and medical ill controls. Information on the child's psychiatric history was obtained from separate Kiddie-SADS interviews with mother and child by different interviewers. In spite of efforts to keep child interviewers blind to maternal diagnosis, violations of the blind occurred in an unspecified proportion of cases. Diagnoses were based on *DSM-III* criteria, although procedures used in assigning diagnoses are not described.

Orvaschel et al. (1988) studied 61 children of 34 parents with recurrent unipolar major depression recruited from a larger pool of subjects enrolled in clinical trials at University of Pittsburgh Western Psychiatric Institute, and 45 children from a random community sample matched on income level and education in which neither parent met any lifetime criteria for major psychiatric illness. School-age subjects ranged in age from 6 to 16 years. *DSM-III* diagnoses were based on separate Kiddie-SADS interviews of mother and child by a single interviewer. It is not stated whether interviewers were blind to parental diagnosis, nor are procedures for reaching diagnostic consensus described.

To avoid the possible confound of treatment-seeking bias on reported rates of psychiatric illness in young offspring of depressed parents, Beardslee et al. (1988) reported on a sample of families randomly selected without knowledge

of psychiatric history from a large pool of those enrolled in a health maintenance organization. Potential subjects were told they would be participating in
a study of psychosocial adjustment, and since results of the research interviews
were not volunteered to parents, selection bias was minimized. Diagnoses in
adults were established by SADS-Lifetime (SADS-L) interviews and RDC.
Subjects consisted of 89 school-age children from 49 families in which one or
both parents had affective illness, 19 children from 11 families in which one or
both parents had nonaffective psychiatric illness, and 45 children from 21
families in which neither parent had a history of psychiatric disorder. The
majority of affectively ill parents suffered from primary unipolar major depression. Consensus *DSM-III* diagnoses in children were based on separate and
independent DICA interviews of parent and child by assessors who were blind
to parental diagnostic status.

In a study by Welner & Rice (1988), rates of psychiatric disorders were
compared in 60 school-age children of parents with affective disorder, mainly
unipolar type, 43 children from unscreened community control families, and 15
children from unscreened medically ill control families. Ill parents were recruited from subjects at the St Louis site of the NIMH Collaborative Study of the
Psychobiology of Depression. Controls were selected from a pool of names
who were acquaintances of first-degree relatives of these subjects, and from
patients treated in the dialysis unit of the Washington University Medical
Center. *DSM-III* diagnoses were based on DICA interviews of parent and child
conducted by different assessors, each of whom was blind to parent diagnosis.
Best estimate diagnoses were determined by consensus judgement of the two
clinicians.

Klein et al. (1988) studied 47 offspring, 14–22 years of age, of 24 primary
unipolar depressives recruited through inpatient services of a large university
medical centre. Two control groups were employed: 33 offspring of 19 adults
with chronic rheumatoid arthritis or orthopaedic disease, and 38 offspring of
adults without any personal or family history of psychiatric illness. Normal
controls were drawn from random sampling of adults living in the same
community as the index depressed families. Offspring were personally and
blindly interviewed with a modification of the lifetime SADS. Final diagnoses
were made blindly by a single interviewer using *DSM-III*, *DSM-III-R*, and RDC.

Sylvester et al. (1988) examined rates of major depression and anxiety
disorders in 125 children, 7–17 years of age, from 72 families. Twenty-seven
were offspring of a parent with major depression, 50 were offspring of a parent
with panic disorder and 48 were from families without psychiatric disorder.
Separate and independent interviews were conducted blind to parental diag-

nosis using the DICA. Procedures used in reaching final diagnoses are not described.

Rates of affective diagnoses among offspring examined in these studies are given in Table 7.1. A wide variation in rates is evident, especially for major depression. This is not unanticipated, given interstudy differences in diagnostic instruments; training and skill of interviewers; procedures for rendering study diagnoses; ascertainment of adult probands; and the inevitable differences among clinicians in thresholds applied for determining caseness. Even so, in the nine studies that include unipolar, or mainly unipolar, disorder in the index adult proband, a clear association between parent and offspring affective disorder is found. The risk of major depression in these offspring ranges from 9 to 47% the average being 25%. For offspring of normal controls, the range is 0–24%, the average being 7%. Moreover, in four of the 11 studies, major depression was nonexistent among offspring of normal controls.

Only three studies employed medically ill controls (Hammen et al., 1987; Klein et al., 1988; Welner & Rice, 1988); none the less, rates of major depression in their offspring are low (17, 0 and 5%, respectively), and they are low, as well, in offspring of mixed psychiatric controls (Klein et al., 1985; Beardslee et al., 1988). On the other hand, two studies indicate widely divergent rates of major depression in offspring of adults with anxiety disorders – 12% in Breslau et al. (1987) compared to 48% in Sylvester et al. (1988). However, this latter figure is not entirely unexpected given evidence of similar genetic liabilities influencing risk of major depression and anxiety disorders (Merikangas, 1990; Kendler et al., 1992).

Taken together, these data suggest that major depression is roughly three to four times more likely in juvenile offspring of adults with unipolar affective disorder in comparison to offspring of normal, medically ill and nonaffective, but psychiatrically ill adults. By contrast, two of the three studies (Gershon et al., 1985; Klein et al., 1985) that included adult probands with bipolar illness found no association with major depression in offspring. An exception is the study by Hammen et al. (1987), in which major depression was nearly three times more prevalent in offspring of bipolars compared to offspring of normal controls, but roughly one-half the rate observed in offspring of unipolar depressed adults.

In the six studies that give rates of dysthymia, an association between parent and offspring affective status is supported. The risk among offspring of unipolar adults ranges from 8 to 32%, compared to 0–6% among offspring of controls. In two studies (Klein et al., 1985; Hammen et al., 1987), dysthymia is reported in 8% of offspring with bipolar illness. Pooling these results, dysthymia is roughly

Table 7.1. Rates/100 of affective disorders among school-age offspring of affectively ill adults and controls by *DSM-III* criteria

Study	Parent diagnosis	Major depression	Dysthymia	Bipolar[a]
Gershon et al., 1985	BP	10		3
	NC	14		0
Klein et al., 1985	BP	3	3	27
	PC	5	0	0
Breslau et al., 1987	MD	16		
	AN	12		
	NC	8		
Beardslee et al., 1987	AD	18	12	
	NC	0	0	
Hammen et al., 1987	UP	47	32	
	BP	25	8	
	MC	17	6	
	NC	9	3	
Weissman et al., 1987	UP	38		
	NC	24		
Beardslee et al., 1988	AD	20	17	
	PC[b]	0	0	
	NC	0	2	
Klein et al., 1988	UP	9	15	6
	MC	0	3	0
	NC	0	0	0
Orvaschel et al., 1988	UP	15	15	2
	NC	0	2	0
Sylvester et al., 1988	MD	37		
	AN[c]	48		
	NC	21		
Welner & Rice, 1988[d]	AD	23		
	MC	5		
	NC	5		

BP, bipolar illness; NC, no psychiatric illness control; PC, psychiatric controls; MD, major depression, polarity unspecified; AN, anxiety disorder; AD, affective disorder, mainly unipolar type; UP, unipolar major depression; MC, medically ill control.

[a] Bipolar I, hypomania; bipolar II, cyclothymia combined.
[b] Majority of adult probands diagnosed panic disorder.
[c] Generalized anxiety.
[d] Rates reported based on psychiatric interview of child.

seven times more prevalent in offspring of affectively ill adults compared to offspring of controls.

Only four studies give rates of bipolar conditions among offspring. In two studies (Gershon et al., 1985; Klein et al., 1985) the index parental diagnosis is bipolar illness, and unipolar depression in the others (Klein et al., 1988; Orvaschel et al., 1988). Most noteworthy is the fact that all cases of bipolar illness occur in offspring of affectively ill parents, the majority of these receiving diagnoses of cyclothymia or hypomania.

Nonaffective conditions among offspring

Although not consistent across studies, rates of nonaffective psychiatric disorders are higher among offspring of affectively ill parents compared to offspring of controls. In seven studies (Beardslee et al., 1987, 1988; Gershon et al., 1985; Hammen et al., 1987; Weissman et al., 1987; Klein et al., 1988; Welner & Rice, 1988), rates of conduct disorder range from 11–47%, compared to 0–17% among offspring of controls – an average fourfold greater risk. Five studies (Gershon et al., 1985; Weissman et al., 1987; Beardslee et al., 1988; Orvaschel et al., 1988; Welner & Rice, 1988) report rates of attention deficit disorder; the rates range from 5–20% in offspring of affectively ill parents compared to 5–8% in offspring of controls – an average twofold increased risk. Substance abuse is reported in five studies (Beardslee et al., 1987, 1988; Hammen et al., 1987; Weissman et al., 1987; Klein et al., 1988) to occur in 10–26% of offspring of affectively ill parents, compared to 3–8% in offspring of control – an average 2.7-fold increased risk. And in seven studies (Hammen et al., 1987; Weissman et al., 1987; Beardslee et al., 1988; Klein et al., 1988; Orvaschel et al., 1988; Sylvester et al., 1988; Welner & Rice, 1988), rates of anxiety disorders in offspring of affectively ill parents ranged from 5 to 47%, compared to 9–27% in offspring of controls – a nearly twofold increased risk.

Unfortunately, these studies do not make clear to what extent these rates reflect comorbidity of affective and nonaffective diagnoses within individual offspring as opposed to clustering of nonaffective diagnoses among the larger group of offspring at risk. The importance of this distinction has been discussed by Merikangas (1990) and by Cloninger et al. (1988, 1990), who show how spurious conclusions about the clinical boundaries of familially transmitted disorders can be reached in genetic epidemiological studies by failing to pay close attention to patterns of diagnostic covariation within individuals and between individuals within families. Thus, the association of affective and nonaffective diagnoses in these offspring studies is open to multiple interpretations: (1) affective illness and certain nonaffective psychiatric disorders in children may reflect variable expressions of a common transmitted liability; (2) one disorder predisposes to another; (3) certain conditions are nonspecific effects of environmental disruption arising from parental depressive illness; and (4) they are aetiologically distinct conditions that aggregate in families because of parental assortative mating for particular diagnostic syndromes.

Considering these possibilities, it is reasonable to assume that fundamentally different mechanisms are operating to a greater or lesser degree in the transmission of risk between parent and child. Thus, in some families a child's depression might signify a true homotypic pattern of genetic inheritance, in others a nonspecific demoralization reaction to parental disease and its sequelae, or to the functional impairment resulting from antecedent nonaffective psychopathology present in the child. In a similar vein, the co-occurrence of depression and substance abuse might be independent of genetic factors, but explained by the frequent use of alcohol and other drugs by depressed adolescents to self-medicate negative affect states. And to the extent that conduct disorders and substance abuse often co-aggregate in families (West & Prinz, 1987), the clustering together of all three diagnoses is not unexpected. However, a common genetic propensity seems unlikely given evidence of independent familial transmission of alcoholism and affective disorders (Merikangas et al., 1985).

By contrast, the co-occurrence of anxiety and depression amongst offspring of depressed parents may well reflect the operation of common, or overlapping, familial–genetic determinants, as previously noted. Along the same lines, longitudinal follow-up data from the Zurich cohort study (Angst et al., 1990) shows that upwards of one-half of subjects who present initially with pure anxiety develop prominent depressive illness over time. In short, certain anxiety and depressive conditions may lie on a common genetic continuum of clinical phenotypes transmitted by affectively ill parents to their children.

Identification of specific risk factors

Several studies provide information about specific familial and parental variables possibly associated with elevated risk for general psychiatric impairment, and depressive disorder in particular. Keller et al. (1986) reported on the power of measures of the severity and chronicity of parental depression, family discord and demographic variables in predicting impairment in a cohort of 72 children with at least one biological parent with a history of depressive disorder. Marital discord and a more severe and chronic course of depression in parents were associated with greater overall functional impairment in their offspring and an increased risk of a *DSM-III* diagnosis of some sort. However, these effects varied by sex of the affected parent; children from families where the mother was depressed exhibited greater functional impairment than did children from families with paternal depression.

With regard to predictors of specific diagnostic outcomes, Orvaschel et al. (1988) found no association between sex of the affected parent and specific diagnosis in the child, nor were number of lifetime episodes of depression in the affected parent or symptom severity at the time of intake into the study related to specific diagnosis in the children. However, positive findings are reported in two studies. In the study by Welner & Rice (1988), maternal depression and paternal alcoholism were associated with elevated risk for depression in off-spring of depressed parents, whereas divorce was a significant predictor of conduct disorder. Klein et al. (1988) showed that the odds of a diagnosis of dysthymia in offspring of unipolar depressed adults were significantly increased if the family contained major affective disorder in the co-parent or in a first-degree relative of the affected parent or unaffected co-parent; chronicity of parental depression; or early onset of parental illness.

Further evidence of the potential importance of parental and familial vari-ables in predicting diagnostic status in the children of unipolar adults is found in an important study by Warner et al. (1992). These investigators examined the rate of new incident cases of depression, time to recovery and risk of recurrence during a 2-year period in offspring of unipolar depressed adults and offspring of normal controls. All of the new incident cases developed in offspring of depressed adults, and were predicted by previous subclinical depressive symp-toms and an antecedent diagnosis of conduct disorder. Within this subset, recurrence was associated with a preexisting diagnosis of dysthymia, whereas time to recovery was more protracted in offspring with prepubertal onset of depression, the majority of whom had parents with multiple episodes of depression.

Todd and colleagues (1996a) sought to identify possible environmental and genetic mechanisms of disease risk by studying the form and distribution of psychiatric illness among 50 juvenile members, age range 6–17 years, of 14 extended pedigrees identified through bipolar probands ascertained for the NIMH Initiative Study of Bipolar Affective Disorder. Nine cases of affective disorder were found among 23 offspring with an affected kindred parent, compared to three cases of illness among the 27 offspring of healthy parents – a statistically significant difference. Within these pedigrees, the degree of off-spring risk for affective disorder varied predictably by genetic relatedness to affected kindred relatives.

In critically evaluating possible reasons for the highly variable expression of psychopathology among offspring of parents with affective illness, Merikangas and colleagues (1988a,b) have called attention to powerful effects of parental concordance for psychiatric disorder on the transmission of specific vulnerabilities. They found that comorbidity and parental assortative mating for alcoholism significantly increased the risk of substance abuse and antisocial conduct in offspring, whereas comorbidity and assortative mating for anxiety disorder in the parent or parental dyad sharply increased the risk for anxiety and depressive disorders among offspring. These findings make it evident that one cannot ignore the nature of parental mating types when attempting to unravel familial mechanisms through which risk of specific pychopathologies are transmitted between generations.

In short, the studies highlighted in this section suggest that general measures of parental illness and quality of marital interaction may predict a broad range of outcomes in overall psychosocial adaptation in children while having little association with nosologically discrete diagnoses. At the same time, certain indices of parent illness and familial liability – whether genetically or environmentally mediated – may be informative predictors of symptom development in high-risk individuals.

Psychiatric illness in adult relatives of affectively ill juveniles

Nine case-control family studies begin with children or adolescents as probands and give rates of affective disorder in adult biological relatives. An important advantage of this so-called bottom-up approach is that the validating index – the form and distribution of illness in pedigrees – is better defined clinically and nosologically.

Livingston et al. (1985) determined rates of psychiatric disorder in 58 first- and second-degree relatives of 11 children with major depression, and 69 relatives of 12 controls with anxiety disorder. The probands ranged in age from 6 to 12 years and were diagnosed by *DSM-III* criteria following structured clinical interviews using the DICA. Although polarity of illness in depressed probands is not defined, it can be assumed that the majority are nonbipolar. Diagnoses of relatives were derived from family history-RDC (FH-RDC) interviews evaluated independently and blindly by two psychiatrists.

A study by Strober et al. (1988) examined lifetime rates of psychiatric illness in 523 first- and second-degree relatives of adolescent-age probands with bipolar illness, and 321 first- and second-degree relatives of 31 carefully matched schizophrenic controls. Proband diagnoses based on RDC criteria were established through SADS interviews and a review of all hospital records. Over

80% of first-degree relatives were interviewed personally using the SADS; family history interviews (FH-RDC; Andreasen et al., 1977) were used to establish diagnoses for second-degree relatives. Interviewers were fully blind to proband diagnosis and the narrative summaries were separately coded to avoid bias from knowledge of familial illness. All diagnoses were determined by a single clinician who assigned best estimate diagnoses according to RDC.

Mitchell et al. (1989) studied 169 parents of 94 probands with major depression and 65 parents of 38 nondepressed psychiatric controls. Probands ranged in age from 7 to 17 years. Diagnoses were based on Kiddie-SADS interviews using RDC; however, polarity of illness in depressed probands is not specified. Diagnoses of controls included: anxiety disorder, 9; conduct disorder, 6; parent–child conflict, 5; attention deficit disorder, 4; gender identity disorder, 1; and adjustment disorder, 13. Virtually all mothers, and slightly more than half the fathers, were directly interviewed using the SADS and RDC; FH-RDC interviews were used to obtain diagnostic information on unavailable relatives. All interviews of relatives were conducted blind to proband status.

Puig-Antich and colleagues (1989) studied 503 first- and second-degree relatives of 48 prepubertal probands with major depression, 165 relatives of 20 nondepressed psychiatric controls and 302 relatives of 27 never-ill controls. Of the 48 depressed probands, five had histories of manic or hypomanic episodes. All probands were assessed using the Kiddie-SADS. The diagnosis of major depression was based on RDC, whereas *DSM-III* criteria were used to diagnose controls. Of the 20 nondepressed controls, 19 had some form of anxiety disorder. Never-ill controls were obtained through random sampling in an urban school whose sociodemographic characteristics resembled those of the depressed probands. Mothers were assessed directly using the SADS and provided FH-RDC information to diagnose fathers and second-degree relatives. Although attempts were made to keep interviewers blind to proband status, this condition was broken in roughly one-third of patient proband families.

Kutcher & Marton (1991) studied 81 first-degree relatives of 23 adolescent probands with bipolar illness, 95 relatives of 26 unipolar depressives, and 83 relatives of 24 normal controls. Patients were assessed using the Kiddie-SADS and diagnosed according to *DSM-III* criteria. Controls were solicited from local church groups and through advertisement. Relatives' diagnoses were based exclusively on the FH-RDC method with mothers serving as the informant in the majority of cases; it is unclear whether or not these interviews were blind to diagnosis of the proband.

Williamson and colleagues (1995) compared lifetime rates of psychiatric illness in 228 first- and 736 second-degree relatives of 76 adolescents with major depression by RDC to 107 first- and 323 second-degree relatives of 34 age-matched normal controls using the FH-RDC method with interviewers blind to proband status. Controls were obtained through advertisement and word of mouth. Diagnoses of probands used the Kiddie-SADS and RDC.

Wozniak et al. (1995) determined rates of lifetime psychiatric illness in 46 first-degree relatives of 16 children 12 years of age or under with a diagnosis of manic illness determined by structured Kiddie-SADS interview and diagnosed by *DSM-III-R* criteria. These rates were compared to those obtained on 305 first-degree relatives of 78 age- and gender-matched control probands with attention deficit and hyperactivity disorder and 200 first-degree relatives of 100 normal controls. Interviews of relatives were conducted blind to clinical diagnosis and ascertainment group of the proband. Best estimate procedures were used by four senior clinicians to establish final consensus diagnoses.

Harrington et al. (1997) reported rates of illness in 399 first- and 635 second-degree relatives of 62 depressed child probands and 69 psychiatric controls followed up on average 18 years after original referral to the Maudsley child psychiatry services. The longitudinal design allowed the use of the probands affective status in both childhood and adulthood (defined as older than 17 years) to generate four proband groups: (1) prepubertal depressive disorder onset (onset aged 6–14 years, $n = 18$); (2) pubescent or postpubertal depressive disorder (onset aged 11–16 years, $n = 33$); (3) adult-onset depressive disorder (i.e. a child psychiatric control group who had an episode of RDC depressive disorder after 17 years of age, $n = 16$); and (4) a child psychiatric control group who had not been depressed in either childhood or adulthood. Pubertal status was chosen as a marker for development rather than age, because increased rates of depression more closely resemble pubertal status than age and because their follow-up study into adult life suggested significant differences between the outcomes of pre- and postpubertal depressed cases (Harrington et al., 1990). Psychiatric status of the proband in adult life was made using a modified version of the SADS-L. In childhood the diagnoses were made from case-note data which included item sheets on depressive signs and symptoms at presentation. At least one first-degree relative was interviewed directly with the SADS-L in 85% of the families, with the family history method employed for the diagnosis of noninterviewed relatives. All diagnoses were rendered blind to diagnosis of the proband.

Kovacs et al. (1997) studied rates of illness in 197 first- and 574 second-degree relatives of 99 probands with unipolar depression, 49 first- and 150 second-degree relatives of 26 probands with bipolar illness, and 116 first- and 298 second-degree relatives of 55 probands with nonaffective psychiatric condi-

Table 7.2. Lifetime rates/100 of unipolar and bipolar affective disorder among adult first-degree relatives of juvenile probands

Study	Proband diagnosis	Unipolar	Bipolar
Livingston et al., 1985	MD	24	0
	AN	30	3
Strober et al., 1988	BP	15	15
	SZ	4	0
Mitchell et al., 1989	MD	46	1
	PC	37	3
Puig-Antich et al., 1989	AD	34	4
	PC	20	2
	NC	16	0
Kutcher & Marton, 1991	BP	19	15
	UP	20	5
	NC	4	1
Williamson et al., 1995	MD	25	0.4
	NC	13	1
Wozniak et al., 1995	BP	23	13
	NC	6	3
Harrington et al., 1997 (includes second-degree relatives)	MD (child–prepubertal)	14.9	0.6
	MD (child–postpubertal)	16.8	2.8
	MDD (adult-onset)	13.3	0
	PC	7.5	0.5
Kovacs et al., 1997	UP	54	5
	BP	71	7
	PC	44	6

MD, major depression, polarity unspecified; AN, anxiety disorder; BP, bipolar illness; SZ, schizophrenia; PC, nonaffectively ill psychiatric controls; AD, affective disorder, mainly unipolar type; NC, normal controls; UP, unipolar depression.

tions. Probands were clinically referred and ranged in age from 8 to 17 years. In most instances, mothers served as informants and were diagnosed by SADS interview using RDC. The family history method was employed for the diagnosis of noninterviewed relatives. All diagnoses were rendered blind to diagnosis of the proband.

Results of these studies appear in Table 7.2, which gives lifetime rates of unipolar and bipolar illness among relatives of probands. Several methodological points must be taken into account in considering the implications of these data, and in comparing results across studies. First, only three studies (Puig-Antich et al., 1989; Kutcher & Marton, 1991; Williamson et al., 1995) include a control group of never-ill probands and their relatives. Second, with one exception (Strober et al., 1988) and one partial exception (Harrington et al., 1997), these studies rely primarily on the family history method for determining illness in relatives – a procedure more prone to imprecision. Third, in three of the studies (Livingston et al., 1985; Puig-Antich et al., 1989; Kutcher & Marton, 1991) interviewers were not blind to diagnosis of the proband, or the blind was broken in a substantial minority of cases.

In spite of these shortcomings, the results indicate that relatives of juvenile probands with major depression or bipolar illness are several times more likely to develop affective disorders than individuals in the general population, where the average lifetime expected morbidity has been estimated at roughly 7% (Tsuang & Faraone, 1990), or in nondepressed psychiatric comparison groups. However, at first glance the results seem to offer only partial support for distinct familial transmission. Two studies (Livingston et al., 1985; Mitchell et al., 1989) failed to find a higher lifetime risk of affective disorder among relatives of index probands compared to relatives of controls. There is, however, a related confound in both: the selection of anxiety disorder as a comparison group in the Livingston et al. study, and the presence of anxiety disorder in one-quarter of the control probands studied by Mitchell et al. This is problematic since, as previously noted, longitudinal and family studies support at least some association between affective and anxiety disorders in aetiological factors. As such, the negative findings are not unanticipated, nor is the lack of differentiation between relatives of depressed probands and relatives of psychiatric controls in rates of affective disorder reported by Puig-Antich et al. (1989) unexpected given the predominance of anxiety disorder diagnoses in control probands. In short, if 'true' cases of affective disorder are nested within anxiety disorder controls then the implications of these data with regard to the specificity of familial transmission are greatly limited.

These caveats aside, evidence of familial transmission is strong in six studies (Strober et al., 1988; Kutcher et al., 1991; Williamson et al., 1995; Wozniak et al., 1995; Harrington et al., 1997: Kovacs et al., 1997). Collectively, these studies show a several-fold increase in rates of affective disorders in relatives of unipolar and bipolar probands compared to controls and increased rates of affection in first- compared to second-degree relatives (Williamson at al., 1995; Kovacs et al., 1997). One study has noticeably higher familial rates of illness in prepubertal compared to adolescent probands (Kovacs et al., 1997) but another found no difference between prepubertal, postpubertal and adult-onset probands (Harrington et al., 1997). The Strober et al. study is noteworthy in that it shows a clear familial separation of bipolar illness and schizophrenia in adolescence, a finding supported by the Harrington study which also indicates clear familial association for bipolar disorder in their postpubertal adolescent group. And, while a lower relative risk is reflected in the comparison between relatives of depressed and normal control probands in the Puig-Antich et al. (1989) study, the rate of affectation among relatives of depressed probands is still twice that of relatives of normals. Moreover, this relative risk increases to 2.5 if the analysis is restricted to depressed probands without concurrent conduct disorder. By contrast, the risk of affective disorders among relatives of depressed probands with conduct disorder is no different from that in relatives of normal controls, lending added support for the nosological separation of depressive syndromes with and without antisocial behaviour.

With regard to bipolar illness, five studies noted in Table 7.2 report rates of manic illness in adult relatives of juvenile bipolar probands. In three (Strober et al., 1988; Kutcher & Marton, 1991; Wozniak et al., 1995), the rates of familial disease exceed those reported in most case-control family–genetic studies of adult bipolar illness (Strober, 1992).

Early age of onset and familial aggregation

As noted, an unusually high density of familial illness appears to be a distinguishing feature of juvenile-onset mood disorders. Disorders with non-Mendelian inheritance and variable age of onset are generally believed to have complex and heterogeneous familial aetiologies. For this reason, there is increasing interest in identifying more discrete subforms of affective illness in order to improve the precision and replicability of genetic analyses. Several reports in the adult literature are germane.

A considerable literature exists on the relationship between age of onset and density of familial loading in both unipolar and bipolar illness (Tsuang & Faraone, 1990; Moldin et al., 1991). In most studies, age 40 is the cut-off used to stratify probands into early- and late-onset subgroups. With some exceptions, they indicate that the lifetime risk of affective disorder is significantly greater among relatives of probands with early-onset disease.

However, recent evidence suggests that this particular stratification results in considerable loss of information in estimating the magnitude of the age effect on familial aggregation. Three recent family studies of unipolar depression show that, as the age cut-off is extended downward, familial morbid risk increases in an almost linear fashion. In studies by Weissman et al. (1984) and

Kupfer et al. (1989), relatives of probands with onset of illness before age 20 had a twofold increased risk for affective illness compared to relatives of probands with later onset. However, the data from the Harrington et al. study (1997) show no significant difference in familial aggregation for unipolar depression between childhood- and adolescent-onset cases. A similar trend has also been detected in the juvenile offspring of depressed parents examined by Weissman et al. (1988) as part of the Yale Family Study. In this study, children aged 6–23 of parents with an onset of major depression before age 20 had 1.5–1.7 times the risk of major depression compared to offspring of parents with later age of onset, and had a 14-fold increased risk of prepubertal onset of depressive disorder.

Concerning bipolar illness, Rice et al. (1987) applied a segregation analysis to family data from 187 bipolar I probands stratified by age of onset into separate liability classes. Transmissible liability was assumed to be inversely related to age of onset and was derived by taking the log age of onset, subtracting the mean for the proband's birth cohort and dividing by the standard deviation. When a mixed multifactorial-autosomal major locus model was examined, ignoring age of onset, major locus transmission was rejected. However, relatives of probands whose age of onset was one standard deviation or more below their cohort-specific mean had twice the morbid risk of bipolar illness compared with relatives of probands in the adjacent liability class. When age of onset in probands was modelled as a covariate in the segregation analysis, single major locus transmission provided a better fit to the data than multifactorial-polygenic inheritance. These authors suggest that age of onset be treated as an important parameter in efforts to reduce aetiological heterogeneity in quantitative and molecular genetic analyses.

In their family study of bipolar adolescent probands, Strober et al. (1988) modelled an age-of-onset effect by subdividing probands on the presence or absence of prepubertal onset of psychiatric abnormality. Two findings of note emerged: there was a very high ratio of bipolar to unipolar cases among affected relatives of probands with prepubertal onset of psychopathology; and relatives of this subgroup had 3.5 times the risk for bipolar illness compared to relatives of probands who had no major signs of psychiatric disorder prior to the onset of their affective illness (29.4% vs. 8.6%). These risk estimates are especially compelling in that they greatly exceed those reported in family–genetic studies of adult bipolar probands (Gershon, 1990; Tsuang & Faraone, 1990).

More recently, an analysis of family morbid risk data from the Amish study of bipolar illness (Pauls et al., 1992) lends additional support to the idea that juvenile onset delimits a more severe or familial subform of disease. In this study, relatives of probands with onset of illness before age 20 had a threefold increase in risk of bipolar I illness compared to relatives of probands with later age of onset, and a 1.6-fold increase in the combined risk of bipolar and unipolar conditions.

Finally, work by Baron et al. (1990) raises the interesting possibility of an association between early-onset bipolar illness and X-linked inheritance. Re-analysing previously published data on five large multiplex pedigrees, the authors compared several clinical parameters of illness in these X-linked pedigrees to general samples of familial bipolar probands reported in the literature. Affected cases from X-linked pedigrees were found to develop their illness at an earlier age and had a higher ratio of bipolar to unipolar-type illness. The authors postulate that an X-linked variant of bipolar illness may be overrepresented among individuals with early onset of disease.

Conclusions

Several different lines of enquiry point to the validity of depressive disorder in children and adolescents. In spite of this, some qualifications to our current knowledge are in order.

Depression is clearly among the most prominent types of psychopathology in offspring of parents with affective disorder, unipolar major depression in particular; however, psychopathology in general is widespread in these samples, thus raising questions about the mechanisms underlying parent–child resemblance for depression and the co-aggregation of affective and nonaffective conditions. Heritability of depressive vulnerability is doubtless one important causal factor; but it may be too rigid a conclusion that depression in children of depressed parents is determined solely by genetic factors when other pathogenic influences are displayed in these families in varying degrees. A more parsimonious view holds that the cumulative impact of these adverse family circumstances may well be sufficient in intensity and chronicity to mediate the development of affect disturbance of some type in certain offspring of depressed parents. But what clinical features, if any, differentiate these environmental phenocopies from genetically transmitted depressive states remains unclear at present. In addition to specific transmissible effects of parental affective disorder, psychiatric outcome in offspring is also heavily influenced by patterns of parental concordance for psychopathology. Parental matings involving depression and anxiety appear significantly to increase liability for both conditions in offspring, whereas parental alcoholism elevates

Endicott, J. & Spitzer, R. L. (1978). A diagnostic interview: the schedule for affective disorders and schizophrenia. *Archives of General Psychiatry*, **35**, 837–44.

Faraone, S. V., Biederman, J., Mennin, D., Wozniak, J. & Spencer, T. (1997). Attention-deficit hyperactivity disorder with bipolar illness: a familial subtype? *Journal of the American Academy of Child and Adolescent Psychiatry*, **36**, 1379–87.

Gershon, E. S. (1990). Genetics. In *Manic-Depressive Illness*, ed. F. K. Goodwin & K. R. Jamison, pp. 373–401. Oxford: Oxford University Press.

Gershon, E., McKnew, D., Cytryn, L. et al. (1985). Diagnosis in school-age children of bipolar affective disorder parents and normal controls. *Journal of Affective Disorders*, **8**, 283–91.

Hammen, C. (1991). *Depression Runs in Families*. New York: Springer-Verlag.

Hammen, C., Gordon, D., Burge, D. et al. (1987). Maternal affective disorders, illness, and stress: risk for children's psychopathology. *American Journal of Psychiatry*, **144**, 736–41.

Hammen, C., Burge, D., Burney, E. & Adrian, C. (1990). Longitudinal study of diagnoses in children of women with unipolar and bipolar affective disorder. *Archives of General Psychiatry*, **47**, 1112–17.

Harrington, R., Fudge, H., Rutter, M., Pickles, A. & Hill, J. (1990). Adult outcomes of childhood and adolescent depression. *Archives of General Psychiatry*, **47**, 465–73.

Harrington, R., Rutter, M., Weissman, M. et al. (1997). Psychiatric disorders in the relatives of depressed probands. I. Comparison of prepubertal, adolescent and early adult onset cases. *Journal of Affective Disorders*, **42**, 9–22.

Herjanic, B. & Reich, W. (1982). Development of a structured psychiatric interview for children: agreement between child and parent on individual symptoms. *Journal of Abnormal Child Psychology*, **10**, 307–24.

Katz, M. & Klerman, G. L. (1979). Introduction: over-view of the clinical studies program. *American Journal of Psychiatry*, **136**, 49–51.

Keller, M., Beardslee, W., Dorer, D. et al. (1986). Impact of severity and chronicity of parental affective illness on adaptive functioning and psychopathology in children. *Archives of General Psychiatry*, **43**, 930–7.

Kendler, K. S., Neale, M. C., Kessler, R. C., Heath, A. C. & Eaves, L. J. (1992). Major depression and generalised anxiety disorder: same genes, (partly) different environments? *Archives of General Psychiatry*, **49**, 716–22.

Klein, D., Depue, R. A. & Slater, J. F. (1985). Cyclothymia in the adolescent offspring of parents with bipolar affective disorder. *Journal of Abnormal Psychology*, **94**, 115–27.

Klein, D., Clark, D., Dansky, L. & Margolis, E. T. (1988). Dysthymia in the offspring of parents with primary unipolar affective disorder. *Journal of Abnormal Psychology*, **97**, 265–76.

Klerman, G. L. & Weissman, M. M. (1989). Increasing rates of depression. *Journal of the American Medical Association*, **261**, 2229–35.

Kovacs, M., Feinberg, T. L., Crouse-Novak, M. et al. (1984). Depressive disorders in childhood. II. A longitudinal study of the risk for a subsequent major depression. *Archives of General Psychiatry*, **41**, 643–9.

Kovacs, M., Devlin, B., Pollock, M., Richards, C. & Mukerji, P. (1997). A controlled family history study of child-hood onset depressive disorder. *Archives of General Psychiatry*, **54**, 613–23.

Kupfer, D. J., Frank, E., Carpenter, L. L. & Neiswanger, K. (1989). Family history in recurrent depression. *Journal of Affective Disorders*, **17**, 113–19.

Kutcher, S. & Marton, P. (1991). Affective disorders in first degree relatives of adolescent onset bipolars, unipolars, and normal controls. *Journal of the American Academy of Child and Adolescent Psychiatry*, **30**, 75–8.

Livingston, R., Nugent, H., Rader, L. & Smith, R. C. (1985). Family histories of depressed and severely anxious children. *American Journal of Psychiatry*, **142**, 1497–9.

Merikangas, K. R. (1990). Comorbidity for anxiety and depression: review of family and genetic studies. In *Comorbidity of Mood and Anxiety Disorders*, ed. J. D. Maser & C. R. Cloninger, pp. 331–48. Washington, DC: American Psychiatric Press.

Merikangas, K. R., Leckman, J. F., Prusoff, B. A., Pauls, D. L. & Weissman, M. M. (1985). Familial transmission of depression and alcoholism. *Archives of General Psychiatry*, **42**, 367–72.

Merikangas, K. R., Prusoff, B. A. & Weissman, M. M. (1988a). Parental concordance for affective disorders: psychopathology in offspring. *Journal of Affective Disorders*, **15**, 279–90.

Merikangas, K. R., Weissman, M. M., Prusoff, B. A. & John, K. (1988b). Assortative mating and affective disorders: psychopathology in offspring. *Psychiatry*, **51**, 48–57.

Mitchell, J., McCauley, E., Burke, P., Calderon, R. & Schloredt, K. (1989). Psychopathology in parents of depressed children and adolescents. *Journal of the American Academy of Child and Adolescent Psychiatry*, **28**, 352–7.

Moldin, S. O., Reich, T. & Rice, J. (1991). Current perspectives on the genetics of unipolar depression. *Behaviour Genetics*, **21**, 211–42.

Nurcombe, B., Seifer, R., Scioli, A. et al. (1989). Is major depressive disorder in adolescence a distinct diagnostic entity? *Journal of the American Academy of Child and Adolescent Psychiatry*, **28**, 333–42.

Orvaschel, H. (1983). Parental depression and child psychopathology. In *Childhood Psychopathology and Development*, ed. S. B. Guze, F. J. Earls & J. E. Barrett, pp. 53–66. New York: Raven Press.

Orvaschel, H., Weissman, M. M., Padian, N. & Lowe, T. L. (1981). Assessing psychopathology in children of psychiatrically disturbed parents: a pilot study. *Journal of the American of Child Psychiatry*, **20**, 112–22.

Orvaschel, H., Walsh-Allis, G. & Ye, W. (1988). Psychopathology in children of parents with recurrent depression. *Journal of Abnormal Child Psychology*, **16**, 17–28.

Pauls, D. L., Morton, L. A & Egeland, J. (1992). Risks of affective illness among first-degree relatives of bipolar I older-order Amish probands. *Archives of General Psychiatry*, **49**, 703–8.

Puig-Antich, J., Goetz, D., Davies, M. et al. (1989). A controlled family history study of prepubertal major depressive disorder. *Archives of General Psychiatry*, **46**, 406–20

Rice, J., Reich, T., Andreasen, N. C. et al. (1987). The familial transmission of bipolar illness. *Archives of General Psychiatry*, **44**, 441–50.

Robins, L. N., Helzer, J. E., Croughan, J. & Ratcliff, K. S. (1981). The National Institute of Mental Health diagnostic interview schedule. *Archives of General Psychiatry*, **38**, 381–7.

Ryan, N. D., Puig-Antich, J., Ambrosini, P. et al. (1987). The clinical picture of major depression in children and adolescents. *Archives of General Psychiatry*, **44**, 854–61.

Seifer, R., Nurcombe, B., Scioli, A. & Grapentine W. L. (1989). Is major depressive disorder in childhood a distinct diagnostic entity? *Journal of the American Academy of Child and Adolescent Psychiatry*, **28**, 935–41.

Spitzer, R. L., Endicott, J. & Robins, E. (1978). Research Diagnostic Criteria: rational and reliability. *Archives of General Psychiatry*, **35**, 773–82.

Strober, M. (1992). Relevance of early age-of-onset in genetic studies of bipolar affective disorder. *Journal of the American Academy of Child and Adolescent Psychiatry*, **31**, 606–10.

Strober, M. (1996). Outcome studies of mania in children and adolescents. In *Mood Disorders Across the Life Span*, ed. K. I. Shulman, M. Tohen & S. P. Kutcher, pp. 149–58. New York: Wiley-Liss.

Strober, M., Morrell, W., Burroughs, J. et al. (1988). A family study of bipolar I illness in adolescence: early onset of symptoms linked to increased family loading and lithium resistance. *Journal of Affective Disorders*, **15**, 255–68.

Sylvester, C. E., Hyde, T. S. & Reichler, R. J. (1988). Clinical psychopathology among children of adults with panic disorder. In *Relatives at Risk for Mental Disorders*, ed. D. L. Dunner, E. S. Gershon & J. E. Barrett, pp. 87–102. New York: Raven Press.

Todd, R. D., Reich, W., Petti, T. A. et al. (1996a). Psychiatric diagnoses in the child and adolescent members of extended families identified through adult bipolar affective disorder probands. *Journal of the American Academy of Child and Adolescent Psychiatry*, **35**, 665–71.

Todd, R. D., Geller, B., Neuman, R., Fox, L. W. & Hickok, J. (1996b). Increased prevalence of alcoholism in relatives of depressed and bipolar children. *Journal of the American Academy of Child and Adolescent Psychiatry*, **35**, 717–24.

Tsuang, M. T. & Faraone, S. V. (1990). *The Genetics of Mood Disorders*. Baltimore, MD: Johns Hopkins University Press.

Warner, V., Weissman, M. M., Fendrich, M., Wickramaratne, P. & Moreau, D. (1992). The course of major depression in the offspring of depressed parents: incidence, recurrence, and recovery. *Archives of General Psychiatry*, **49**, 795–801.

Weissman, M. M. (1988). Psychopathology in the children of depressed parents: direct interview studies. In *Relatives at Risk for Mental Disorders*, ed. D. L. Dunner, E. S. Gershon & J. E. Barrett, pp. 143–59. New York: Raven Press.

Weissman, M. M. (1990). Evidence for comorbidity of anxiety and depression: family and genetic studies of children. In *Comorbidity of Mood and Anxiety Disorders*, ed. J. D. Maser & C. R. Cloninger, pp. 349–66. Washington, DC: American Psychiatric Press.

Weissman, M. M., Wickramaratne, P., Merikangas, K. R. et al. (1984). Onset of major depression in early adulthood: increased familial loading and specificity. *Archives of General Psychiatry*, **41**, 1136–43.

Weissman, M. M., Gammon, G. D., John, K. et al. (1987). Children of depressed parents: increased psychopathology and early onset of major depression. *Archives of General Psychiatry*, **44**, 847–53.

Weissman, M. M., Warner, V., Wickramaratne, P. & Prusoff, B. A. (1988). Early-onset major depression in parents and their children. *Journal of Affective Disorders*, **15**, 269–78.

Welner, Z. & Rice, J. (1988). School-aged children of depressed parents: a blind and controlled study. *Journal of Affective Disorders*, **15**, 291–302.

West, M. O. & Prinz, R. J. (1987). Parental alcoholism and childhood psychopathology. *Psychological Bulletin*, **102**, 204–18.

Williamson, D. E., Ryan, N. D., Birmaher, B. et al. (1995). A case-control family history study of depression in adolescents. *Journal of the American Academy of Child and Adolescent Psychiatry*, **34**, 1597–607.

Wozniak, J., Biederman, J., Mundy, E., Mennin, D. & Faraone, S. V. (1995). A pilot family study of childhood-onset mania. *Journal of the American Academy of Child and Adolescent Psychiatry*, **34**, 1577–83.

8

Life events: their nature and effects

Ian M. Goodyer

Introduction

A life event is an environmental circumstance that has an identifiable onset and ending and may carry the potential for altering an individual's present state of mental or physical well-being. Such circumscribed happenings should be discriminated from other forms of longer-term ongoing experiences which may carry the same or similar effects but do not have readily identifiable onsets and endings. When either of these two forms of environmental experience are considered undesirable and exert a negative impact in the days and weeks after exposure they carry the potential for increasing the liability for mental and behavioural symptoms and syndromes and psychosocial impairment. Twentieth-century psychosocial theories of depression were founded on the assumptions that undesirable social experiences, such as loss of a loved one, result in enduring psychological change for some individuals that give rise to the negative cognitions and related signs and symptoms that characterize depressive disorders. Whilst there is now considerable evidence that undesirable life events do precede and increase the risk for depression in adolescents and adults, how they exert their effects remains unclear.

Evaluating events and difficulties

It is now widely accepted that event evaluation should include a description of the nature and characteristics of the circumstance to include qualitative differences in the content of life experiences between persons (Brown & Harris, 1978; Paykel, 1978). Brown & Harris (1978) demonstrated that, by doing this, the latent psychological effects of socially differing events between individuals can be reliably and validly compared. This semistructured approach to event measurement requires face-to-face assessments and is probably best for life experiences that have happened in the recent past – generally between 12 and 24 months. Major events and some of their personally salient details can however be reliably recalled over a 5-year period. A few highly memorable experiences such as major disasters, deaths and permanent separations can be recalled over a lifetime. These methods have been adapted for use in children and adolescents, with the additional feature of taking the child's developmental status into account (Goodyer et al., 1985, 1997a; Sandberg et al., 1998, 1993). Determining the degree of undesirability of such experiences can be made by the subject, a relative such as the parent of a child or by panel raters, generally mental health research workers, blind to the behavioural status of the child. Mental health professionals evaluate the degree of negative impact or personal threat to well-being carried by the event from the descriptive characteristics obtained at the time of interview. When gathering what is generally referred to as the contextual information of a life event, an interviewer is required to edit the subjective bias inherent in such descriptions such that ratings can be made on the facts (in so far as that is possible).

For example, in case-control studies, panel ratings are advisable as ratings by the subject or parents of patients may inflate the liability to record retrospective events as more negative than they actually were. This appears somewhat more likely in adults with severe illnesses with psychotic symptoms or severe cognitive distortion of reality rather than milder outpatient-based disorders of emotions and behaviour. In milder common disorders of young people and in prospective community studies, ratings of the impact of events on the self made by the adolescent and panel ratings are in fact highly correlated (Goodyer, 1996). This suggests that, for most research circumstances involving community populations, the former can be used, and this is more efficient and less time-consuming.

Social descriptions of events can still be recorded by the child or adolescent and be used to subtype these experiences according to *a priori* definitions. Currently there are four subtypes of interest when investigating the relations between life events and emotional disorders:

1. Danger to self: where there is a clear expectation or occurrence of physical threat to the child such as illness or accidents, involvement in a household or community disaster or becoming the subject of a personal attack.
2. Danger to others: similar events where the person exposed is a parent, sibling, friend or significant other (e.g. teacher, first-degree relative, neighbour).
3. Personal disappointments: the failure of a previously held set of expectations and/or hopes (e.g. to the self includes breakdown of boyfriend–girlfriend relationship, examination failure; to another includes loss of job, new financial difficulties, extramarital affair).
4. Loss: the permanent state of no further contact with a valued other, which includes only death and permanent separation.

The incorporation of concurrent measurement of longer-term difficulties over the child's lifetime, together with recent life events, has been an important recent advance in the evaluation of a broader range of environmental experiences (Sandberg et al., 1993, 1998). The advantage of incorporating evaluations of different types of life experiences is that the relative contribution of recent life events to the onset or maintenance of depression can only be understood if the contribution of other ongoing social adversities has been taken into account both to the liability for having events as well as to the risk for psychopathology.

Precedence of experience to disorder

Using semistructured interviews with children, adolescents and their parents also allows interviewers to determine the timing of onset of experiences with a reasonable degree of validity. Distinguishing between events and difficulties that precede onset of disorder from those that follow inception of a syndrome is a crucial issue if causal links are being investigated between antecedent happenings and depressive disorders. This includes the separation of events that are dependent on the personal behaviour (even if they precede onset) of the subject and those that are truly independent, occurring either by chance or through circumstances clearly outside personal influence. Distinguishing between events that are brought about by a person's own actions and those that are independent happenings improves the chances of eliciting causal processes and their associated mechanism of action. Dependent events may not exert true causal effects if concurrent measurement of the behaviours that result in their inception is also carried out. By contrast, if truly independent events precede onset of disorder and are not correlated with personal behaviour or preexisting long-term social difficulties, then they are likely to exert a degree of causal effect on the liability for depression.

A further important methodological issue is the timing of social adversities in relation to onset of disorder. Having established that events and difficulties precede onset, it is necessary to establish the time frame of occurrence of the event or difficulty. The current procedures are mainly concerned with determining at what point exposure to the experience began. Correlations are generally reported between onset of event and disorder. Few studies have reported off-set correlations, that is, the period between when the exposure to a circumscribed event or experience ceased, and the subsequent onset of depression. Whether the risk for depression is related to exposure time of an event is unclear, as the consequences of events rated as 'undesirable to the self' are only counted as such if by definition they carry effects in terms of 'at least days or weeks'. How many days or weeks is generally not included in the measure.

These components of life events and difficulties measurement result in three different types of quantitative and qualitative measurement. The number of undesirable events occurring before disorder can be determined and the total burden of negative experiences to onset can be evaluated. Classifying events according to a set of social or psychological characteristics obtained from the subject's description and assigning these to dependent or independent categories of personal experiences will clarify the types of experiences to onset. Recording how close to the onset of disorder events occur will provide an estimate of the importance of temporal proximity between the environmental stimulus and the abnormal response.

It would also be possible to investigate if recent events and more ongoing experiences occurring prior to onset are themselves connected circumstances. Connectivity may occur in two broad ways. First, a prior set of experiences may correlate with the same type of happening recurring at a later point in time. This suggests a potentially specific association between experiences. Second, prior adverse experiences may increase the general liability for further but different negative events in a child's life, indicating a more nonspecific effect of adversities on the liability of onset. These two forms of connectivity should be distinguished from the independent cumulation of disparate negative experiences occurring by chance, where subjects may accrue undesirable circumstances and happenings arising from quite distinct origins, such as exposure to sudden death in the family and disappointing experiences within a peer group.

Why measure the social environment?

Environmental causation of depression

What is the theoretical basis for undertaking quantitative investigations of individual social experience of time? Theorists have consistently emphasized the role of negative experiences in childhood creating a psychological vulnerability that is enduring but remains latent (i.e. out of consciousness and exerting no immediate pathogenic effect) until a second similar experience occurs that reactivates the original exposure. This notion of 'double hit', occurring many years later, was part of the original psychoanalytic ideas concerning the onset of depression (Abraham, 1927). These theorists were particularly focused on personal disappointments in love during childhood being reactivated by similar disappointments in adult life. If true, then depression will only be seen in subjects with a relatively recent disappointing love event but who also had a matching experience in early childhood (theoretically, loss of maternal love in infancy). There have been many refinements of this position with the more relation-based theory of Bowlby (1980) being particularly influential. Bowlby postulated that deficiencies in early child relations with primary care-giving resulted in a negative developmental trajectory in childhood, leading to unsatisfactory social relations which by adult life would result in a failure of intimate personal relations and subsequent emotional disorder. Bowlby's theoretical refinements meant that there should be a measurable connectivity of negative interpersonal experience between infancy, childhood and adult life. This reformulated social model would not merely be a 'double hit' of the same type of experiences with no discernible difficulties in between, but a series of interpersonal disappointments in relations, with potentially mutually reinforcing effects. Bowlby's theorizing also allowed individuals to escape from the effects of early infant difficulties if positive social environments became available, thereby ameliorating the effects of early emotional neglect on mental and behavioural development . This addition of a restitutional component to psychopathology theory was an important psychological advance and has led to the further postulate that some children are resilient in the face of social adversities (Rutter, 1985, 1994).

These social processes have been postulated to operate via psychological mechanisms, thereby proposing a crucial role for social environmental factors in determining and shaping the notion of the self (knowing and evaluating who we are). (See Chapters 2 and 3 for a full account of the developmental psychopathology of self-understanding and its relation to depression.) It has been convincingly argued that depression arises when a negative view of ourself is dominant over other self-beliefs. If this view is taken as true by the individual, then responding to this internal view of the self in overt behavioural ways may be maladaptive. Two influential psychological perspectives on how negative events result in distortions of the self are relevant to interpreting the associations between events and depression. Both follow the earlier theories in proposing that early adversities within the primary care-giver result in a negative cognitive set about the self. First, Aaron Beck proposed that early negative experience results in an enduring triad of negative cognitions about the self, the world and the future which become embedded as a latent negative schema and is activated by subsequent events (Beck, 1979; Teasdale & Barnard, 1993). This formulation indicates that some individuals are sensitized to subsequent negative reactions.

Brown & Harris (1978) originally suggested a narrow and specific social model that the death of the mother in childhood leads to an enduring (but not latent) cognitive attitude that one's own efforts are useless. These models predict that recent events alone would only be associated with the onset of depression if they were associated with a lowered sense of self-esteem, an index of the degree to which a person has a negative view of him- or herself. Brown has argued that this is indeed the case, at least for adult women, where the risk for depression is only increased in those who are exposed to a severe personally threatening recent life event to the self and who also have a history of long-standing social difficulties and low self-esteem (Brown et al., 1990a,b). Recent events alone without the other two variables carry no increase in risk for psychopathology. The origins of long-term personal difficulties and low self-esteem remain somewhat unclear, and in Brown's model there is no clear place for the notion of a latent psychological vulnerability, i.e. subjects appear fully aware of their vulnerabilities. In addition there has as yet been no adequate test as to whether or not low self-esteem arises in childhood as a consequence of failures in maternal care-giving. This highly influential group have however shown that lack of maternal care in early life is what they term a vulnerability factor for subsequent major depression (Bifulco et al., 1987). Brown's findings go some way to supporting the notion that long-term adverse experiences have negative consequences for self-perception in adults (Brown & Harris, 1993). It is also clear that a recent life event (i.e. one that occurs within a few weeks of onset) provokes onset of depression in such sensitized women but not in those without such vulnerabilities.

A second influential psychological theory may also be of importance. Seligman (1978) and Abramson et al. (1978) have proposed that frequent exposure to uncontrollable and unpredictable events leads to an enduring loss of adaptive behaviours. The end-stage of this process Seligman called learned helplessness, implying permanent deficits in cognitive and emotional processes. If Seligman is correct, then recent events occurring close to onset would not have a more provoking role in depression than other social adversities in people's lives, such as constant stress at work, chronic marital difficulties, poor physical health. The effects of recent life events would merely be one measurable component in a multiple social pathway through which individuals' level of resilience in the face of adversity was no longer sufficient.

Seligman's model makes no reference to the importance of early experience as such and thereby allows the notion of learned helplessness to be applicable across the life span, even in subjects who received adequate maternal care in childhood. For example, a child with a positive early family environment may still develop learned helplessness if exposed to multiple long-term difficulties and events from adolescence through to early adult life. It is unclear how long someone needs to be exposed to such adversities before developing disorder but it is probably years rather than weeks or months. Individual variation in time to onset of disorder will be determined by nonsocial factors such as genetic vulnerability to depression, hypothalamic–pituitary axis activity, and the nature and characteristics of memory function.

The evidence for this more long-standing psychosocial process influencing the liability for depression is strong. Thus, the majority of depressions occur in individuals with long-standing difficulties in their lives but only about 50% of depressive episodes in adolescents are preceded by highly proximal undesirable life events (Lewinsohn et al., 1994, 1995; Goodyer et al., 2000a). The remainder show slower onsets over time, often with onsets occurring following rising levels of depressive symptoms. Longitudinal studies suggest that, even for the 'event-driven' cases, there is a significant relationship between previous and current experience and the level of intercurrent negative views of the self and depressive symptoms (Reuter et al., 1999). It seems that the learned helplessness model makes an important contribution to understanding how social adversities result in depressive disorders.

Genetic influences on life events and depression

Psychiatric genetic research has reported significant heritability not only for depressive symptoms and some types of depressive disorder, but also for the liability to experience life events, particularly amongst postpubertal girls (Silberg et al., 1999). Heritability appears to be greater for self-reports compared to parent reports, suggesting that genetic influences may operate through cognitive appraisal of events (Thapar & McGuffin, 1996). Interestingly, as a group, girls report being exposed to more threatening events in the recent past than boys (Brooks-Gunn, 1991; Brooks-Gunn & Petersen, 1991; Petersen et al., 1991). It may be that this reflects a genetically sensitive gender bias in the negative appraisal of recent social experiences.

This suggests that a correlation between recent events and depression may reflect a genetic susceptibility to both these phenomena, making the interpretation that events cause depression less likely. In such circumstances it seems that both events and disorders may have been brought about by genetically mediated person–environment interactions. A recent twin study has shown, however, that recent stressful life events that are independent of an individual's behaviour do have a substantial causal relationship with onset of major depression (Kendler et al., 1999). Findings from adolescent twin data have reached similar conclusions, but further suggest that there are two somewhat different genetic influences: first, a direct effect increasing the risk for depression independent of social experiences; and, second, increasing the liability for experiencing life events (Silberg et al., 1999). Whether these findings indicate two different sets of genes operating through different functional processes remains to be determined. Because of the low rates of depressive disorder in the twin samples, these data rely on analysing self-reported depressive symptoms and have recorded life events using checklists rather than semistructured interviews. As a result, the relationship of the genetic findings to major depressive disorder is unclear.

Nevertheless, these data argue for a partly genetically mediated general liability to experience undesirable life events that arise through the adolescent's own behaviour. The nonsocial nature of this observed genetic risk is also an important area for further research. As already noted, some individuals, perhaps more girls than boys and amongst postpubertal rather than prepubertal children, are rendered more liable to negative affective and cognitive appraisals of ordinary life experiences. Genetic effects are also likely to operate at a physiological and/or neural level, resulting in individual differences in response to the environmental demands. Further studies of brain–behaviour–environment relations are required to understand the bidirectional relations between events and the individual. This requires a greater multidisciplinary neuroscientific effort than has occurred hitherto in determining what social adversities do to people.

The characteristics of undesirable events

Classifying the nature of undesirable experiences

Brown and colleagues attempted to improve the specificity between recent negative events and major depression by refining the latent psychological construct from the social characteristics of the experience (Brown et al., 1987). First, events that were viewed as carrying long-term threat were dichotomized into upper and lower, indicating whether a threat was imminent or had already occurred. Second, six types of loss were considered: (1) death; (2) separation; (3) unemployment; (4) physical illness; (5) disappointment; and (6) loss of a cherished idea. The first four of these classes of loss are identifiable from the recorded social characteristics. The last two are more latent constructs; disappointments are relatively easily inferred from the social information, defined as an undesirable and unexpected revision of a previously held expectation about the outcome of the event. Loss of a cherished idea was defined as disruption of an expectation of trust, faithfulness or commitment which may lead individuals to question these qualities in themselves. The latter experience excludes a consideration of previous experiences and is made on the basis of undesirable changes to ideas, and reflects an attempt to measure the symbolic aspects of appraisal of life experiences.

The concept of danger was also divided into present and anticipated danger, the latter suggesting effects in the near future as a consequence of a current negative experience. Miller and colleagues (Miller et al., 1987; Miller & Surtees, 1993) also reclassified events on six psychological dimensions (loss, personal threat, social action, hopeless situation, uncertain outcome, choice of action).

Both these groups demonstrated that these social psychological character-istics provided a better correlate with major depression than the more global concept of negative impact on undesirability. The greatest effects appear to occur between ratings of personal disappointments, loss and depression. Brown's data suggested that dangerous events were specifically associated with anxiety rather than depressive disorders (Finlay-Jones & Brown, 1981). Brown's extensive indepth life interviews also allowed a comparison of long-term past experiences with recent events. This group showed that an episode was more likely when recent experiences matched a past undesirable experience in terms of their social characteristics. This suggests that the early psychoanalytic notion of 'double hit', with the first exposure occurring in early life (but not infancy, more like before the age of 12 years), may have some validity but without a prospective repeat measures design, taking multiple events into account over a number of years, the issue remains unclear.

The hypothesis that a negative appraisal of the recent event appears more likely when there has been double exposure to such disappointing experiences is important, as it reflects an indirect test of the notion that early disappointing experiences may bias an individual to think (and feel) more negatively about recent experiences (Teasdale & Barnard, 1993).

Brown's group also suggested that childhood sexual abuse increased the risk of depression in adult life. Interestingly, the association between early sexual abuse, later disappointments and depression in adult life was entirely accounted for by the presence of a depressive episode close to the abusive experience in childhood or adolescence (Bifulco et al., 1991, 1998). Once this history of affective disorder was taken into account there was no association between childhood sexual abuse and adult depression. This does not mean that abuse does not have negative effects – the theoretical point is that there is no enduring psychological effect from the childhood experience *per se* that specifically relates to the development of major depression in adult life.

Matching experiences and psychological activation of depressive features

Parker and colleagues also examined the postulate that in early childhood adverse social experiences can establish a psychological vulnerability that is activated by a subsequent matching social experience in later life (Parker et al., 1998). Using retrospective survey methods in a large series of patients, Parker adopted the term 'lock and key' to denote a pathogenic process whereby early adverse experiences were 'locked' in an assumed negative cognitive schema that was opened by a recent matched event, operating as a 'key'. Parker infers that the key experience serves to maintain the ongoing cognitive schema. The hypothesis is a variation of the 'double hit' theme, present throughout the century, and continues the tradition of utilizing scientifically based social analysis methods to investigate the notion that there is a direct line of risk for depression between two events, one early and the other later in life, regardless of the intervening experiences. The study focused on relatively factual early events, including parental death and sexual abuse, rather than experiences open to subjective interpretation, such as recall of rejecting parents. The 'early years' included all the childhood years under 16 and the information was gathered retrospectively from interviews with 270 clinically depressed adults.

Overall, around a third of the depressed adults in their sample described a developmental 'lock' and a recent activating 'key' process. Lack of emotional support at a time of crisis was the most common matched 'lock and key' theme. This replicated the findings by Brown and colleagues, who proposed that poor emotional and social support in a time of crisis is the dominating depressogenic stressor in working-class women (Brown et al., 1986, 1987). For two-thirds of this sample there were no specific 'lock and key' themes, with specific matched links (at least on the basis of descriptive characteristics of relatively factual events) appearing unlikely. These depressed adults appear to have experienced a rather general set of earlier social vulnerabilities described under the generic heading of insecure parenting, that was linked to a range of subsequent 'key' life events. Some specificity was noted between recall of abusive parenting and abusive and personally dangerous subsequent events but no evidence linking parental loss with any key event. These latter links were not frequent enough to be clearly associated in any meaningful way with depression of any particular type (i.e. nonmelancholic vs. melancholic). Parker et al. (1998), acknowledging the limitations of a cross-sectional retrospective study in clinically referred adults, concluded that depressive disorder may be more a reaction to a salient rather than a severe stressor, and that early adverse experiences may variably establish specific and nonspecific patterns of vulnerability to having depression triggered by exposure to a salient mirroring life event.

Overall, the retrospective adult studies attempting to link early vulnerabilities with recent adverse experiences have had some limited success in noting that a significant proportion of depressive onsets occur in individuals with both past and recent social adversities matched on certain social characteristics. There is, however, no overwhelming support that a specific model of matched events occurring in early life and again in adulthood leads to major depression. Neither is there evidence that 'lock and key' or 'vulnerability and provoking' social activation processes account for the majority of depressive onsets at any age. There may be some depressive onsets that are brought about in this way, but it is rather more likely that ongoing social vulnerabilities in childhood will exert generalized nonspecific effects on the risk for psychopathology.

One of the key features for later disorder appears to be the nature of the psychological reaction proximal to the original developmental stressor. As noted above, the work of Bifulco and Brown showed that childhood abusive experiences are only associated with major depression in those who developed depression in adolescence (Bifulco et al., 1998). If the childhood reactions to inadequate parenting were predominantly behavioural or anxious, would there be continuity for these forms of disorder? Although evidence for continuity for some forms of anxiety disorders and for conduct disorder and antisocial personality disorder is beginning to emerge (Caspi et al., 1995; Silove et al., 1995; Manicavasagar et al., 1998), specific associations with different forms of early parenting or family adversities appear to be no more frequent for these disorders than they have for depression.

The replicated observation that it is the personal salience rather than the nonspecific negative intensity of adverse experiences that is important for depression illustrates the importance of evaluating the emotional and cognitive processes that are activated by different types of social experience. For example, Brown's observation that 'poor emotional support' is the most depressogenic factor at a time of crisis demonstrates that this appears to be so when a woman is already in a negative emotional state. This points to the central importance of negative mood in the processes and mechanisms of what makes personally salient adverse life events 'mentally toxic'. Without the internal components of emotional and cognitive appraisal, it is not possible to explain how recent events exert their effects.

The notion that undesirable events of sufficient severity will result in emotional psychopathology, or that onset will occur if there is an increasing burden of such events (depression will not arise simply as a strain of the multiple numbers of events) regardless of current mental function is not supported by any research to date. From the perspective of depressive disorders it seems most likely that recent negative life experiences will only be depressogenic if they are immediately salient to the individual who is already in a nonclinical low mood state which activates negative cognitions.

Studies of children and adolescents

The connected nature of life experiences

In childhood and adolescent case-control studies the findings have been broadly similar. There is relatively good evidence that recent personally threatening events that are generically undesirable are associated with the onset of an episode of major depression (Goodyer et al., 1985; Berden et al., 1990; Berney et al., 1991; Williamson et al., 1995, 1998). The associations are strongest for events that are personally salient and carry a moderate to severe degree of negative impact. This association appears particularly apparent for negative events that are dependent or partially dependent on the young person's own behaviour but may also include events that affect others and are independent of child behaviour. There is no suggestion that depression in adolescents is associated with any particular patterning of events, as defined by their social characteristics such as marital, physical illnesses, bereavements or community disasters (Goodyer, 1991). There is however an increased level of long-term difficulties as well as events in the social circumstances of most mentally ill and behaviourally disturbed young people, indicating that depressed young people are exposed to considerable social adversity (Jensen et al., 1991; Sandberg et al., 1993, 1998). The association seems to be rather nonspecific if events and difficulties are measured simply as personally threatening experiences (Sandberg et al., 1998). These findings also suggested that preceding recent events may be less causal in clinically referred populations than considered hitherto. In the study by Sandberg et al. about one-third of all severe events and one-quarter of chronic difficulties were considered likely to have been brought about by the child's own behaviour. Unfortunately, sample size constraints made it unclear whether this was more likely in behavioural rather than emotional, and specifically depressive, disorders. It does appear that some young people are acting in ways that put them at much increased risk for events. Such 'person-dependent' events do seem likely to arise from ongoing family activities where the child may be an active participant, or as a result of social disadvantages actively brought about by disenfranchised young people with narrow opportunities and limited choices.

A significant proportion of child-focused events occur as a result of other environmental factors in their lives. Family-focused experiences such as parental psychiatric disorder and family difficulties such as marital disharmony may increase the risk for psychopathology and for further negative experiences focused on the child, such as abusive experiences, school nonattendance and divorce. It is increasingly apparent that some families are life event-prone, increasing the exposure of their offspring to personally undesirable events (Goodyer et al., 1993b). This chain of connected experiences provides a more cogent explanation of how social risk process (regardless of their origins) increases the liability for disorder than theories built on any one social element alone.

Loss and depression

The classical theories for the formation of depression in adults suggest that loss of a loved one in childhood is a prerequisite factor. If such losses were to result in psychopathology close to the loss itself, then the risk for subsequent depression may in fact be through those immediate psychiatric consequences.

There have been substantive investigations of loss experiences in young people, which has clearly shown that brief separations (days or a few weeks) from parents and other care-givers does not carry a long-term risk for psychiatric disorder in middle childhood and adolescence (Goodyer, 1991). Permanent separations do however exert adverse behavioural effects in many children both close to and at a distance in time from the event, although the most apparent feature is the diversity of response: some children are markedly resilient in the fact of this adversity, even in the long term (Hetherington, 1989; Hetherington et al., 1989; Hetherington & Stanley-Hagan, 1999).

Whilst children who suffer bereavement in early life are at increased risk for higher levels of emotional symptoms, they do not appear to be particularly sensitized through this single experience alone for subsequent onsets of major depression (Van Eerdewegh et al., 1982). Bereavement in the school age, but not preschool years, may however be more closely associated with depressive disorders than separations or other types of loss events occurring at the same time period (Berney et al., 1991).

Lifetime recall of permanent separations and deaths is reliable and not subject to distortions of recall that are potentially serious confounders of the descriptions of prior experience. What evidence there is suggests that a significant association exists between depression and multiple losses (two or more) or separations but no association with a single such experience (Goodyer & Altham, 1991a,b). In this case-control study of 200 subjects (100 depressed and 100 controls), nearly twice as many depressed children had been exposed to two or more such exit events compared with controls (45% vs. 25%), controlling for age, as risk for exposure to loss increases with time. Such evidence provides tentative support for a matching social process for school-aged depressed subjects who have been doubly exposed to parental loss. Exposure to double loss is however neither necessary nor specific to account for depression, as a quarter of the controls were exposed to multiple losses. A longitudinal catch-up study comparing rates of depression and other psychopathologies in adolescents exposed to bereavement, divorce and separation separately or as multiple experiences would considerably illuminate the question of specificity between types of loss and psychiatric outcome.

In studies of adults, the loss or absence of a confiding relationship has been taken to mean a deficiency of emotional support, increasing the risk for subsequent depression (Paykel, 1992). The absence of social support in adults appears to act as an independent risk factor from that of recent life events and is related to a longer course of the episode. In children and adolescents, a positive confiding relationship with parents has been noted to decrease the risk of psychopathology in general (Radke-Yarrow & Brown, 1993; Rutter, 1994; Tiet et al., 1998). The role of confiding relationships with peers in relation to the risk for psychopathology in children and adolescents remains remarkably under-studied (Cairns et al., 1995). What little evidence there is suggests that impairments in the availability, adequacy and intimacy of close friends are potentially different risk processes from those produced through family-focused events and difficulties (Goodyer et al., 1990). Whether particular deficits in friendships such as peer popularity, the presence of a best friend and the use of peers as confidants influence the onset of major depression is not known. The origins of such friendship difficulties are themselves complex and it is likely that children are involved in bringing about peer group dysfunction (Berndt & Keefe, 1995; Cairns et al., 1995; Bukowski et al., 1996). This would indicate that such problems may not operate as independent casual processes in the onset of depression, although they may exert additive effects in the presence of other known risks, such as difficult temperament, poor personal achievement, social isolation or bullying. Current evidence suggests that, rather than the overall character of the larger peer group *per se*, it is when dyadic peer relations are personally disappointing that emotional disorders may occur, but the issue is in urgent need of more detailed research.

Longitudinal studies

An important longitudinal study from New Zealand has clearly indicated that general risks for psychopathology and maladaptive behaviour in adolescents are a consequence of interactions between past and current adversities (Fergusson et al., 1990; 1995; Fergusson & Lynskey, 1995; Nicholson et al., 1999). A striking feature of this and other similar studies is the importance of personal attributes, particularly general intelligence and a sociable temperament, within the adolescent in mediating the impact of risk following exposure to adverse circumstances (Masten et al., 1990; Radke-Yarrow & Brown, 1993; Fergusson & Lynskey, 1996; Tiet et al., 1998).

Lewinsohn and colleagues investigated the specificity of a wide array of psychosocial factors that preceded the onset of major depression (*DSM-III-R* and *-IV* criteria: American Psychiatric Association, 1994) in adolescents 14–18 years of age. Diagnostic and psychosocial assessments were made on 1507 randomly selected students on two occasions 12 months apart. Adolescents who experienced an episode of depression during that year were exposed to significantly more negative life events than controls or subjects with substance abuse disorder (Lewinsohn et al., 1995). Lewinsohn and colleagues noted that episodes of major depression were specifically more likely in adolescents with past histories of suicide attempts, previous depressive episodes, past anxiety disorder, a desire for greater emotional support from others and greater reports of physical ill health in the previous year. This suggests that a significant proportion of adverse social experiences may indeed be a consequence of the adolescent's own behaviour and/or of previous episodes of clinical depression. Interestingly, tobacco use and academic difficulties were specific to substance use disorder. Conflict with parents was common risk for both groups of disorders.

A comparison of the occurrence of different types of life events between first episode and recurrent depressives demonstrated that a romantic break-up predicted first episodes but not a second or chronic recurrent disorder (Lewinsohn et al., 1998). However, the exact nature of the association between this form of personal disappointment and disorder is unclear. For example, the negative salience to the subject is assumed rather than measured, even though some break-ups may be desirable, affording relief from a dysfunctional interpersonal relationship.

The findings from this longitudinal study do suggest, however, that the relationship between personally threatening life events and difficulties and the onset of major depression may be different between first episode and recurrent disorders (Rohde et al., 1994; Lewinsohn et al., 1999). First episode disorders are more sensitive to events and difficulties than recurrent disorders, suggesting potentially different mechanisms based on frequency rather than just the nature of the disorder. Post (Post et al., 1986; Post & Weiss, 1997) has theorized that first-onset depressions occur following social sensitization but recurrences require increasingly less environmental provocation. The implication that less severe and possibly less personally salient minor events may be responsible for recurrent onsets because of alterations in the underlying brain substrate which is responsible for responses to the environment is intriguing, but as yet untested. Lewinsohn's study is again informative here. The Oregon data suggest that dysphoric symptoms and negative dysfunctional thinking are significantly associated with recurrent depressives, compared with those having had their first episode of depression, whereas major life stress is more significantly associated with the onset of first episodes (Lewinsohn et al., 1999). These findings suggest that episodes of major depression can alter psychological states, increasing the liability for further episodes and that this may reflect altered brain function.

Social and nonsocial factors and the onset of major depression

In a recent prospective study, Goodyer and colleagues investigated the antecedent role of social, cognitive and endocrine measures in the onset of a first episode of major depression in 13–16-year-olds (Goodyer et al., 2000a,b).

This study demonstrated that almost all episodes of major depression occurred in subjects with high preexisting levels of depressive symptoms who were also at high psychosocial risk for psychopathology (Goodyer et al., 2000a). Thirty (97%) out of 31 episodes of major depression over a 12-month period occurred in subjects exposed to two or more psychosocial risks, consisting of: marital disharmony, parental psychiatric disorder, two or more lifetime exit events (permanent separations and/or death), two or more recent undesirable life events and the temperamental style of high emotionality (adolescents who respond intensely to social stimuli and who score >80th percentile on this behavioural-style subscale of a measure of temperament: Goodyer et al., 1993a).

This collection of risk factors and processes was chosen because each, on its own or in combination, has been reported as a risk correlate for psychiatric disorder. Interestingly, in this prospective sample all five of these risks contributed to the liability for the onset of disorder. This suggests that there is a necessary set of long-standing adversities present in the life of an adolescent that result in affective psychopathology. The need for all five of these factors suggests that there are multiple aetiological processes involved in the onset of major depression in young people. The risk profile was not influenced by age of the subjects at entry to the study, but more girls reported experiencing recent life events than boys (Goodyer et al., 2000a). Interestingly, in this high-risk population neither sex nor age contributed to the liability for onset of depression. At first sight, this suggests that the increased rates of depression in adolescent girls compared to boys may be because more girls report being exposed to negative life events than boys. A closer inspection of the timing and the type of life events in relation to the onset of depression (defined as an observable increase in personal impairment and the presence of *DSM-IV* major depression) revealed that only events in the month before disorder were associated with onset. There was no association for events occurring between the second and 11th month before onset. Importantly, there were no sex differences in the recall of undesirable events in the 1-month period before onset of disorder, indicating that truly provoking events are equally as likely to be reported by boys as they are by girls. The observation that significantly more girls reported being exposed to negative life events is only true for those events not provoking depressive disorder suggests that the well-established sex bias in reporting of events in the community at large (Brooks-Gunn, 1991) may not be a sufficient explanation for the increased rates of female depressives in the adolescent years.

When the types of events in that 1-month period were examined, personal disappointments and losses (permanent separations and/or deaths) made independent contributions to the onset of major depression, whereas dangerous events to the self or others did not. Disappointments involve adolescents in interpersonal behaviours and are therefore dependent events, whereas all the losses measured were outside the adolescent's control, making them independent events. It appears that both types of events make a contribution to onset and that adolescents who are already at high risk are liable to develop a major episode of depression within a few days or weeks of exposure to a particular type of provoking undesirable life event. This social model is broadly in agreement with longitudinal studies of women at high risk.

However, 47% of the adolescents who developed depression did not experience either a loss or a disappointment in the month before onset. This indicates that such provoking events are neither necessary nor sufficient for the onset of depression. It also indicates that a substantial proportion of cases have a slower onset arising from a background of chronic or longer-term adversities.

Overall, these short-term longitudinal studies suggest that there may be two broad groups of major depressive disorder: slow-onset cases without any apparent social provocation, where adolescents appear to slide into major depression; and rapid-onset cases, where such personally salient and negative social experiences result in the onset of disorder. Evidence for a slow-onset group has recently been forthcoming from a longitudinal study of 303 families assessed face-to-face at yearly intervals for 4 years (Reuter et al., 1999). The findings showed that persistent escalating life events, such as parental disagreements, over this time period were indirectly increasing the risk for internalizing disorder onset through their direct association with high or increasing depressive symptom levels. Chronically high or increasing symptom levels directly increased the risk for internalizing disorder. In those adolescents with slowly increasing levels of depressive symptoms, the prodromal phase was drawn out over time.

Equally intriguing from Goodyer's findings was that approximately a quarter of high-risk subjects who did experience a provoking event in that 1 month period did not develop major depression. This raises two crucial issues: first, are other factors required to increase the liability for disorder beyond the provoking effects of recent life events and ongoing difficulties? Second, what processes result in some adolescents being resilient in the face of adversity?

First, it appears that, as with Lewinsohn's study and in the majority of studies on adults, it is those adolescents with higher self-report scores for depression at entry who are somewhat more likely to develop depression independently of the effects of proximal life events. However, as one might predict from the work of Rueter and colleagues (1999), there was an interaction between social risk and higher depressive symptoms at entry, suggesting that the origins of high subclinical depressive symptoms relate to the presence of long-standing adverse environments.

Second, individuals with extreme daily levels (>80th percentile of the sex-related mean) of dehydroepiandrosterone and cortisol were at significantly raised risk of depression. Interestingly, these endocrine variables were not correlated with any risk factor, including provoking life events, nor with elevated self-reported scores of negative mood and feelings (Goodyer et al., 2000a,b). These are very intriguing findings, suggesting a potentially causal effect involving psychoendocrine processes, the origins of which may be through a more distal environment (for example, in earlier childhood or infancy) or via genetic influences. Angold has noted from epidemiological studies (see Chapter 6) that testosterone and oestrogen may be more relevant for depressive disorders in girls than dehydroepiandrosterone (Angold et al., 1999). Whether sex hormones in adolescence exert effects independently of social factors that precede onset of disorder is unclear. Currently, the precise behavioural functions in humans of cortisol, dehydroepiandrosterone and sex hormones remain unclear and there may be important differences in their behavioural functions that require a clearer understanding before firm conclusions can be reached regarding the precise nature of hormone depression relations (see Chapters 4, 6 and 9 for a fuller discussion of endocrine influences).

Could there be an early neural vulnerability in some children indexed by higher circulating levels of steroids and arising from the early environment? If so, are proximal events activating negative cognitions that are related to such early predispositions? These are highly speculative statements at this stage of knowledge, and as yet we do not have the tools to examine the direct effects of hormones on the developing human brain. There is however a degree of evidence that the brain is shaped by early social experiences such as maternal care in infancy, the social context of a child's surroundings and the nature of early peer group function (Gunnar, 1998). Early maternal deprivation in rodents results in an alteration of the structure and function of the hippocampus – a part of the brain that is crucial for adequate memory function (Vazquez, 1998). High cortisol levels are associated with impaired social functioning in nonhuman primates and involution of the dendrites in the hippocampus (McEwen, 1995; McEwen & Sapolsky, 1995; Sapolsky, 1989, 1994; Sapolsky et al., 1997). In adult human volunteers, high levels of circulating cortisol are associated with impairments in conscious declarative memory such as recall of previously (but recently) rehearsed words, but have no discernible effect on unconscious implicit memory which stores rules and procedural elements of behaviour (Newcomer et al., 1999).

Whilst there are some preliminary findings that there are individual differences in cortisol characteristics in young children, we know very little about how dehydroepiandrosterone, or testosterone contributes. To date, small sample sizes or the lack of a representative community population and the absence of longitudinal data, including measures of memory and social function as well as hormones, have yet to be carried out in adequately designed studies. If we are to understand what social experiences do to brain and mind through childhood and adolescence and to examine how the characteristic core deficits of depression arise, then future studies will need to be more inclusive at the level of measurement. Selecting populations who have been exposed to different types of life events and difficulties, both in the recent and the distant past, together with incorporating experimental procedures to activate the neural and affective-cognitive processes of interest, may result in elucidating the mechanisms through which personally salient undesirable life events result in depressive disorders.

Life events and the maintenance of depression

Studies on adults

A body of research has investigated how life events, good and bad, may influence the course of depressive disorders. Tennant and colleagues (1981) examined the relationship between life events and the remission of neurotic disorders in adults and concluded that 30% of all remissions were due to a neutralizing life event, defined as an event which specifically neutralized the impact of an earlier threatening life event. This appeared to be true for anxious and depressive conditions. Miller and colleagues suggested that the duration, course and nature of depression were related to the form and timing of the life event (Miller et al., 1987). Events rated as likely to be of uncertain outcome were associated with illnesses of relatively longer duration, whereas events involving impaired interpersonal relations were associated with continuing illnesses. Events containing neither of these factors were associated with transient disorders of a few weeks' duration only.

Brown and colleagues (1988, 1992) suggested that some events may exert a positive influence on the outcome of disorder because they intrinsically alter the person's appraisal of his or her life circumstances for the better through the instillation of hope for the future. Such events have been referred to as 'fresh start' events. The hedonic qualities of 'fresh start' events do not indicate their effects. Thus, such events may often possess undesirable qualities in themselves, such as a serious personal accident, sudden unemployment or divorce. In such circumstances some individuals appear to use this negative experience for the better. In an important and imaginative randomized clinical trial, Harris and colleagues demonstrated that volunteer befriending significantly improved recovery of chronically depressed women and that 'fresh start' events contributed to this improvement above any effects of other treatments (Harris et al., 1999a,b). These studies all suggest that events with positive functions, apparent or latent, occurring after the onset of major depression may shorten the course of depressive disorder occurring in women in the community and that social interventions designed to increase the supporting social context and encourage 'fresh starts' are effective therapeutic interventions.

In adults, events which result in a failure to meet expectations are associated with longer episodes of illness. By contrast, events which instil hope for the future appear to improve the opportunity of recovery. A reappraisal of one's own life may occur through private experiences of illnesses and personal failures. To date there is no evidence that such a set of processes is important for children or adolescents.

It is also apparent, however, that in many severely depressed cases in adults, events that precede or follow onsets of depression do not markedly influence the course of disorder (Paykel, 1992). A host of other factors may modify individual differences in response to events and outcome of disorder. These include both genetic and other environmental factors, ranging from biochemical through to family and other social experiences, temperament and coping strategies.

Studies in childhood and adolescence

The duration of an episode of major depression in young people is highly variable, with episodes lasting from a few weeks to as long as 18 months (McCauley & Myers, 1992; Sanford et al., 1995; Goodyer et al., 1997b). A number of studies have investigated whether this variability in course is influenced by factors in the current environment of the child and its family.

In a 12-month follow-up study of a sample of anxious and depressive disorders attending a child psychiatry clinic, neither the reduction in exposure to undesirable life events nor the improvement in maternal confiding predicted the child's recovery (Goodyer et al., 1991). Failure to recover was predicted, however, by friendship difficulties occurring *after* onset of disorder, particularly for those with a diagnosis of depression. The possibility that an episode of depression increases the risk for *subsequent* friendship difficulties is suggested by these findings. In other words, psychopathology appears to increase the likelihood of children promoting, through their own behaviour, difficulties in their peer group environment.

Family dysfunction may also be implicated in the time to recovery. Concurrent family difficulties reflecting impaired family problem-solving, communication and level of critical comment may be more closely associated with depressive conduct disorders than other depressive subtypes (Asarnow et al., 1993; Puig-Antich et al., 1993; Tamplin et al., 1997).

In a second study, greater attention was paid to classifying the nature of recent life events and difficulties. Events at the time of presentation were classified into loss (deaths or permanent separations), personal disappointments and physical danger to self or to others. In addition, measures of ongoing family dysfunction and chronic background adversities (financial problems, housing difficulties, safety in the locality, chronic marital problems) were measured. Systematic evaluation of the clinical characteristics of the depressed population was made, including severity, comorbid syndromes and duration of current episode. The findings showed that, at 36 weeks after presentation four adversities were associated with persistence of psychiatric disorder: the mother lacking a confiding relationship with her partner; family dysfunction; poor friendships at presentation; and disappointing events between presentation and follow-up (Goodyer et al., 1997a,b).

Interestingly, current family difficulties were specifically associated with comorbid oppositional defiant or conduct disorder, itself a predictor of non-recovery, but not persistent depression *per se* (Tamplin et al., 1997). A striking feature of this short-term follow-up study was that no combination of long-term or recent life events or difficulties was specifically associated with persistent depression, suggesting that nonsocial factors may be implicated in the maintenance of disorder. When the endocrine status of depressed subjects at entry was examined it was noted that those with a high evening cortisol/dehydroepiandrosterone ratio at entry were more likely to be depressed at 36-weeks follow-up than those without, even when severity of depression and comorbidity at presentation were taken into account (Goodyer et al., 1997c). Of some interest was the finding that this altered hormone ratio was associated with an increase in personally disppointing events during the folow-up period. This suggests a further putative psychoendocrine effect increasing the occurrence of undesirable life events dependent on the adolescent's behaviour.

It is a striking feature of two follow-up studies that person-related disappointments and friendship difficulties are associated with persistent depression. These findings also suggest that nonsocial factors may need to be taken into account specifically to explain the phenotypic persistence of major depression disorder in first-episode nonrecovered cases within a year of presentation.

Clinical implications

These longitudinal findings on clinical populations indicate the importance of interpersonal interventions aimed at improving the quality of peer relations and perhaps thereby decreasing the risk for subsequent disappointing experiences. High levels of intimacy between small groups of peers is important for the emerging normative psychological characteristics of adolescents (Berndt & Keefe, 1995), indicating that ameliorating poor friendships should be an important treatment focus for developmental as well as psychopathological reasons. Establishing whether peer group problems are indeed real and seen as such by identified friends, or whether they represent sensitive thinking by the patient is an important first step in such cases. Perhaps in depressed adolescents even small misinterpretations of the peer environment may increase the risk for disappointments to occur. Psychoeducational approaches, explaining in straightforward terms the nature and characteristics of depression and its effect on friendships to the peer group, as well as to first-degree relatives, may prove to be an important early component of a comprehensive treatment strategy. If this can be achieved within the naturalistic setting of a child's social group, perhaps the need for formal befriending strategies may be avoided.

Conclusions

Specificity of life events and depression

A striking feature of the findings discussed in this chapter is the lack of any clear specific associations between any one pattern of social adversities and the subsequent onset or outcome of major depression. To date, the findings indicate that an onset of major depression may occur as a consequence of a range of recent life events and difficulties from either the familial or peer group domain. From the narrow perspective of recent life events, personal losses and disappointments are more specifically associated with the subsequent onset of major depression than other forms of emotional disorder, but only in the context of adolescents who are already at high risk for psychopathology. The patterns of social risk elucidated so far fail to predict either the form (combination of clinical feaures) or type (e.g. first versus recurrent episode or familial versus nonfamilial) of disorder. There is compelling evidence to consider the quality of peer group experiences and the child's perception of his or her own social worth as particularly important in the outcome of depression, but the precise role of such features in onset remains unclear. Whilst much remains to be established, currently there is no clearcut evidence that dysfunctional family processes specifically precede and predict the onset of major depression. By contrast, personal assaults, such as child abuse, clearly have the capacity to produce major depression in adolescents but the specificity and consequences of that relationship are not known and most certainly require further investigation.

Some depressed young people are at risk for recurrent major depression, perhaps through impairments of the capacity for evolving confiding relationships in adolescence and young adult life. There is also clearcut evidence that, for some individuals, major depression is bad for subsequent well-being, resulting in persistent psychological and perhaps neural vulnerabilities. The reason that 'double hits' or multiple adverse events of similar experiences over time may be less theoretically important than considered hitherto is that, following an episode some individuals are quite different psychologically, with an increased set of dysfunctional emotional and cognitive processes. This does not appear to be the outcome for all adolescents with a history of depression. A major research task for the future is to determine which first-episode depressives are more at risk for these internal vulnerabilities.

The findings on both prospective community and longitudinal clinical studies that have carried out concurrent hormone measurement implicate non-psychosocial processes in the onset and maintenance of depression. These physiological abnormalities may indicate the role of genetic and/or early environmental factors in the origins of a vulnerable endocrine environment that increases the liability for subsequent major depression.

Future research clearly requires a combined approach both in terms of the design of studies and collaboration between behavioural and neuroscientists. The importance of psychological (temperament, emotion regulation, negative cognitions, general intelligence) and physiological (steroids and monoamines) factors as agents in the nature, course and outcome of major depression via their interrelationships with the environment is likely to be more important than considered hitherto.

Acknowledgements

Ian Goodyer's research, quoted in this chapter, has been supported by project and programme grants from the Wellcome Trust.

REFERENCES

Abraham, K. S. (1927). Notes on the psychoanalytic investigation and treatment of manic-depressive insanity and allied conditions. In *Selected Papers on Psycho-analysis*, pp. 137–56. London: Hogarth Press.

Abramson, L., Seligman, M. & Teasdale, J. (1978). Learned helplessness in humans: critique and reformulation. *Journal of Abnormal Psychology*, **87**, 49–74.

American Psychiatric Association (1994). *Diagnostic and Statistical Manual for Mental and Behavioral Disorders*, vol. IV. Washington, DC: American Psychiatric Association.

Angold, A., Costello, E. J., Erkanl, A. et al. (1999). Pubertal changes in hormone levels and depression in girls. *Psychological Medicine*, **29**, 1043–53.

Asarnow, G., Goldstein, M., Tompson, M. et al. (1993). One year outcomes of depressive disorders in child psychiatric in-patients: the evaluation of a brief measure of expressed emotion. *Journal of Child Psychology and Psychiatry*, **34**, 129–38.

Beck, A. T., Rush, A. J., Shaw, B. F. & Emery, G. (1979). *Cognitive Therapy of Depression*. New York: Guilford Press.

Berden, G. F. M. G., Althaus, M. & Verhulst, F. (1990). Major life events and changes in the behavioural functioning of children. *Journal of Child Psychology and Psychiatry*, **31**, 949–60.

Berndt, T. & Keefe, K. (1995). Friends' influence on adolescents' adjustment at school. *Child Development*, **66**, 1312–29.

Berney, T., Bhate, S., Kolvin, I. et al. (1991). The context of childhood depression: the Newcastle childhood depression project. *British Journal of Psychiatry*, **159** (Suppl. 11), 28–35.

Bifulco, A. T., Brown, G. W. & Harris, T. O. (1987). Childhood loss of parent, lack of adequate parental care and adult depression: a replication. *Journal of Affective Disorder*, **12**, 115–28.

Bifulco, A., Brown, G. W. & Adler, Z. (1991). Early sexual abuse and clinical depression in adult life. *British Journal of Psychiatry*, **159**, 115–22.

Bifulco, A., Brown, G. W., Moran, P. et al. (1998). Predicting depression in women: the role of past and present vulnerability. *Psychological Medicine*, **28**, 39–50.

Bowlby, J. (1980). *Attachment and Loss*, vol. 3: *Loss, Sadness and Depression*. New York: Basic Books.

Brooks-Gunn, J. (1991). How stressful is the transition to adolescence in girls? In *Adolescent Stress: causes and consequences*, ed. M. Colton & S. Gore, pp. 131–49. Hawthorne, New York: Aldine de Gruyter.

Brooks-Gunn, J. & Petersen, A. C. (1991). Studying the emergence of depression and depressive symptoms during adolescence. *Journal of Youth and Adolescence*, **20**, 115–19.

Brown, G. W. & Harris, T. (1978). *Social Origins of Depression: a study of psychiatric disorder in women*. London: Tavistock Publications.

Brown, G. W., Andrews, B., Harris, T., Adler, Z. & Bridge, L. (1986). Social support, self esteem and depression. *Psychological Medicine*, **16**, 813–31.

Brown, G. W. & Harris, T. O. (1993). Aetiology of anxiety and depressive disorders in an inner-city population. 1. Early adversity. *Psychological Medicine*, **23**, 143–54.

Brown, G. W., Bifulco, A. & Harris, T. (1987). Life events, vulnerability and the onset of depression: some refinements. *British Journal of Psychiatry*, **150**, 30–42.

Brown, G. W., Adler, Z. & Bifulco, A. (1988). Life events, difficulties and recovery from chronic depression. *British Journal of Psychiatry*, **152**, 487–98.

Brown, G. W., Bifulco, A. & Andrews, B. (1990a). Self-esteem and depression III. Aetiological issues. *Social Psychiatry and Psychiatric Epidemiology*, **25**, 235–43.

Brown, G. W., Bifulco, A., Veiel, H. O. et al. (1990b). Self-esteem and depression II. Social correlates of self esteem. *Social Psychiatry and Psychiatric Epidemiology*, **25**, 225–34.

Brown, G. W., LeMyre, L. & Bifulco, A. (1992). Social factors and recovery from anxiety and depressive disorders. *British Journal of Psychiatry*, **152**, 44–54.

Bukowski, W., Newcomb, A. & Hartup, W. (eds) (1996). *The Company they Keep: friendships in childhood and adolescence*. Cambridge: Cambridge University Press.

Cairns, R., Leung, M.-C., Buchanan, L. et al. (1995). Friendships and social networks in childhood and adolescence: fluidity, reliability and interrelations. *Child Development*, **66**, 1330–45.

Caspi, A., Henry, B., McGee, R. O. et al. (1995). Temperamental origins of child and adolescent behavior problems: from age three to age fifteen. *Child Development*, **66**, 55–68.

Fergusson, D. M. & Lynskey, M. T. (1995). Childhood circumstances, adolescent adjustment, and suicide attempts in a New Zealand birth cohort. *Journal of the American Academy of Child and Adolescent Psychiatry*, **34**, 612–22.

Fergusson, D. M. & Lynskey, M. T. (1996). Adolescent resiliency to family adversity. *Journal of Child Psychology and Psychiatry*, **37**, 281–92.

Fergusson, D. M., Horwood, L. J. & Lawton, J. M. (1990). Vulnerability to childhood problems and family social background. *Journal of Child Psychology and Psychiatry*, **31**, 1145–60.

Fergusson, D. M., Horwood, L. J. & Lynskey, M. T. (1995). Maternal depressive symptoms and depressive symptoms in adolescents. *Journal of Child Psychology and Psychiatry*, **36**, 1161–78.

Finlay-Jones, R. & Brown, G. W. (1981). Types of stressful life event and the onset of anxiety and depressive disorders. *Psychological Medicine*, **11**, 803–15.

Goodyer, I. M. (1991). *Life Events, Development and Childhood Psychopathology.* Chichester: John Wiley.

Goodyer, I. M. (1996). Recent undesirable life events: their influence on subsequent psychopathology. *European Child and Adolescent Psychiatry*, **5** (Suppl. 1), 33–7.

Goodyer, I. M. & Altham, P. M. E. (1991a). Lifetime exit events in anxiety and depression in school age children I. *Journal of Affective Disorders*, **21**, 219–28.

Goodyer, I. M. & Altham, P. M. E. (1991b). Lifetime exit events in anxiety and depression in school age children II. *Journal of Affective Disorders*, **2**, 229–38.

Goodyer, I. M., Kolvin, I. & Gatzanis, S. (1985). Recent undesirable life events and psychiatric-disorder in childhood and adolescence. *British Journal of Psychiatry*, **147**, 517–23.

Goodyer, I. M., Wright, C. & Altham, P. M. E. (1990). The friendships and recent life events of anxious and depressed school-age children. *British Journal of Psychiatry*, **156**, 689–98.

Goodyer, I. M., Germany, E., Gowrusankur, J. et al. (1991). Social influences on the course of anxious and depressive disorders in school-age children. *British Journal of Psychiatry*, **158**, 676–84.

Goodyer, I. M., Ashby, L., Altham, P. M. E. et al. (1993a). Temperament and major depression in 11–16 year olds. *Journal of Child Psychology and Psychiatry*, **34**, 1409–23.

Goodyer, I. M., Cooper, P. J., Vize, C. et al. (1993b). Depression in 11 to 16 year old girls: the role of past parental psychopathology and exposure to recent undesirable life events. *Journal of Child Psychology and Psychiatry*, **34**, 1103–17.

Goodyer, I. M., Herbert, J., Tamplin, A. et al. (1997a). Short term outcome of major depression: II. Life events, family dysfunction and friendship difficulties as predictors of persistent disorder. *Journal of the American Academy of Child and Adolescent Psychiatry*, **36**, 474–80.

Goodyer, I. M., Herbert, J., Secher, S. et al. (1997b). Short term outcome of major depression: I. Comorbidity and severity at presentation as predictors of persistent disorders. *Journal of the American Academy of Child and Adolescent Psychiatry*, **36**, 179–87.

Goodyer, I. M., Herbert, J. & Altham, P. M. E. (1997c). Short term outcome of major depression. III. A high cortisol/DHEA ratio and subsequent disappointing life events predict persistent depression. *Psychological Medicine*, **28**, 265–73.

Goodyer, I. M., Herbert, J., Tamplin, A. et al. (2000a). First episode major depression in adolescents: affective, cognitive and endocrine characteristics of risk status and predictors of onset. *British Journal of Psychiatry*, **176**, 142–49.

Goodyer, I., Herbert, J. Tamplin, A. et al. (2000b). Recent life events, cortisol and DHEA in the onset of major depression amongst 'high risk' adolescents. *British Journal of Psychiatry* (in press).

Gunnar, M. R. (1998). Quality of early care and buffering of neuroendocrine stress reactions: potential effects on the developing human brain. *Preventative Medicine*, **27**, 208–11.

Harris, T., Brown, G. W. & Robinson, R. (1999a). Befriending as an intervention for chronic depression among women in an inner city. 1: Randomised controlled trial. *British Journal of Psychiatry*, **174**, 219–24.

Harris, T., Brown, G. W. & Robinson, R. (1999b). Befriending as an intervention for chronic depression among women in an inner city. 2: Role of fresh-start experiences and baseline psychosocial factors in remission from depression. *British Journal of Psychiatry*, **174**, 225–32.

Hetherington, E. M. (1989). Coping with family transitions: winners, losers, and survivors. *Child Development*, **60**, 1–14.

Hetherington, E. M. & Stanley-Hagan, M. (1999). The adjustment of children with divorced parents: a risk and resiliency perspective. *Journal of Child Psychology and Psychiatry*, **40**, 129–40.

Hetherington, E. M., Stanley-Hagan, M. & Anderson, E. R. (1989). Marital transitions. A child's perspective. *American Psychology*, **44**, 303–12.

Jensen, P., Richters, J. & Ussery, T. (1991). Child psychopathology and environmental influences: discrete life events versus ongoing adversity. *Journal of the American Academy of Child and Adolescent Psychiatry*, **30**, 303–9.

Kendler, K. S., Karkowski, L. M. & Prescott, C. A. (1999). Causal relationship between stressful life events and the onset of major depression. *American Journal of Psychiatry*, **156**, 837–41.

Lewinsohn, P. M., Roberts, R. E., Seeley, J. R. et al. (1994). Adolescent psychopathology: II. Psychosocial risk factors for depression. *Journal of Abnormal Psychology*, **103**, 302–15.

Lewinsohn, P. M., Gotlib, I. & Seeley, J. R. (1995). Adolescent psychopathology: IV. Specificity of psychosocial risk factors for depression and substance abuse in older adolescents. *Journal of the American Academy of Child and Adolescent Psychiatry*, **34**, 1221–9.

Lewinsohn, P. M., Rohde, P. & Seeley, J. R. (1998). Major depressive disorder in older adolescents: prevalence, risk factors, and clinical implications. *Clinical and Psychological Review*, **18**, 765–94.

Lewinsohn, P. M., Allen, N. B., Seeley, J. R. et al. (1999). First onset versus recurrence of depression: differential processes of psychosocial risk. *Journal of Abnormal Psychology*, **108**, 483–9.

Manicavasagar, V., Silove, D. & Hadzi-Pavlovic, D. (1998). Subpopulations of early separation anxiety: relevance to risk of adult anxiety disorders. *Journal of Affective Disorders*, **48**, 181–90.

Masten, A., Morison, P., Pellegrini, D. et al. (1990). Competence under stress: risk and protective factors. In *Risk and Protective Factors in the Development of Psychopathology*, ed. J. Rolf, A. Masten, D. Cicchetti et al., pp. 236–56. Cambridge: Cambridge University Press.

McCauley, E. & Myers, K. (1992). *The Longitudinal Clinical Course of Depression in Children and Adolescents*, vol. 1. Philadelphia: W. B. Saunders.

McEwen, B. (1995). Stressful experience, brain and emotions: developmental, genetic and hormonal influences. In *The Cognitive Neurosciences*, ed. M. Gazzaniga, pp. 1117–35. Massachusetts: MIT Press.

McEwen, B. S. & Sapolsky, R. M. (1995). Stress and cognitive function. *Current Opinions in Neurobiology*, **5**, 205–16.

Miller, P. M. & Surtees, P. G. (1993). Partners in adversity: II. Measurement and description of stressful event sequences ('complexes'). *European Archives of Psychiatry and Clinical Neuroscience*, **242**, 233–9.

Miller, P. M., Ingham, J. G., Kreitman, N. B. et al. (1987). Life events and other factors implicated in onset and in remission of psychiatric illness in women. *Journal of Affective Disorders*, **12**, 73–88.

Newcomer, J. W., Selke, G., Melson, A. K. et al. (1999). Decreased memory performance in healthy human induced by stress-level cortisol treatment. *Archives of General Psychiatry*, **56**, 527–33.

Nicholson, J. M., Fergusson, D. M. & Horwood, L. J. (1999). Effects on later adjustment of living in a stepfamily during childhood and adolescence. *Journal of Child Psychology and Psychiatry*, **40**, 405–16.

Parker, G., Gladstone, G., Roussos, J. et al. (1998). Qualitative and quantitative analyses of a 'lock and key' hypothesis of depression. *Psychological Medicine*, **28**, 1263–73.

Paykel, E. S. (1978). The contribution of life events to the causation of psychiatric illness. *Psychological Medicine*, **8**, 245–53.

Paykel, E. S. (1992). *Handbook of Affective Disorders*, 2nd edn. Edinburgh: Churchill Livingstone.

Petersen, A. C., Sarigiani, P. A. & Kennedy, R. E. (1991). Adolescent depression: why more girls? *Journal of Youth and Adolescence*, **20**, 247–71.

Post, R. M. & Weiss, S. R. (1997). Emergent properties of neural systems: how focal molecular neurobiological alterations can affect behavior. *Development and Psychopathology*, **9**, 907–29.

Post, R., Rubinow, D. & Ballenger, J. (1986). Conditioning and sensitisation in the longitudinal course of affective illness. *British Journal of Psychiatry*, **149**, 191–201.

Puig-Antich, J. Kauffman, J. & Ryan, N. (1993). The psychosocial functioning and family environment of depressed children. *Journal of the American Academy of Child and Adolescent Psychiatry*, **32**, 244–54.

Radke-Yarrow, M. & Brown, E. (1993). Resilience and vulnerability in children of multiple risk families. *Development and Psychopathology*, **5**, 581–92.

Rohde, P., Lewinsohn, P. M. & Seeley, J. R. (1994). Are adolescents changed by an episode of major depression? *Journal of the American Academy of Child and Adolescent Psychiatry*, **33**, 1289–98.

Rueter, M. A., Scaramella, L., Wallace, L. E. et al. (1999). First onset of depressive or anxiety disorders predicted by the longitudinal course of internalizing symptoms and parent–adolescent disagreements. *Archives of General Psychiatry*, **56**, 726–32.

Rutter, M. (1985). Psychosocial resilience and protective mechanisms. In *Risk and Protective Factors in the Development of Psychopathology*, ed. J. Rolf, M. Masten, D. Cicchetti et al., pp. 181–214. Cambridge: Cambridge University Press.

Rutter, M. (1994). Stress research: accomplishments and the tasks ahead. In *Stress, Risk and Resilience in Children and Adolescence*, ed. R. Haggert, L. Sherrod, N. Garmezy et al., pp. 354–86. Cambridge: Cambridge University Press.

Sandberg, S., McGuinness, D., Hillary, C. et al. (1998). Independence of childhood life events and chronic adversities: a comparison of two patient groups and controls. *Journal of the American Academy of Child and Adolescent Psychiatry*, **37**, 728–35.

Sandberg, S., Rutter, M., Giles, S. et al. (1993). Assessment of psychosocial experiences in childhood: methodological issues and some illustrative findings (published erratum appears in

Journal of Child Psychology and Psychiatry 1994; **35**, 397). *Journal of Child Psychology and Psychiatry*, **34**, 879–97.

Sanford, M., Szatmari, P., Spinner, M. et al. (1995). Predicting the one year course of adolescent major depression. *Journal of the American Academy of Child and Adolescent Psychiatry*, **34**, 1618–28.

Sapolsky, R. (1989). Hypercortisolism among socially subordinate wild baboons originates at the CNS level. *Archives of General Psychiatry*, **46**, 1047–51.

Sapolsky, R. M. (1994). The physiological relevance of glucocorticoid endangerment of the hippocampus. *Annals of the New York Academy of Science*, **746**, 294–304.

Sapolsky, R. M., Alberts, S. C. & Altmann, J. (1997). Hypercortisolism associated with social subordinance or social isolation among wild baboons. *Archives of General Psychiatry*, **54**, 1137–43.

Seligman, M. E. (1978). Learned helplessness as a model of depression. Comment and integration. *Journal of Abnormal Psychology*, **87**, 165–79.

Silberg, J., Pickles, A., Rutter, M. et al. (1999). The influence of genetic factors and life stress on depression among adolescent girls. *Archives of General Psychiatry*, **56**, 225–32.

Silove, D., Harris, M., Morgan, A. et al. (1995). Is early separation anxiety a specific precursor of panic disorder-agoraphobia? A community study. *Psychological Medicine*, **25**, 405–11.

Tamplin, A., Goodyer, I. & Herbert, J. (1997). Family function and parent general health in families of adolescents with major depressive disorders. *Journal of Affective Disorders*, **48**, 1–13.

Teasdale, J. D. & Barnard, P. J. (1993). *Affect, Cognition and Change: remodelling depressive thought.* Hillsdale, NJ: Lawrence Erlbaum.

Tennant, C., Bebbington, P. & Hurry, J. (1981). The role of life events in depressive illness. Is there a substantive causal relation? *Psychological Medicine*, **11**, 379–89.

Thapar, A. & McGuffin, P. (1996). Genetic influences on life events in childhood. *Psychological Medicine*, **26**, 813–20.

Tiet, Q. Q., Bird, H. R., Davies, M. et al. (1998). Adverse life events and resilience. *Journal of the American Academy of Child and Adolescent Psychiatry*, **37**, 1191–200.

Van Eerdewegh, M., Bieri, M., Parrilla, R. & Clayton, P. (1982). The bereaved child. *British Journal of Psychiatry*, **140**, 23–9.

Vazquez, D. M. (1998). Stress and the developing limbic–hypothalamic–pituitary–adrenal axis. *Psychoneuroendocrinology*, **23**, 663–700.

Williamson, D. E., Birmaher, B., Anderson, B. P. et al. (1995). Stressful life events in depressed adolescents: the role of dependent events during the depressive episode. *Journal of the American Academy of Child and Adolescent Psychiatry*, **34**, 591–8.

Williamson, D. E., Birmaher, B., Frank, E. et al. (1998). Nature of life events and difficulties in depressed adolescents. *Journal of the American Academy of Child and Adolescent Psychiatry*, **37**, 1049–57.

9

Adolescent depression: neuroendocrine aspects

Stephen Sokolov and Stan Kutcher

Introduction

The development of criterion-based diagnostic systems has been an impetus for the investigation of the neurobiological underpinnings of psychiatric disturbance in children and adolescents. Although, to date, insufficient knowledge exists specifically to identify the aetiologies of various disorders, studies of clinical and normative populations have led to a veritable explosion of knowledge about the neuroendocrine aspects of psychiatric disorders. As a result of these investigations, the specificity of current diagnostic systems has been questioned, the pathophysiology of various psychiatric disorders has been explored and simplistic models which previously have been invoked to explain both normal and pathological behaviour (for example: adolescent turmoil is due to hormones) are no longer tenable (Buchanan et al., 1992).

Neuroendocrine studies in adolescent depression have arisen from the influence of similar research in adult populations, and some of the earliest work in this field was an attempt to determine if the neurobiological features found in adult depressives would also be present in children and adolescents. Similar findings, it was argued, would provide further evidence for the presence of depressive disorders in younger populations and thus lend credibility to the diagnostic classification of child and adolescent depression. This work of pioneering investigators has been further developed by the realization of the different central nervous system (CNS) and neurohormonal aspects of adolescents compared to adults (Buchanan et al., 1992).

Furthermore, adolescent neuroendocrinology, with its developmentally determined differences that occur rapidly during a few years of the life cycle, give an added dimension of complexity that is not usually addressed in studies of adult populations. Thus, the study of the neuroendocrinology of adolescent mood disorders has become an important area of investigation in its own right.

This importance is further substantiated by the recent realization that depressive disorders are, by and large, adolescent-onset disorders (Christie et al., 1989; Weissman & Klerman, 1992). The prevalence rate of major depression changes with age from about 1% prepubertally to levels of between 5% and 8% by age 19, with lower rates for boys compared to girls postpubertally (see Chapter 6). That the onset of this disorder occurs during a phase of a major CNS reorganization concurrently with the onset of puberty suggests that an understanding of these issues may advance our knowledge of the aetiology of depression, an idea that receives further support from the well-known relationship between organic disorders of the central nervous and endocrine systems and depression.

Neuroendocrine studies of depression in the adolescent population have some advantages over studies of adult populations, including the likelihood of studying subjects free from the confounds of prolonged antidepressant treatments and previous episodes. There are however changes in neural functioning as a result of development and life experience (Gunnar, 1998), and neuroendocrine abnormalities may be a consequence rather than a cause of depressive disorders. Hormonal indices of CNS dysregulation may therefore be different in those exposed to early environmental adversities, such as maternal deprivation and neglect, regardless of age of onset. There may also be differences between those with recurrent or persistent disorders and those with first episodes in later life compared to adolescent-onset disorders (Post et al., 1986; Post & Weiss, 1997). Developmentally sensitive studies are required which focus on charcterziting neuroendocrine function in different types of depressive disorders at different ages and stages of development.

Neuroendocrine studies in adolescent depression have two complementary but different purposes. First, they are an attempt to determine the biological aetiology of depression. According to this model, depression is the symptomatic expression of a final common pathway of CNS dysfunctions that may involve a number of neurotransmitter systems (Siever & Davis, 1985). The systems most commonly postulated to be involved include the noradrenergic, serotonergic, cholinergic and dopaminergic systems, with disturbances possibly occurring at the level of deficiencies or excesses of specific neurotransmitters, functioning of various receptors, or in second messenger systems (Coppen, 1967; Heninger & Charney, 1987; Charney et al., 1990). Second, neuroendocrine strategies provide a 'window on the brain' model (a method of indirectly assessing CNS functioning) which is useful in the study of putative CNS disturbances by assessing differences in neuroendocrine functioning between depressed adolescents and normal controls. Significant differences in peripheral measures of neuroendocrine variables between depressed teenagers and normal controls are postulated to reflect differences in CNS functioning between groups. These presumed CNS differences are then further proposed to reflect CNS dysregulation associated with the depressed state or trait.

As such, neuroendocrine strategies have inherent limitations. Measurements of monoamine metabolities in peripheral fluids are not exact reflections of monoamine metabolism in the CNS. Nor are they necessarily reflections of metabolism or function within the specific areas in the CNS putatively involved in depression. For example, only about 50% of dopamine metabolites measured in the urine and up to 30% of noradrenaline metabolites measured in plasma originate in the CNS (Kopin et al., 1983; Riddle et al., 1986). Even further removed from presumed CNS pathology are baseline and challenge paradigm evaluations of thyroid and growth hormone, cortisol, prolactin and other hormones. These studies are even more problematic as, in addition to the developmental changes in hormone secretions, the effect of diet, physical activity, baseline levels of arousal, difficulties in laboratory measurement and the generalized stress response may all influence the findings or interpretation (Johnson et al., 1992). However, given these limitations, such studies still advance our understanding of the neurobiology of depression in the adolescent population. These studies may also provide clues as to pharmacological treatments or physiological parameters that may aid in diagnosis, predicting treatment outcome or relapse.

This chapter will review the current literature on various neuroendocrine studies in adolescent depression. Wherever possible, it will also briefly summarize relevant physiological information about various endocrine systems and also, succinctly review selected adult findings in similar areas of investigation, to highlight similarities and differences to adolescent studies in findings where they occur.

Growth hormone

The hypothalamic–pituitary–growth hormone (HPGH) axis provides a good model for evaluating CNS functioning. The HPGH axis is under serotonin, histamine, acetylcholine, noradrenaline and dopamine control at the level of the hypothalamus (Checkley, 1980; Dieguez et al., 1987). Growth hormone (GH) release from the pituitary is regulated by the interplay of the above neurotransmitters, either by direct hypothalamic action or through their effect on intermediate compounds such as growth hormone-releasing hormone (GHRH) or somatostatin. Thus, disturbances in various parameters (basal secretion and stimulated secretion) of the HPGH axis, if found in adolescents with major depression, could be understood as reflecting disordered CNS neurotransmission, and would be best viewed as a downstream marker of CNS dysfunction.

GH secretion from the anterior pituitary is controlled by an intricate balance of CNS peptides, including somatostatin and GHRH. While somatostatin is widely distributed in the CNS, GHRH is primarily localized in the arcuate and ventromedial nuclei of the hypothalamus. GH is released from the pituitary in a pulsatile pattern, primarily in response to the interaction between somatostatin and GHRH, with somatostatin acting to decrease the GHRH-stimulated GH release by signalling the offset of each secretory phase. Additionally, adrenocortical hormones and corticotrophic releasing hormone (CRH) play a modulating role on somatotropin functioning. Furthermore, nocturnal GH secretion may be under different monoamine influences (primarily serotonergic) than daytime GH secretion (primarily noradrenergic). Thus, clinical evaluation of the GH axis may involve time-of-day effects, with studies conducted during the day to evaluate CNS control mechanisms that differ from those that are active nocturnally.

Basal GH secretion declines significantly with age. The daily pattern of GH secretion also changes, with significantly fewer GH peaks and a lower night-to-day secretory ratio occurring with increased age (Finkelstein et al., 1972; Zadik et al., 1985). Furthermore, recent studies have shown similar age effects in growth hormone-binding protein (GHBP) with progressive increases in GHBP during the first two decades of life (Daughaday & Trivedi, 1991) and decreases in GHBP beginning some time in the third decade of life (Hattori et al., 1991). The response of GH to GHRH, however, is relatively consistent throughout life, suggesting that GH basal secretion is due to changes in the secretory patterns of GHRH or somatostatin occurring at the hypothalamic level (Gelato & Merriam, 1986).

Basal growth hormone secretion

Basal GH secretory studies in depressed adults do not show consistent findings, with reports of nocturnal hypersecretion (Schilkrut et al., 1975), hypersecretion over a 24-hour period (Mendlewicz et al., 1985) and hypersecretion prior to sleep onset (Linkowski et al., 1987a,b). However, Jarrett et al. (1990) reported a reduction in GH secretion occurring during the initial 3 hours following sleep onset and Rubin et al. (1990) were not able to determine any differences in 24-hour secretory profiles between adult depressives and controls. In Rubin's study, however, both male and female depressives had much higher GH secretory peaks during the 24:00 to 02:00 hour period compared to controls. The lack of significance in this report may be due to the large standard deviation of serum GH values in the sample.

Studies of basal GH secretion in adolescent samples have also been contradictory. Kutcher et al. (1989, 1991) have reported that adolescents with major depressive disorder hypersecrete GH at night, with the period between 24:00 and 02:00 hours showing the greatest difference compared to normal controls. This difference occurred independently of sleep disturbances and the amount of slow-wave sleep prior to the first rapid eye movement (REM) period. These findings parallel those reported by Puig-Antich et al. (1984a,c) in depressed children. However, Dahl et al. (1992b) did not find significant differences in nocturnal GH secretion between depressed teenagers and controls. The reasons for the discrepant findings are not clear but may reflect different patient populations, different comorbid conditions or different study techniques.

Stimulated growth hormone secretion

Studies of GH stimulation in depressed adults have shown a variety of results, usually with blunting of GH reported to a variety of stimuli, including insulin-induced hypoglycaemia; clonidine, dextroamphetamine and desmethylimipramine (Sachar et al., 1971; Gregoire et al., 1977; Checkley et al., 1981; Charney et al., 1982; Siever et al., 1982; Amsterdam et al., 1987a,b). However, not all investigators have found this pattern in either insulin-induced hypoglycaemia (Koslow et al., 1982; Amsterdam & Maislin, 1991) or dextroamphetamine stimulation (Halbreich et al., 1982). Finally, a number of studies have demonstrated GH blunting to GHRH (Lesch et al., 1987; Risch et al., 1988), although not all investigators have demonstrated this (Eriksson et al., 1988; Thomas et al., 1989).

Studies of GH stimulation in depressed children have generally demonstrated GH blunting to both insulin-induced hypoglycaemia (Puig-Antich et al., 1984b) and clonidine challenge (Jensen & Garfinkel, 1990). On the other hand, Brambilla et al. (1994) failed to demonstrate a difference in GH response to either clonidine or GHRH in prepubertal children and normal controls. However, this study involved a very small sample size ($n = 9$ per cell). In the largest study to date, Ryan et al. (1994) found a blunted GH response to insulin-induced hypoglycaemia and GHRH but not clonidine.

In depressed adolescents, Jensen & Garfinkel (1990) demonstrated a similar blunted GH response to clonidine stimulation. Ryan et al. (1988) showed GH blunting in response to intramuscular desipramine challenge in teens with major depression, with maximal blunting found in the most suicidal of the depressives. Waterman et al. (1991) did not find any significant differences between depressed adolescents and normal controls in the GH response to dextroamphetamine. There are no reports to our knowledge of GH responses to GHRH in depressed teenagers.

Somatostatin and growth hormone

Somatostatin has been reported to be decreased in adult depressives but has not been evaluated in depressed adolescents (Rubinow et al., 1983; Agren & Lundqvist, 1984). However, low somatostatin levels fit the paradigm of high nocturnal GH secretion reported by Kutcher et al. (1989, 1991) and blunted GH responses to a variety of stimulation tests, including GHRH, on the basis of reduced daytime pituitary reserve secondary to nocturnal hypersecretion. In any case, although the studies are not conclusive, the available evidence suggests that depressed adolescents exhibit a disturbance of the GH axis that is probably reflective of CNS dysregulation, possibly primarily in the serotonin system (Kutcher et al., 1991).

Thyroid hormone

The hypothalamic–pituitary–thyroid axis has been studied in response to historical observations of mood alteration in the presence of thyroid disease and as a putative window on CNS processes in depression (Bauer & Whybrow, 1988; Joffe, 1990; Joffe & Sokolov, 1994). While there is a voluminous literature on the thyroid and adult mood disorders, the adolescent literature is more limited.

Neuronal regulation of the thyroid axis at the hypothalamic and pituitary level is not well understood in humans. On the basis of animal studies, it is known that the hypothalamus receives neuronal input via dopaminergic, noradrenergic and serotonergic pathways originating in the midbrain. In animals, dopamine seems to play a stimulatory role in thyroid-releasing hormone (TRH) secretion mediated through dopamine type 2 (D_2) receptors.

In the pituitary, noradrenergic fibres stimulate thyroid-stimulating hormone (TSH) release through activation of the adenylate cyclase system. Dopamine, somatostatin and glucocorticoids inhibit TSH release by decreasing pituitary response to TRH stimulation (Scanlon, 1991; Larsen & Ingbar, 1992). The role of the central serotonergic system has been reviewed elsewhere, with reports of both an inhibitory and stimulatory effect on TSH secretion (Krulich, 1982; Scanlon, 1991). This may reflect the plethora of serotonin receptor subtypes and the observation that different serotonin subsystems may have opposite physiological effects.

At the level of the thyroid gland, noradrenergic, cholinergic and peptidergic nerves innervate and terminate along the follicles and the blood vessels supplying them. Adrenergic fibres activate the adenylate cyclase system, promoting colloid droplet formation and thyroid hormone release. Noradrenaline stimulates thyroid hormone secretion under basal conditions and inhibits thyroid hormone release under conditions of TSH stimulation. Acetylcholine inhibits TSH-induced thyroid hormone secretion while vasoactive intestinal peptide (VIP), a peptidergic neurotransmitter, stimulates basal thyroid hormone secretion and potentiates thyroid hormone secretion in response to TSH. To complicate matters further, VIP and acetylcholine may coexist in nerves in the thyroid and the two may be released together when these nerves are stimulated. However, at this time, the exact role of neural mechanisms of thyroid regulation in depression remains unclear (Ahren, 1986; Larsen & Ingbar, 1992).

TSH response to TRH stimulation increased linearly with age in prepubertal children. Although present in both sexes, the increase by age was most marked in girls.

Overall developmental considerations may apply when assessing thyroid function in the paediatric or adolescent age group and this reinforces the necessity for utilizing age- and sex-matched controls. In a recent study by Garcia et al. (1991), TSH response to TRH stimulation increased linearly with age in prepubertal children. Although present in both sexes, the increase by age was most marked in girls.

Basal thyroid secretion

Numerous reports of basal thyroid hormone levels in adult depression exist in the literature with the most consistent findings being elevated (but within the euthyroid range) levels of thyroxine (T_4) in depressives relative to controls with or without an elevation of some measure of free T_4, thought to be secondary to increased T_4 production. Additionally, studies that have followed thyroid indices through the course of the depressive episode demonstrate a decrease in T_4 and/or free T_4 with antidepressant or electroconvulsive therapy. It has been reported that the magnitude of the decrease in T_4 has been correlated with the magnitude of the treatment response to these modalities (Dewhurst et al., 1968; Whybrow et al., 1972; Hatotami et al., 1974; Kirkegaard et al., 1975, 1977, 1990; Linnoila et al., 1979; Gold et al., 1981; Kirkegaard, 1981; Kirkegaard & Faber, 1981, 1991; Baumgartner et al., 1988; Joffe & Singer, 1990; Styra et al., 1991).

Thus, findings with respect to basal thyroid function in the adult literature suggest that major depression in this age group is associated with relative thyroid overactivity and that this resolves with recovery.

Reports of basal thyroid function in adolescent depression have been few.

Carstens et al. (1990) reported that basal values of free T_4 in patients and controls were within the normal laboratory range but were significantly elevated in depressed subjects compared to normal controls (Carstens et al., 1990). Sokolov et al. (1994) assessed baseline thyroid function in a group of adolescents with DSM-III-R (American Psychiatric Association, 1987) major depressive disorder and bipolar disorder, manic phase at the time of their first psychiatric hospitalization. Depressed and bipolar subjects were found to have a significantly elevated total T_4 when compared to normal controls. All thyroid indices, however, were within the normal range. Kutcher et al. (1991) described no significant group differences between depressed adolescents and normal controls in nocturnal secretions of T_4 or free T_4. Nocturnal TSH, however, was significantly elevated in about one-third of the depressed group, suggesting that a suprapituitary mechanism may be implicated in the findings of thyroid axis dysregulation. Finally, Sokolov et al. (1996) compared thyroid function in acutely ill depressed adolescents prior to and following treatment with desipramine 200 mg/day for 6 weeks. Similar to findings in adult depressives, desipramine responders were found to have larger pretreatment levels of T_4 and, with treatment, larger decreases were observed in responders versus nonresponders. Therefore, despite a more limited adolescent literature, findings within this age group also seem to support an association between overactivity of the thyroid axis and depression.

Stimulated TSH secretion

The TRH Stimulation Test has been used extensively in numerous studies of depressed adult patients and has been reviewed elsewhere (Kirkegaard, 1981; Loosen, 1986; Bauer & Whybrow, 1988; Joffe, 1990; Joffe & Sokolov, 1994). Despite some inconsistencies in methodology, a blunted TSH response to TRH stimulation has been generally noted in 25–30% of depressed adults. However, certain exogenous and endogenous factors are known to influence the TSH response to TRH. These factors include age, sex and caloric intake (Larsen & Ingbar, 1992). What is more, a blunted TSH response to TRH stimulation is not specific to major depression and may be found in individuals without psychiatric illness or in persons with anorexia nervosa (Gold et al., 1980), alcoholism (Loosen, 1986), borderline personality disorder (Garbutt et al., 1983) and schizophrenia (Baumgartner, 1986).

Although the pathophysiology is unclear, a blunted TSH response in depression may represent overactivity of the thyroid axis. This may be understood as follows. First, the TSH response to TRH is sensitive to feedback inhibition by elevated levels of thyroid hormone. A blunted TSH response may then result from the higher levels of T_4 in patients with depression (Joffe & Sokolov, 1994). Second, elevated TRH in the cerebrospinal fluid has been observed in patients with endogenous depression (Kirkegaard et al., 1979; Banki et al., 1988). Since repeated injections of TRH result in a progressively more blunted TSH response to TRH stimulation (Linnoila et al., 1979; Winokur et al., 1984), a blunted TSH response in depression may in fact arise from chronic exposure of the pituitary to excessive TRH secretion. This would presumably result in either receptor downregulation at the pituitary level, depletion of pituitary stores of TSH, or both. Therefore, it can be taken that studies of stimulated TSH secretion in depressed adults, along with studies of basal thyroid function, provide further evidence of an association of relative thyroid overactivity with depressive illness.

Investigations of the TSH response to TRH in adolescent depression are few. Chabrol et al. (1983) noted that only two out of 20 adolescent outpatients referred for suicidal ideation exhibited a blunted TSH response to TRH (Chabrol et al., 1983). However, none of these patients met *DSM-III* criteria for major depressive disorder. Kahn (1987) reported that 33% of adolescents with major depression showed TSH blunting compared to 43% of substance abusers and 17% of psychiatric controls (Kahn, 1987). In another study, Kahn (1988) reported that 37% of adolescents with major depressive disorder (MDD) showed a blunted TSH response to TRH. However, high rates of TSH blunting were again present in adolescents with substance abuse, conduct disorders and adjustment disorders. No significant differences were found between diagnostic groups. Brambilla et al. (1989) studied a small group of medication-free dysthymic children and adolescents. Compared to controls, dysthymics did not differ with respect to TSH responses to TRH stimulations. Carstens et al. (1990) reported that 17% of his study population showed a blunted TSH response to TRH, an insignificant difference from controls. Taken together, these findings suggest that up to one-third of adolescent depressions may show TSH blunting to TRH, a frequency comparable to findings in adults. The specificity and significance of these findings, however, remain unclear.

As in the adult literature, patterns of basal thyroid dysfunction in the absence of thyroid illness have been found in some adolescents with depression as well as other psychiatric disorders. With respect to TSH response to TRH stimulation, findings are inconsistent in children and adolescents. This may be due in part to variations in the dose of TRH employed as well as due to age and sex effects (Garcia et al., 1991). Furthermore, the evidence to date suggests that the TRH stimulation test is of little diagnostic utility in this age group. Of interest, however, is that in both basal secretion and in response to TRH stimulation, about one-third of adolescent depressives may show deranged TSH parameters. Whether this constitutes a specific subgroup or other particular features of adolescent depression remains a question for further study.

Cortisol

Interest in cortisol function has stemmed from observations suggestive of overactivity of the hypothalamic–pituitary–adrenal (HPA) axis and the role of this axis in the mediation of stress response in humans. This has led to speculation, followed by biochemical evidence (Heim et al., 1997), that early stressful life events predispose to the development of depression and anxiety disorders.

CRH, originating mainly in the paraventricular nucleus of the hypothalamus, causes an immediate and dose-dependent release of adrenocorticotrophic hormone (ACTH) from the anterior lobe of the pituitary, and is considered to be the major regulator of pituitary secretory ACTH activity (Rivier & Plotsky, 1986). Glucocorticoids, secreted from the adrenals under the influence of ACTH, and ACTH itself, exert a complicated pattern of inhibition on CRH-induced ACTH release through a variety of feedback mechanisms that exhibit both immediate and long-term effects (Axelrod & Reisine, 1984; Aguilera et al., 1987). Both acute and chronic stress intimately affect the HPA axis, with direct effects on the amount and patterns of circulating glucocorticoids (Hauger et al., 1989; Johnson et al., 1992). Additionally, studies of primates and other species have suggested that significant stresses occurring during the neonatal period may alter HPA responses to stress occurring later in life and that these responses may reflect developmentally induced susceptibility to depression (Thomas et al., 1968; Gold et al., 1988; Kalin & Takahashi, 1988). These features of the HPA axis, particularly its role in the stress response, make evaluation of its function in depression somewhat problematic as a variety of stressors that may be nonspecific to depression can affect the functioning of this system. However, given these caveats, the evaluation of the HPA axis in depression may have some utility.

Neurotransmitter regulation of CRH is exceedingly complex and involves the input of the cholinergic, catecholaminergic, indolaminergic systems and other substances such as γ-aminobutyric acid, histamine and angiotensin II (Pepper & Krieger, 1984; Johnson et al., 1992). Plasma ACTH and cortisol levels exhibit a diurnal variation; highest amounts are found during the early morning just prior to awakening and the nadir is located in the late afternoon or early evening. Episodic secretory spikes are superimposed on this daily rhythm (Krieger et al., 1971). This circadian rhythm of HPA activity is thought to be driven by an endogenous CNS pacemaker located in the suprachiasmatic nucleus of the hypothalamus (Moore & Eichler, 1972; Stokes & Sikes, 1987) and this pattern apparently persists throughout the life cycle.

A significant set of associations has been reported between blood and cerebrospinal fluid levels of cortisol and other neuroactive steroids, dehydroepiandrosterone (DHEA) and its sulphate (DHEA-S), taken within 10 minutes of each other from 62 subjects fitted with ventriculoperitoneal or lumbar peritoneal shunts for a variety of diagnoses (Guazzo et al., 1996). The proportional levels of cortisol and DHEA in the cerebrospinal fluid were around 5% of those in the blood, with the figure for DHEA-S being much lower (0.15%). There are also highly significant correlations between salivary and blood cortisol and DHEA, with salivary levels representing about 5% of those in the blood, similar to the cerebrospinal fluid (Goodyer et al., 1996). Whilst no studies have directly measured steroids in the brain, these latter findings provide some supportive evidence that peripheral salivary and blood measures, frequently used in studies of child and adolescent outpatients, reflect centrally active levels.

Basal cortisol secretion

Studies assessing cortisol activity in both urine and serum have described 24-hour hypersecretion of cortisol, with increased numbers of secretory episodes and a loss of the afternoon/early-evening nadir, with a resulting flattening of the circadian curve in many but not all adult depressives. Additionally, a phase advance of 1–3 hours in the early-morning cortisol rise has been described (Doig et al., 1966; Sachar et al., 1973; Stokes et al., 1984; Linkowski et al., 1987a,b). Although some studies report contradictory results, this increase in cortisol secretion may be secondary to an increased incidence of daily ACTH pulses (Holaday et al., 1977; Kirkegaard & Carroll, 1980; Nasr et al., 1983; Follenius et al., 1987; Mortola et al., 1987; Krishnan et al., 1990). Cortisol and CRH levels in the cerebrospinal fluid have been reported as elevated in some adult depressives (Traskman et al., 1980; Nemeroff et al., 1984; Stokes et al., 1984) and, while not all investigators have demonstrated this phenomenon (Jimmerson et al., 1980), it can be generally concluded that many depressed adults show perturbations in the basal tone of the HPA axis during the depressive episode.

Studies of basal cortisol secretion in adolescent depressives are few. Dahl et al. (1989) failed to find any significant differences in the 24-hour cortisol secretory profiles of teenage depressives compared to normal controls. In another report using a similar study methodology, Dahl et al. (1991) found that some depressed adolescents showed significantly elevated cortisol levels compared to normal controls but only near the time of sleep onset. Of interest is that most of these differences were accounted for by a subgroup of suicidal inpatient adolescents. Kutcher et al. (1991) were not able to demonstrate any significant differences in nocturnal cortisol secretion between adolescent depressives and normal controls. Similarly, Kutcher & Marton (1989), using a neuroendocrine day-study paradigm, reported that elevated afternoon cortisol secretion occurred in less than one-third of depressed adolescents. Goodyer et al. (1996) demonstrated evening cortisol hypersecretion and morning DHEA hyposecretion in a sample of 82 8–16-year-olds with major depression compared to controls. A close examination of the relations between the comorbid characteristics of these depressed subjects and the hormone profiles showed that cortisol hypersecretion was significantly associated with 'double depression', i.e. major depressive disorder superimposed on chronic dysthymia (Herbert et al., 1996). In addition, depressive disorders comorbid for acute phobic or panic disorder were not associated with any endocrine abnormality. Finally, Goodyer & Herbert also noted that higher evening cortisol/DHEA ratios were specifically associated with obsessive-compulsive disorder amongst this already depressed population. These influences of comorbidity on the associations with cortisol and DHEA abnormalities suggest that specific endocrine disturbances may be associated with different clinical subtypes of major depression in adolescent depressives. Although there was a psychiatric and community control group in these latter studies, analysing comorbid subtypes results in small sample sizes and these findings require replication. Ideally, future studies should compare depressive subtypes categorized by nondepressive comorbid disorder with psychiatric comparison groups of dysthymia, panic, phobic and obsessive-compulsive disorder presenting as the primary condition. This would determine the effect of major depression on the hormone functions of interest in the presence of other psychopathologies.

Finally, Kutcher et al. (1991) reported that fewer than 10% of depressed adolescents showed any individual abnormalities in their nocturnal cortisol secretion profiles. Those who demonstrated nocturnal hypersecretion showed elevated serum cortisol levels beginning early in the morning, suggesting a phase advance in the cortisol secretory rise. Of interest is that these patients were characterized by severe guilty ruminations, suggesting a differential HPA effect in those depressed teenagers who exhibited quasidelusional symp-tomatology. Goodyer et al. (1991), using sophisticated mathematical modelling, demonstrated in a small number of subjects that 24-hour cortisol rhythms may change following recovery from depression. Although no control groups were available for comparison, these findings taken together suggest that subtle alterations in baseline cortisol secretion may occur in adolescent depressives, particularly in subgroups, but further detailed investigations are needed. A striking feature of studies examining the correlations between steroids and psychopathology is the nonlinear nature of the relationship. In the main the greatest magnitude of the association is seen with extreme hormone values. It is possible that the majority of studies to date on adolescent popula-tions have had insufficient power to take this into account.

DHEA has been overlooked in studies of psychopathology and requires further investigation. Both DHEA and its sulphate, DHEA-S, are classified amongst a group of steroids known as neurosteroids because they can be synthesized *de novo* in the CNS (Kroboth et al., 1999). Indeed, concentrations of these two hormones are considerably higher in the brain than in any other organ. Unlike cortisol in humans, DHEA and DHEA-S concentrations vary with age and with gender. DHEA concentrations decline from the first few months of life until 5 years of age and then rise rapidly from age 7 in girls and around 9 in boys, until concentrations reach their peak between the ages of 20 and 30 years of age. Levels begin to decline again from the fourth decade, reaching their nadir by the sixth. DHEA and DHEA-S have been noted to have wide systemic activity in both health and disease, including preliminary sugges-tions of antidepressant action, perhaps most apparent in major depressives with cortisol hypersecretion (Kroboth et al., 1999; Wolkowitz et al., 1999). DHEA is measurable by salivary assay and should be a part of hormone assays in further studies of depressed adolescents.

HPA axis stimulation tests
Dexamethasone suppression test
Nonsuppression of serum cortisol by dexamethasone has frequently been reported in depressed adults (Carroll et al., 1976, 1981; Brown & Shuey, 1980; Brown, 1984; Rubin et al., 1987), but the specificity of this test has not been demonstrated and recent investigations have raised questions about the exact mechanism of dexamethasone suppression itself (Miller et al., 1992). For example, cortisol escape from suppression by dexamethasone is strongly pre-dicted by the additive effects of basal cortisol levels and increasing age (Maes et

al., 1991). Current consensus, however, is that the dexamethasone suppression test (DST) has little diagnostic validity (Holsboer et al., 1986) in this population. An application, however, may be in its use as a state marker which has utility in assessing treatment response. For example, adult depressives who show initial DST nonsuppression tend to show DST normalization on clinical recovery. Persistent DST nonsuppression despite symptomatic improvement may be associated with impending relapse (Greden et al., 1983; Holsboer et al., 1983; Kutcher & Shulman, 1985; Grunhaus et al., 1987; Charles et al., 1989; Coryell, 1990).

Studies of DST secretion in children with depression have not shown HPA axis dysregulation of a similar nature to adult depressives (Puig-Antich et al., 1989; Birmaher et al., 1992b; Dahl et al., 1992a).

Studies of DST in adolescent depressives have been the most frequently reported of the neuroendocrine evaluations in this population, partly perhaps because of the ease in administration of this procedure. Unfortunately, most reports do not provide an assessment of basal cortisol dynamics so the relationship of the DST to basal cortisol secretion cannot be evaluated. Taken as a whole, DST nonsuppression in depressed adolescents has been reported in 14–80% (Extein et al., 1982; Robbins et al., 1982, 1983; Targum & Capodanno, 1983; Ha et al., 1984; Klee & Garfinkel, 1984; Freeman et al., 1985; Emslie et al., 1987; Evans et al., 1987; Kahn, 1987; Woodside et al., 1987; Appleboom-Fondu et al., 1988; Casat & Powell, 1988; Birmaher et al., 1992a; Dahl et al., 1992a) of the populations studied. Taken together, the findings from these studies suggest that the sensitivity of the DST for adolescent depression is about 40%. Specificity estimates are difficult to determine because of a lack of studies utilizing nondepressed psychiatric control groups. Thus, the DST in adolescent depression has little diagnostic utility.

However, there are suggestions that the DST may identify specific subgroups of adolescent depressives. Chabrol et al. (1983), Robbins & Alessi (1985) and Kutcher et al. (1991) have reported that DST nonsuppression in depressed teenagers is associated with suicidal behaviours. These findings are similar to those reported by Pfeffer et al. (1991) in a sample of prepubertal patients in whom suicidality, regardless of a depressive diagnosis, was associated with DST nonsuppression. Whether this test indeed defines a depressive subtype with a distinct HPA axis difference or is merely a reflection of the increased arousal or physiological stresses associated with a suicide attempt, however, is not clear.

Furthermore, Dahl et al. (1992a), in a carefully controlled study of 27 adolescents with MDD and 34 normal controls, were not able to demonstrate any relationship between DST nonsuppression and suicidality; thus, this issue awaits further study. The same is true for other potential DST nonsuppression and specific MDD characteristics such as clinical status, endogenous MDD subtype and premorbid state (Robbins et al., 1983; Klee & Garfinkel, 1984; Freeman et al., 1985; Dahl et al., 1992a).

Finally, at this time, there has been insufficient evaluation of the potential utility of the DST in the assessment of the state aspects of adolescent depression. Specifically, it is not clear whether persistence of DST nonsuppression concurrently with symptomatic recovery is predictive of early relapse, if DST nonsuppression predicts response to antidepressant treatment, or if DST non-suppression may be a marker of a specific subtype of depressive disorder in teenagers.

Corticotrophin-releasing hormone stimulation test

CRH stimulates ACTH release from the anterior pituitary. Studies of adult depressives have shown blunted ACTH responses to CRH regardless of serum cortisol levels (Gold et al., 1984; Amsterdam et al., 1987a,b; Holsboer et al., 1987). These findings, taken together with elevated serum cortisol level and elevated cerebrospinal fluid CRH levels, suggest that a suprapituitary abnormality is responsible for the derangements of the HPA axis found in adult depressives.

CRH stimulation studies have been reported in childhood but only to a limited extent in adolescent depressives. Dorn et al. (1996) found no difference in ACTH response to ovine CRH stimulation in depressed versus nondepressed adolescents. Thus, the HPA axis has been insufficiently studied in terms of the CNS control factors of HPA axis functioning in depressed teens. As would be expected, findings are similar to the basal cortisol secretions and DST nonsuppression studies, in that CRH stimulation of ACTH in adolescents has not shown the same blunting of ACTH reported in adult studies.

Certainly, CNS developmental factors or repeated depressive episode effects may be at issue in comparing adolescent to adult HPA findings. Accumulated stress effects associated with increasing age may impair HPA axis responses to new stressors, thus older patients may show DST nonsuppression when younger patients do not. Furthermore, some evidence exists to suggest that, even when age effects are controlled for, patients with repeated episodes of depression show increased basal cortisol secretion (Halbreich et al., 1984) and abnormal cortisol responses to the combined DST-CRH stimulation tests (von Bardeleben & Holsboer, 1991), compared to same-age normal controls. This suggests that multiple depressive episodes may themselves impact on the functioning of the HPA axis.

The findings of HPA axis abnormalities in studies of adolescent depressives may reflect either an age-dependent CNS maturational issue or the lack of previous depressive episodes. In this scenario, the HPA axis abnormalities found in studies of adult depressives may not reflect primary abnormalities of CNS function, but may instead be the consequences of repeated episodes of the illness on the CNS modulating the subsequent responsiveness of the HPA axis to further undesirable events. This raises the question: are there HPA vulnerabilities to psychopathology that precede the onset of disorder that are not accounted for by other known risk factors? A recent study by Goodyer and colleagues suggests that there may be such an endocrine parameter (Goodyer et al., 2000a). In a prospective study of 181 adolescents at high risk for psychopathology and with no previous history of major depression, early-morning (0800 h) hypersecretion of DHEA predicted subsequent onset of major depression at 12-month follow-up independently of high levels of depressive symptoms or recent life events. Closer inspection of the patterns of hormone secretion suggests that it may be subjects with extreme daily levels of DHEA and/or cortisol measured at 0800 h that are 'at risk' for subsequent episodes (Goodyer et al., 2000b).

This study suggests that closer attention needs to be paid to both the timing and the characteristics of the hormone measurement if putative causal associations are to be made between endocrine abnormalities and psychopathology. The traditional observation of loss of evening diurnal rhythm may be the wrong parameter for investigating causal effects. This emphasis on morning hypersecretion appears to be in agreement with the types of cortisol differences found when (morning) levels are compared in human infants and young children in 'stressful' and 'nonstressful' circumstances (Gunnar et al., 1997; Gunnar, 1998). A striking difference, however, is that the hormone abnormalities in Goodyer's study show a total lack of association between extreme hormone values and recent life events. The implication is that the origins of these endocrine risks are indeed from the early environment, as suggested by the developmental literature, or from genetic influences, or both. There is very little known about the genetics of steroids other than preliminary data that there are genetic effects on cortisol secretory patterns (Linkowski et al., 1993). There is also some preliminary evidence suggesting a familial aggregation of abnormal response to the combined DST-CRH stimulation test in the first-degree relatives of adult probands with a history of major depression (Holsboer et al., 1995).

Overall, these findings suggest that there are sufficient reasons to presume a potential aetiological effect for HPA axis abnormalities in the onset of first-episode major depression in adolescents. This also raises the possibility that the abnormalities seen in cortisol secretion during a first episode in an adolescent (which occur less frequently than in adult depressives, most of whom have recurrent disorder) may be more likely in such 'hormone-vulnerable' subjects. This speculative hypothesis, whilst intriguing, requires considerable further investigation before firm conclusions about the causative role of HPA axis abnormalities can be reached.

Melatonin

Interest in the retino–hypothalamic–pineal axis in depression has stemmed from clinical observations that depressed patients exhibit sleep disruptions and the hypothesis that these may reflect disturbances of sleep regulation associated with pineal gland light/dark cycle rhythmicity. Further interest stems from the observation that melatonin secretion may be negatively correlated with cortisol secretion and is under noradrenergic control. Melatonin has then been investigated as a potential indicator of both noradrenergic disturbance in depression and of circadian rhythm disturbance.

The pineal gland is a small CNS structure embryologically derived from cells of the roof of the third ventricle and located posterior to the posterior commisure. In mammals the pineal receives light input originating from the retina. The retina transmits information pertaining to light and dark via the retinohypothalamic tract to the superchiasmatic nucleus (SCN) which is located in the hypothalamus and acts as a pacemaker for a number of hormonal rhythms. Fibres from the SCN descend to regulate preganglionic neurons in the lateral cell columns of the spinal cord. From there, postganglionic nerves from the superior cervical ganglia (SCG) convey impulses to the pineal gland (Reiter, 1989; Reichlin, 1992). Without light input, pineal rhythms will persist as driven by the SCG pacemaker. However, these rhythms are no longer synchronized to the light/dark cycle. There is evidence that, in some vertebrates, the pineal also receives input from thalamic, hypothalamic, epithalamic and mesencephalic areas (Reiter, 1989).

Melatonin is the principal hormonal product of pineal gland metabolism (Lerner et al., 1958). Melatonin secretion follows a diurnal profile, with most being synthesized and secreted at night. The principal rate-limiting step is the conversion of serotonin to melatonin by serotonin-N-acetyl transferase (NAT). Concentrations of NAT may vary 100-fold within a few minutes and parallel the rise and fall in plasma melatonin content. Melatonin synthesis and secretion are activated within minutes of exposure to darkness and stopped by exposure to light. The route by which melatonin reaches the pituitary and hypothalamus is not entirely clear (Reiter, 1989; Reichlin, 1992) but, at least in primates, it is secreted into the blood.

At the site of the pituitary and hypothalamus, melatonin appears to have antigonadotrophic effects, but the precise end-organ effects of this hormone are still not completely known. Administration of melatonin is known to inhibit luteinizing hormone (LH) and GH secretion. Behavioural effects of melatonin include sleepiness, increased REM sleep, increased number of α-waves on electroencephalogram (Reichlin, 1992) and possibly an exacerbation of dysphoric symptoms in patients with existing depression (Carman et al., 1976).

Neurotransmitter regulation of melatonin secretion is complicated and not fully understood. The nocturnal rise in melatonin is mediated by noradrenaline via sympathetic innervation from the superior cervical ganglia. Adrenergic receptors of α_1 and β_1 subtypes are found on pinealocyte membranes. In rats and probably humans, the number of pineal β_1-adrenoreceptors increase at night. This is most likely to allow maximal stimulation of melatonin production by noradrenaline. In humans, the role of pineal α-adrenergic receptors is unclear but may serve to potentiate β-adrenergic-mediated melatonin production.

Other factors that may affect pineal melatonin production include extremely low-frequency electrical fields, age, sex, calcification of the pineal, stress and ingestion of alcohol (Wilson, 1988; Reiter, 1989; Reichlin, 1992). Developmentally, melatonin secretion decreases with advanced age (Reiter, 1989). Animal studies suggest that nighttime, more reliably than daytime, melatonin secretion is blunted by stress and that this mechanism appears to be mediated by cortisol (Joshi et al., 1986; Troiani et al., 1987, 1988).

Basal melatonin secretion

In the investigation of the role of melatonin in adult depression, plasma melatonin, urinary melatonin and urinary 6-sulphatoxy melatonin (its principal metabolite) have been studied. However, studies have generally included patients taking a variety of medications, used different assay techniques, and did not use closely matched controls, which makes generalization from them problematic.

Some cross-sectional data suggest a 'low melatonin syndrome' in depressive illness characterized by low nocturnal melatonin secretion inversely related to serum cortisol levels. Claustrat et al. (1984) reported that depressed adults showed a significantly lower amplitude of nocturnal melatonin secretion than controls. Nair et al. (1984) found that depressed patients had a nocturnal melatonin secretion that was lower in magnitude when compared to normal controls. Beck-Friis et al. (1985) reported significant correlations between a low maximal nocturnal melatonin secretion and retardation symptoms, parental loss before the age of 17 and absence of suicidal behaviour in depressed adults. Thompson et al. (1985) and McIntyre et al. (1986) described lower nocturnal melatonin secretion in depressives than controls. Wetterberg et al. (1979, 1982, 1984) reported that adult depression was characterized by an elevation of nocturnal cortisol secretion and a decrease in melatonin secretion. Taken together, these studies suggested that disturbances in the HPA axis and the retino–hypothalamic–pineal axis in depression might be of diagnostic utility and may provide evidence of noradrenergic disturbance associated with depression.

However, recently, contradictory studies have been reported. Thompson et al. (1988) and Rubin et al. (1992) were not able to demonstrate lower nocturnal or 24-hour melatonin secretion in depressed adults compared to rigorously matched normal controls. Their studies suggest that the previous findings of decreased secretion of melatonin in depression may be related to factors that influence melatonin secretion independent of the presence of depressive illness. Studies of melatonin secretion using a within-subjects design and comparing basal melatonin secretion during the depressed state to the recovery state have been contradictory. Mendlewicz et al. (1980) and Wetterberg et al. (1984) found no differences, while Halbreich et al. (1981) reported that depressives improving with desipramine treatment showed lower daytime melatonin levels than nonresponders. Thompson et al. (1985) and Kennedy & Brown (1992), however, reported elevated serum melatonin and urinary 6-sulphatoxy melatonin in desipramine-treated depressives, suggesting a direct noradrenergic stimulation of melatonin secretion secondary to desipramine effect. Thus, at this time the understanding of basal melatonin secretion in adult depression is not yet clear.

Melatonin: longitudinal studies

Several investigators have studied melatonin secretion in patients in the acutely ill and later in the recovered phase. Mendlewicz et al. (1980) reported results on four depressed women whose 24-hour pattern of melatonin secretion was measured first in the depressed phase and then after treatment with amitriptyline (Mendlewicz et al., 1980). Nocturnal melatonin secretion was not elevated from daytime secretion in three of the depressed women in either the depressed or well state. Halbreich et al. (1981) studied 32 patients with a Research Diagnostic Criteria diagnosis of endogenous depression treated with desipramine. After treatment, responders had significantly lower levels of daytime melatonin compared to nonresponders. In both responders and nonresponders, serum melatonin levels correlated negatively with plasma levels of desipramine. Responders showed a stronger negative correlation than nonresponders. This inverse relationship was thought to be related to pineal β-adrenergic receptor downregulation in response to desipramine. Patients studied by Wetterberg et al. (1984) on remission showed no difference in nocturnal melatonin secretion compared to the acutely ill phase. Souetre et al. (1989) investigated melatonin secretion in 16 endogenously depressed patients and 15 of them in the recovered (antidepressant-treated) state. In the recovered state, nocturnal peaks of TSH and melatonin were significantly lower in depressed patients versus normals.

Investigations of basal melatonin secretion in the child and adolescent literature are few. Cavallo et al. (1987) studied a group of five early/mid pubertal and four prepubertal depressed boys who were medication-free for at least 3 months and 10 male controls. Mean 24-hour and mean overnight plasma melatonin were significantly lower in depressed patients versus normal. In contrast, Shafii et al. (1990) compared overnight melatonin secretion in a sample of 6–16-year-olds with primary and secondary depression. Overnight melatonin secretion was found to be elevated in patients with primary depression but not in those with secondary depression or normal controls. Waterman et al. (1992) studied nocturnal 6-hydroxymelatonin sulphate levels in 31 prepubertal depressed subjects and showed no significant difference in this melatonin metabolite compared to normal controls. Recently, Shafii et al. (1996) attempted to replicate their findings in drug-free children and adolescents with depression in dim light conditions. Overall, nocturnal melatonin secretion was elevated in depressed subjects compared to controls while asleep but not while awake in dim light conditions.

Given the limited literature regarding children and adolescents, it is difficult to determine the significance of the retino–hypothalamic–pineal axis in this population. Nevertheless, recent trends in the adult literature seem to question previous hypotheses of a 'low melatonin syndrome' in relation to noradrenergic hypoactivity in depression in well-controlled studies. Clearly, more rigorously controlled studies need to be performed in the adolescent population as well.

Nonsystem-specific challenge tests

A number of studies in adult depressives, using a variety of probes, have evaluated a multiple hormone response to CNS stimulation (Checkley, 1980;

Siever & Uhde, 1984; Lopez-Ibor et al., 1989;). Although Ryan et al. (1992) have demonstrated decreased cortisol and increased prolactin responses to 5-hy-droxy-L-tryptophan (L-5HTP) in children with major depressive disorder compared to normal controls, no similar studies have been reported in adolescents. Ryan et al. (1992) argue that their findings are consistent with CNS serotonin dysregulation in this population. More recently, Birmaher et al. (1997) found that decreased cortisol and increased prolactin responses to L-5HTP were also found in children who were not depressed but at risk of depression compared to low-risk normal controls (with the prolactin findings limited to female at-risk children).

Cholinergic system challenges have only rarely been reported in the depress-ed adolescent population. Sitaram et al. (1987) found that some young family members of depressed adults, particularly those with a history of depression themselves, showed a supersensitive REM sleep response to cholinergic stimu-lation that was similar to that found in adults with major depressions. How-ever, Dahl et al. (1989), using an arecoline challenge, failed to note this response in depressed children, while McCracken et al. (1991) reported an exaggerated REM response to scopolamine in depressed adolescents. Given the confusing state of reported results in baseline REM sleep measures of adolescent depress-ives (Kutcher & Williamson, 1992), however, these findings are difficult to evaluate.

Other peripheral markers

Rogeness et al. (1985) measured whole-blood serotonin and platelet mono-amine oxidase activity in depressed children and found no differences in comparison to normal controls. In an uncontrolled study of inpatient adoles-cents, Modai et al. (1989), reported lower serotonin platelet uptake V_{max} values in affectively disordered teenagers compared to other psychiatric disorders, including schizophrenia. Imipramine binding studies conducted in depressed adolescents have shown increased B_{max} of imipramine binding (Carstens et al., 1988). Furthermore, Carstens et al. (1988) have reported increased α_2- and β-adrenoceptors on platelets and lymphocytes respectively in depressed teens and children. The difficulties with these studies, apart from lack of replication, is that the peripheral models (platelet and lymphocyte) may not accurately reflect CNS receptor functioning and studies of these parameters in adult depressives are inconsistent and contradictory (Elliott, 1991). Thus, the inter-pretation of these studies awaits further investigation.

Studies of peripheral metabolites of noradrenaline, which is thought to be implicated in the aetiology of depression, have been few. Kahn (1987) and de Villiers et al. (1989) found no differences in peripheral measures of 3-methoxy-4-hydroxyphenylglycol (MHPG: a metabolite of noradrenaline) in depressed teens compared to normal controls. However, since only about 10–30% of peripheral MHPG may have its origin in the CNS, measurement of peripheral MHPG is unlikely to reflect accurately possible subtle changes that may be occurring centrally.

Thus, the various studies of peripheral measures noted above stand in relative isolation and at this time contribute little towards our understanding of the neurobiology of adolescent depression. Obviously, further systematic assessment of these aspects is necessary.

Conclusions

Neuroendocrine studies of adolescent depression are still in their early formative years. They developed from similar approaches which had been utilized in studies of depressed adults and have moved from a simple attempt to replicate adult findings to a systematic study of the uniquely adolescent neuroendocrine aspects of depression. As such, they are still in the pioneering stage and require much further detailed investigation of a variety of neuroendocrine systems before their utility in determining aetiology or defining state or trait markers of the disorder is realized. However, to date, the accumulated evidence suggests that, neurobiologically at least, adolescent and adult depressions are not identical. The neuroendocrine perturbations which have been identified in adolescent depressives have generally been consistent with dysregulations within CNS serotonin system functioning, with less evidence of noradrenergic system dysfunctioning. This suggests, in part, that depressions onsetting in the adolescent years may primarily reflect dysregulation of the indolamine system, with noradrenergic and possibly cholinergic disturbances arising later in the course of the illness, as a result of repeated episodes, or a reflection of the CNS effect of antidepressant medications, or a result of CNS-regulated homeostatic activity. While the serotonin hypothesis of depression is not new (Coppen et al., 1972; Murphy et al., 1978), it may be best studied in the adolescent population at the time when the disorder first occurs, and the subjects and the psychopathology are relatively free from the confounds noted above. Further research into the multiple aspects of serotonergic functioning should be a priority in the future development of neuroendocrine strategies in the assessment of adolescent depression.

REFERENCES

Agren, H. & Lundqvist, G. (1984). Low levels of somatostatin in human CSF mark depressive episodes. *Psychoneuroendocrinology*, **9**, 233–48.

Aguilera, G., Millan, M. A., Hauger, R. L. et al. (1987). Corticotropin-releasing factor receptors: distribution and regulation in brain, pituitary, and peripheral tissues. *Annals of the New York Academy of Science*, **12**, 48–66.

Ahren, B. (1986). Thyroid neuroendocrinology: neural regulation of thyroid hormone secretions. *Endocrine Reviews*, **7**, 149–55.

American Psychiatric Association (1987). *Diagnostic and Statistical Manual of Mental Disorders*, 3rd edn revised. Washington, DC: American Psychiatric Association.

Amsterdam, J. D. & Maislin, G. (1991). Hormonal responses during insulin-induced hypoglycemia in manic-depressed, unipolar depressed, and healthy control subjects. *Journal of Clinical Endocrinology and Metabolism*, **73**, 541–8.

Amsterdam, J. D., Maislin, G., Winokur, A. et al. (1987a). Pituitary and adrenocortical responses to the ovine corticotropin releasing hormone in depressed patients and healthy volunteers. *Archives of General Psychiatry*, **44**, 775–81.

Amsterdam, J. D., Schweizer, E. & Winokur, A. (1987b). Multiple hormonal responses to insulin induced hypoglycemia in depressed patients and normal volunteers. *American Journal of Psychiatry*, **144**, 170–5.

Appleboom-Fondu, J., Kerkhofs, M. & Mendlewicz, J. (1988). Depression in adolescents and young adults: polysomnographic and neuroendocrine aspects. *Journal of Affective Disorders*, **14**, 35–40.

Axelrod, J. & Reisine, T. D. (1984). Stress hormones: their interaction and regulation. *Science*, **224**, 452.

Banki, C. M., Bissette, G. Arato, M. & Nemeroff, C. B. (1988). Elevation of immunoreactive CSF TRH in depressed patients. *American Journal of Psychiatry*, **145**, 1526–31.

Bauer, M. S. & Whybrow, P. C. (1988). Thyroid hormones and the central nervous system in affective illness: interactions that may have clinical significance. *Integrated Psychiatry*, **6**, 75–100.

Baumgartner, A. (1986). Central thyroid stimulation in severely in depressed, manic and schizophrenic patients. *Biological Psychiatry*, **21**, 417–21.

Baumgartner, A., Graf, K. J., Kurten, I. & Meinhold, H. (1988). The hypothalamic–pituitary–thyroid axis in psychiatric patients and healthy subjects: parts 1–4. *Psychiatry Research*, **24**, 271–331.

Beck-Friis, J., Kjellman, B. F., Aperia, B. et al. (1985). Serum melatonin in relation to clinical variables in patients with major depressive disorder and a hypothesis of a low melatonin syndrome. *Acta Psychiatrica Scandinavica*, **71**, 319–30.

Birmaher, B., Dahl, R. E., Ryan, N. D. et al. (1992a). Dexamethasone suppression test in adolescent outpatients with major depressive disorder. *American Journal of Psychiatry*, **149**, 1040–5.

Birmaher, B., Ryan, N. D., Dahl, R. E. et al. (1992b). Dexamethasone suppression test in children with major depressive disorder. *Journal of the American Academy of Child and Adolescent*

Psychiatry, **31**, 291–7.

Birmaher, B., Kaufman, J., Brent, D. A. et al. (1997). Neuroendocrine response to 5-hydroxy-L-tryptophan in prepubertal children at high risk of major depressive disorder. *Archives of General Psychiatry*, **54**, 1113–19.

Brambilla, F., Musetti, C., Tacchini, C. et al. (1989). Neuroendocrine investigation in children and adolescents with dysthymic disorders: the DST, TRH and clonidine tests. *Journal of Affective Disorders*, **17**, 279–84.

Brambilla, F., Guareschi-Cazzullo A., Tacchini C. et al. (1994). Growth hormone response to growth hormone releasing hormone and to clonidine stimulation in peripubertal patients with major depressive disorder. *Biological Psychiatry*, **36**, 51–6.

Brown, W. (1984). Use of dexamethasone suppression test in depression. In *Neurobiology of Mood Disorder*, ed. R. Post & O. Ballanger. London: Williams & Wilkins.

Brown, W. A. & Shuey, I. (1980). Response to dexamethasone and subtype of depression. *Archives of General Psychiatry*, **37**, 747–51.

Buchanan, C. M., Eccles, J. S. & Becker, J. B. (1992). Are adolescents the victims of raging hormones: evidence for activational effects of hormones on moods and behavior at adolescence. *Psychological Bulletin*, **111**, 62–107.

Carman, J. S., Post, R. M., Buswell, R. & Goodwin, F. K. (1976). Negative effects of melatonin on depression. *American Journal of Psychiatry*, **133**, 1181–6.

Carroll, B. J., Curtis, G. C. & Mendels, J. (1976). Neuroendocrine regulation in depression. II. Discrimination of depressed from non-depressed patients. *Archives of General Psychiatry*, **33**, 1051–8.

Carroll, B. J., Feinberg, M., Greden, J. F. et al. (1981). A specific laboratory test for the diagnosis of melancholia. Standardization, validation, and clinical utility. *Archives of General Psychiatry*, **38**, 15–22.

Carstens, M. E., Engelbrecht, A. H., Russell, V. A. et al. (1988). Biological markers in juvenile depression. *Psychiatry Research*, **23**, 77–88.

Carstens, M. E., Taljaard, J. F. F. & Van Zyl, A. M. (1990). The adrenoceptor and endocrine abnormalities in juvenile depression. *South African Medical Journal*, **77**, 360–3.

Casat, C. & Powell, K. (1988). Utility of the dexamethasone suppression test in children and adolescents with major depressive disorder. *Journal of Clinical Psychiatry*, **49**, 390–3.

Cavallo, A., Holt, K. G., Hejazi, M. S. et al. (1987). Melatonin circadian rhythm in childhood depression. *Journal of the American Academy of Child and Adolescent Psychiatry*, **26**, 395–9.

Chabrol, H., Claverie, J. & Moron, P. (1983). DST, TRH test, and adolescent suicide attempts. *American Journal of Psychiatry*, **140**, 265.

Charles, G. A, Schittecatte, M., Rush, A. J. et al. (1989). Persistent cortisol non-suppression after clinical recovery predicts symptomatic relapse in unipolar depression. *Journal of Affective Disorders*, **17**, 271–8.

Charney, D. S., Heninger, G. R. & Ternberg, D. E. (1982). Adrenergic receptor sensitivity in depression: effects of clonidine in depressed patients and healthy subjects. *Archives of General Psychiatry*, **39**, 290–4.

Charney, D., Southwick, S., Delgado, P. et al. (1990). Current status of the receptor sensitivity hypothesis of antidepression action: implications for the treatment of severe depression. In *Pharmacotherapy of Depression*, ed. J. Amsterdam, pp. 13–34. Basel: M. Dekker.

Checkley, S. A. (1980) A neuroendocrine study of adrenoceptor function in endogenous depression. *Acta Psychiatrica Scandinavica*, **61** (Suppl. 280), 211–17.

Checkley, S. A., Slade, A. P. & Shur, E. (1981) Growth hormone and other responses to clonidine in patients with endogenous depression. *British Journal of Psychiatry*, **138**, 51–5.

Christie, K., Burke, J., Reiger, D. et al. (1989). Epidemiologic evidence for early onset of mental disorders and higher risk of drug abuse in young adults. *American Journal of Psychiatry*, **145**, 971–5.

Claustrat, B., Chazot, G., Brun, J. et al. (1984). A chronobiological study of melatonin and cortisol secretion in depressed subjects: plasma melatonin, a biochemical marker in major depression. *Biological Psychiatry*, **19**, 1215–28.

Coppen, A. (1967) The biochemistry of affective disorders. *British Journal of Psychiatry*, **113**, 1237–64.

Coppen, A., Prange, A. J., Whybrow, P. C. & Noguera, R. (1972). Abnormalities of indoleamines in affective disorder. *Archives of General Psychiatry*, **26**, 474–8.

Coryell, W. (1990). DST abnormality as a predictor of course in major depression. *Journal of Affective Disorders*, **19**, 163–9.

Dahl, R. E., Puig-Antich, J., Ryan, N. D. et al. (1989) Cortisol secretion in adolescents with major depressive disorder. *Acta Psychiatrica Scandinavica*, **80**, 18–26.

Dahl, R. E., Ryan, N. D., Puig-Antich, J. et al. (1991). 24 hour cortisol measures in adolescents with major depression: a controlled study. *Biological Psychiatry*, **30**, 25–36.

Dahl, R. E., Kaufman, J., Ryan, N. et al. (1992a). The dexamethasone suppression test in children and adolescents: a review and a controlled study. *Biological Psychiatry*, **32**, 109–26.

Dahl, R. E., Ryan, N. D., Williamson, D. et al. (1992b). Regulation of sleep and growth hormone in depressed adolescents. *Journal of the American Academy of Child and Adolescent Psychiatry*, **31**, 615–21.

Daughaday, O. O. & Trivedi, O. O. (1991). Clinical aspects of GH binding proteins. *Acta Endocrinologica*, **124**, 27–32.

de Villiers, A., Russell, V. & Carstens, M. (1989). Noradrenergic function and hypothalamic–pituitary–adrenal axis activity in adolescents with major depressive disorder. *Psychiatry Research*, **27**, 101–9.

Dewhurst, K. E., El Kabir, D. T., Exley, D. et al. (1968). Blood levels of TSH, protein-bound iodine and cortisol in schizophrenia and affective states. *Lancet*, **ii**, 1160–2.

Dieguez, C., Page, M. D. & Scanlon, M. F. (1987). Growth hormone neuroregulation and its alteration in disease states. *Clinical Endocrinology*, **27**, 109–43.

Doig, R. J., Mummery, R. V., Wills, M. R. & Elkes, A. (1966). Plasma cortisol levels in depression. *British Journal of Psychiatry*, **112**, 1263–7.

Dorn, L. D., Burgess, E. S., Susman, E. J. *et al.* (1996). Response to oCRH in depressed and nondepressed adolescents: does gender make a difference? *Journal of the American Academy of Child and Adolescent Psychiatry*, **35**, 764–73.

Elliott, J. M. (1991). Peripheral markers in affective disorders. In *Biological Aspects of Affective*

Disorders, ed. R. W. Horton & C. L. E. Katona, pp. 95–144. London: Academic Press.

Emslie, G., Weinberg, W., Rush, A. J. et al. (1987). Depression and dexamethasone suppression testing in children and adolescents. *Journal of Child Neurology*, **2**, 31–7.

Eriksson, E., Balldin, J., Linstedt, G. & Modigh, K. (1988). Growth hormone responses to the alpha 2 adrenoceptors against guanifacine and to growth hormone releasing hormone in depressed patients and controls. *Psychiatry Research*, **26**, 59–67.

Evans, D., Nemeroff, C., Haggerty, J. & Perdersen, C. (1987). Use of the dexamethasone suppression test with DSM-III criteria in psychiatrically hospitalized adolescents. *Psychoneuroendocrinology*, **12**, 203–9.

Extein, I., Rosenberg, G., Pottash, A. & Gold, M. (1982). The dexamethasone suppression test in depressed adolescents. *American Journal of Psychiatry*, **139**, 1617–19.

Finkelstein, J. W., Roffwarg, H. P., Boyar, R. M. et al. (1972). Age related change in the twenty-four-hour spontaneous secretion of growth hormone. *Journal of Clinical Endocrinology and Metabolism*, **35**, 665–70.

Follenius, M., Simon, C., Brandenberger, G. & Lenzi, P. (1987). Ultradian plasma corticotropin and cortisol rhythms. Time series analysis. *Journal of Endocrinological Investigations*, **10**, 261–6.

Freeman, L., Pozanski, E., Grossman, J. et al. (1985). Psychotic and depressed children: a new entity. *Journal of the American Academy of Child Psychiatry*, **24**, 195–202.

Garbutt, J. C., Loosen, P. T., Tipermas, A. & Prange, A. J. Jr (1983). The TRH test in patients with borderline personality disorder. *Psychiatry Research*, **9**, 107–13.

Garcia, M. R., Ryan, N. D., Rabinovitch, H. et al. (1991). Thyroid stimulating hormone response to thyrotropin in prepubertal depression. *Journal of the American Academy of Child Adolescent Psychiatry*, **30**, 398–406.

Gelato, M. C. & Merriam, G. R. (1986). Growth hormone releasing hormone. *Annual Review of Physiology*, **48**, 569–91.

Gold, M. S., Pottash, A. L. & Martin, D. et al. (1980). Thyroid stimulating hormone and growth hormone responses to thyrotropin-releasing hormone in anorexia nervosa. *Journal of Psychiatric Medicine*, **10**, 51–7.

Gold, M. S., Pottash, A. L. & Extein, I. (1981). Hypothyroidism and depression. 1. Evidence from complete thyroid function evaluation. *Journal of the American Academy of Child and Adolescent Psychiatry*, **245**, 1919–22.

Gold, P. W., Chrousos, G., Kellner, C. et al. (1984). Psychiatric implications of basic and clinical studies with corticotropin-releasing factor. *American Journal of Psychiatry*, **141**, 619–27.

Gold, P. W., Goodwin, F. K. & Chrousos, G. P. (1988). Clinical and biochemical manifestations of depression. *New England Journal of Medicine*, **319**, 348–420.

Goodyer, I., Herbert, J., Moor, S. & Altham, P. (1991). Cortisol hypersecretion in depressed school-aged children and adolescents. *Psychiatry Research*, **37**, 237–44.

Goodyer, I., Herbert, J., Altham, P. M. E. et al. (1996). Adrenal secretion during major depression in 8- to 16-year-olds, I. Altered diurnal rhythms in salivary cortisol and dehydroepiandrosterone (DHEA) at presentation. *Psychological Medicine*, **26**, 245–56.

Goodyer, I. M., Herbert, J. Tamplin, A. et al. (2000a). First episode major depression in adolescents: affective, cognitive and endocrine characteristics of risk status and predictors of onset. *British Journal of Psychiatry*, **176**, 142–9.

Goodyer, I. M., Herbert, J., Tamplin, A. et al. (2000b). Recent life events, cortisol and DHEA in the onset of major depression amongst 'high-risk' adolescents. *British Journal of Psychiatry* (in press).

Greden, J. F., Gardner, R., King, D. et al. (1983). Dexamethasone suppression tests in antidepressant treatment of melancholia – the process of normalization and test–retest reproducibility. *Archives of General Psychiatry*, **40**, 493–500.

Gregoire, F., Branman, G., DeBuck, R. & Corvilain, J. (1977). Hormone release in depressed patients before and after recovery. *Psychoneuroendocrinology*, **2**, 303–12.

Grunhaus, L., Zelnik J., Albala, A. A. et al. (1987). Serial dexamethasone suppression tests in depressed patients treated only with electroconvulsive therapy. *Journal of Affective Disorders*, **13**, 233–40.

Guazzo, E. P., Kirkpatrick, P. J., Goodyer, I. M. et al. (1996). Cortisol, dehydroepandrosterone (DHEA), and DHEA sulfate in the cerebrospinal fluid of man: relation to blood levels and the effects of age. *Journal of Clinical Endocrinology and Metabolism*, **81**, 3951–60.

Gunnar, M. R. (1998). Quality of early care and buffering of neuroendocrine stress reactions: potential effects on the developing human brain. *Preventative Medicine*, **27**, 208–11.

Gunnar, M. R., Tout, K., de Haan, M. et al. (1997). Temperament, social competence, and adrenocortical activity in preschoolers. *Developmental Psychobiology*, **31**, 65–85.

Ha, H., Kaplan, S. & Foley, C. (1984). The dexamethasone suppression test in adolescent psychiatric patients. *American Journal of Psychiatry*, **141**, 421–3.

Halbreich, U., Weinberg, U., Stewart, J. et al. (1981). An inverse correlation between serum levels of desmethylimipramine and melatonin-like immunoreactivity in DMI-responsive depressives. *Psychiatry Research*, **4**, 109–13.

Halbreich, U., Sachar, E., Asnis, G. et al. (1982). Growth hormone response to dextroamphetamine in depressed patients and normal subjects. *Archives of General Psychiatry*, **39**, 189–92.

Halbreich, U., Asnis, G. M,. Zumoff, B. et al. (1984). Effect of age and sex on cortisol secretion in depressives and normals. *Psychiatry Research*, **13**, 221–19.

Hatotami, N., Nomura, J., Yamaguchi, T. et al. (1974). Clinical and experimental studies of the pathogenesis of depression. *Psychoneuroendocrinology*, **2**, 115–30.

Hattori, N., Kurahachi, H., Ikekubo, K. et al. (1991). Effects of sex and age on serum GH binding protein levels in normal adults. *Clinical Endocrinology*, **35**, 295–7.

Hauger, R. L., Risch, S. C., Millan, M. et al. (1989). Corticotropin-releasing factor regulation of the pituitary–adrenal axis and the central nervous system. In *Psychiatry: psychobiological foundations of clinical psychiatry*, vol. 3, ed. R. Michels, pp. 1–22. New York: J. B. Lippincott.

Heim C., Owens, M. J., Plotsky, P. M. & Nemeroff, C. B. (1997). 1. Endocrine factors in the pathophysiology of mental disorders. Persistent changes in corticotropin releasing factor systems due to early life stress: relationship to the pathophysiology of major depression and post-traumatic stress disorder. *Psychopharmacology Bulletin*, **33**, 185–92.

Heninger, G. & Charney, D. (1987). Mechanism of action of antidepressant treatments: implications for the etiology and treatment of depressive disorders. In *Psychopharmacology: the third generation of progress*, ed. H. Meltzer, pp. 535–44. New York: Raven Press.

Herbert, J., Goodyer, I. M., Altham, P. M. E. et al. (1996). Adrenal secretion and major depression in 8 to 16 year olds, II. Influence of co-morbidity at presentation. *Psychological Medicine*, **26**, 257–63.

Holaday, J. W., Martinez, H. M. & Natelson, B. H. (1977). Synchronized ultradian cortisol rhythms in monkeys: persistence during corticotropin infusion. *Science*, **198**, 56–8.

Holsboer, F., Steiger, A. & Maier, W. (1983). Four cases of reversion to abnormal dexamethasone suppression test response as indicator of clinical relapse: a preliminary report. *Biological Psychiatry*, **18**, 911–16.

Holsboer, F., Phillip, M., Steiger, A. & Gerken, A. (1986). Multisteriod analysis after DST in depressed patients – a controlled study. *Journal of Affective Disorders*, **10**, 241–9.

Holsboer, F., Gerken, A. & Stalla, G. K. (1987). Blunted aldosterone and ACTH release after human CRH administration in depressed patients. *American Journal of Psychiatry*, **144**, 229–31.

Holsboer, F., Lauer, C. J., Schreiber, W. et al. (1995). Altered hypothalamic–pituitary–adrenocortical regulation in healthy subjects at high familial risk for affective disorders. *Neuroendocrinology*, **62**, 340–7.

Jarrett, D. B., Miewald, J. M. & Kupfer, D. J. (1990). Recurrent depression is associated with a persistent reduction in sleep-related growth hormone secretion. *Archives of General Psychiatry*, **47**, 113–18.

Jensen, J. B. & Garfinkel, B. D. (1990). Growth hormone dysregulation in children with major depressive disorder. *Journal of the American Academy of Child and Adolescent Psychiatry*, **29**, 295–301.

Jimmerson, D. C., Post, R. M., von Kommen, D. P. et al. (1980). Cerebrospinal fluid cortisol levels in depression and schizophrenia. *American Journal of Psychiatry*, **137**, 979–80.

Joffe, R. T. (1990). A perspective on the thyroid and depression. *Canadian Journal of Psychiatry*, **35**, 754–8.

Joffe, R. T. & Singer, W. (1990). The effect of tricyclic antidepressants on basal thyroid hormone levels in depressed patients. *Pharmacopsychiatry*, **23**, 67–9.

Joffe, R. T. & Sokolov, S.T.H. (1994). Thyroid hormones, the brain and affective illness. *Critical Reviews in Neurobiology*, **8**, 45–63.

Johnson, O. E., Kamilaris, T. C., Chrousos, G. P. & Gold, P. W. (1992). Mechanisms of stress: a dynamic overview of hormonal and behavioural homeostasis. *Neuroscience and Biobehavioural Reviews*, **16**, 115–30.

Joshi, B. N., Troiani, M. E., Milin, J. et al. (1986). Adrenal-mediated depression of N-acetyltransferase activity and melatonin levels in the rat pineal gland. *Life Science*, **38**, 1573–80.

Kahn, A. U. (1987). Biochemical profile of depressed adolescents. *Journal of the American Academy of Child and Adolescent Psychiatry*, **26**, 873–8.

Kahn, A. U. (1988). Sensitivity and specificity of TRH stimulation test in depressed and nondepressed adolescents. *Psychiatry Research*, **25**, 11–17.

Kalin, N. H. & Takahashi, L. K. (1988). Altered hypothalamic–pituitary–adrenal regulation in animal models of depression. In *The Hypothalamic–Pituitary–Adrenal Axis*, ed. P. W. Gold & G. Chrousos, pp. 67–70. New York: Raven Press.

Kennedy, S. H. & Brown, G. M. (1992). Effect of chronic antidepressant treatment with adinazolam and desipramine on melatonin output. *Psychiatry Research*, **43**, 177–85.

Kirkegaard, C. (1981). The thyrotropin response to thyrotropin-releasing hormone in endogenous depression. *Psychoneuroendocrinology*, **6**, 189–212.

Kirkegaard, C. & Carroll, B. J. (1980) Dissociation of TSH adrenocortical disturbances in endogenous depression. *Psychiatry Research*, **3**, 253–64.

Kirkegaard, C. & Faber, J. (1981). Altered serum levels of thyroxine, triiodothyronines and diiodothyronines in endogenous depression. *Acta Endocrinologica (Copenhagen)*, **96**, 199–207.

Kirkegaard, C. & Faber, J. (1991). Free thyroxine and 3,3′,5′-triiodothyronine levels in cerebrospinal fluid in patients with endogenous depression. *Acta Endocrinologica (Copenhagen)*, **124**, 166–7.

Kirkegaard, C., Bjorum, N., Cohn, D. et al. (1977). Studies in the influence of biogenic amines and psychoactive drugs on the prognostic value of the TRH stimulation test in endogenous depression. *Psychoneuroendocrinology*, **2**, 131–6.

Kirkegaard, C., Norlern, N., Lauridsen, U. B. et al. (1975). Protirelin stimulation test and thyroid function during treatment of depression. *Archives of General Psychiatry*, **32**, 1115–18.

Kirkegaard, C., Faber, L., Hummer, L. & Rogowski, P. (1979). Increased levels of TRH in cerebrospinal fluid from patients with edogenous depression. *Psychoneuroendocrinology*, **4**, 227–35.

Kirkegaard, C., Korner, A. & Faber, J. (1990). Increased production of thyroxine and inappropriately elevated serum thyrotropin in levels in endogenous depression. *Biological Psychiatry*, **27**, 472–6.

Klee, S. & Garfinkel, B. (1984). Identification of depression in children and adolescents: the role of the dexamethasone suppression test. *Journal of the American Academy of Child and Adolescent Psychiatry*, **23**, 410–15.

Kopin, I. J., Gordon, E. K. & Jimmerson, D. (1983). Relation between plasma and cerebrospinal fluid levels of 3-methoxy-4-hydroxyphenethyleneglycol. *Science*, **291**,73–6.

Koslow, S. H., Stokes, P. E., Mendels, J. et al. (1982). Insulin tolerance test: human growth hormone response and insulin resistance in primary unipolar depressed, bipolar depressed and control subjects. *Psychological Medicine*, **12**, 45–55.

Krieger, D. T., Allen, W., Rizzo, F. & Krieger, H. P. (1971). Characterization of the normal temporal pattern of plasma corticosteroid levels. *Journal of Clinical Endocrinology and Metabolism*, **32**, 266–84.

Krishnan, K. R. R., Ritchie, J. C., Saunders, W. et al. (1990). Nocturnal and early morning secretion of ACTH and cortisol in humans. *Biological Psychiatry*, **38**, 47–57.

Kroboth, P. D., Salek, F. S., Pittenger, A. L., Fabian, T. J. & Frye, R. F. (1999). DHEA and DHEA-S: a review. *Journal of Clinical Pharmacology*, **39**, 327–48.

Krulich, L. (1982). Neurotransmitter control of thyrotropin secretion. *Neuroendocrinology*, **35**, 139–47.

Kutcher, S. P. & Marton, P. (1989). Parameters of adolescent depression. *Psychiatric Clinics of North America*, **12**, 895–918.

Kutcher, S. & Shulman, K. (1985). Dexamethasone suppression test normalization and treatment outcome in elderly depressives. *British Journal of Psychiatry*, **147**, 453–4.

Kutcher, S. P. & Williamson, P. (1992). REM latency in endogenously depressed adolescents. *British Journal of Psychiatry*, **161**, 399–402.

Kutcher, S. P., Williamson, P., Silverberg, J. et al. (1989). Nocturnal growth hormone secretion in depressed older adolescents. *Journal of the American Academy of Child and Adolescent Psychiatry*, **27**, 751–4.

Kutcher, S. P., Malkin, D., Silverberg, J. et al. (1991). Nocturnal cortisol, thyroid stimulating hormone and growth hormone secreting properties in depressed adolescents. *Journal of American Academy of Child Adolescent Psychiatry*, **30**, 407–14.

Larsen, P. & Ingbar, S. (1992). The thyroid gland. In *Williams Textbook of Endocrinology*, ed. J. Wilson & D. Foster, pp. 257–87. Philadelphia: W. B. Saunders Company.

Lerner, A. B., Case, J. D., Takahashi, Y. et al. (1958). Isolation of melatonin, the pineal gland factor that lightens melanocytes. *Journal of the American Chemistry Society*, **80**, 2587.

Lesch, K. P., Erb, A., Pfuller, H. et al. (1987). Attenuated growth hormone response to growth hormone-releasing hormone in major depressive disorder. *Biological Psychiatry*, **22**, 1495–9.

Linkowski, P., Mendlewicz, J., Kerkhofs, M. et al. (1987a). 24-hour profile of adrenocorticotropin, cortisol and growth hormone in major depressive illness: effect of antidepressant treatment. *Journal of Clinical Endocrinology and Metabolism*, **65**, 141–51.

Linkowski, P., Mendlewicz, J., LeClerq, R. et al. (1987b). The 24-hour profile of ACTH and cortisol in major depressive illness. *Journal of Clinical Endocrinology and Metabolism*, **61**, 429–38.

Linkowski, P., Van Onderbergen, A., Kerkhofs, M. et al. (1993). Twin study of the 24-h cortisol profile: evidence for genetic control of the human circadian clock. *American Journal of Physiology*, **264**, E173–81.

Linnoila, M., Lamberg, B. A., Rosberg, G. et al. (1979). Thyroid hormones and TSH, prolactin and LH responses to repeated TRH and LRH injections in depressed patients. *Acta Psychiatrica Scandinavica*, **59**, 536–44.

Loosen, P. T. (1986). Thyroid function in affective disorders and alcoholism. *Endocrinology Metabolic Clinics of North America*, **17**, 55–82.

Lopez-Ibor, J. J., Saiz-Ruiz, J. & Iglesias, L. M. (1989). Neuroendocrine challenges in the diagnosis of depressive disorders. *British Journal of Psychiatry*, **154** (Suppl. 4), 73–6.

Maes, M., Minner, B., Suy, E. et al. (1991). Cortisol escape from suppression by dexamethasone during depression is strongly predicted by basal cortisol hypersecretion and increasing age combined. *Psychoneuroendocrinology*, **16**, 295–310.

McCracken, J. T., Poland, R. E., Tondo, L. et al. (1991). Cholinergic dysregulation in adolescent depression: preliminary comparisons with adult depression. *Proceedings of the 144th Annual Meeting of the American Psychiatric Association*. New Orleans: American Psychiatric Association.

McIntyre, I. M., Judd, F. K., Norman, T. R. & Burrows, G. D. (1986). Plasma melatonin concentrations in depression. *Australian and New Zealand Journal of Psychiatry*, **20**, 381–3.

Mendlewicz, J., Branchey, L., Weinberg, U. et al. (1980). The 24 hour pattern of plasma melatonin in depressed patients before and after treatment. *Community Psychopharmacology*, **4**, 49–55.

Mendlewicz, J., Linkowski, P., Kerhofs, M. et al. (1985). Diurnal hypersecretion of growth hormone in depression. *Journal of Clinical Endocrinology and Metabolism*, **60**, 505–12.

Miller, A., Spencer, R. & Pulera, M. (1992). Adrenal steroid receptor activation in rat brain and pituitary following dexamethasone: implications for the dexamethasone suppression test. *Biological Psychiatry*, **32**, 850–69.

Modai, I., Apter, A., Meltzer, M. et al. (1989). Serotinin uptake by platelets of suicidal and aggressive adolescent psychiatric inpatients. *Neuropsychobiology*, **21**, 9–13.

Moore, R. Y. & Eichler, V. B. (1972). Loss of a circadian adrenal corticosterone rhythm following suprachiasmatic lesions in the rat. *Brain Research*, **42**, 201–6.

Mortola, J. F., Liu, J. H., Gillin, J. C. et al. (1987). Pulsatile rhythms of adrenocorticotropin (ACTH) and cortisol in women with endogenous depression: evidence for increased ACTH pulse frequency. *Journal of Endocrinology and Metabolism*, **65**, 962–8.

Murphy, D. L., Campbell, I. C. & Costa, J. L. (1978). The brain serotonergic system in the affective disorders. *Progress in Neuropsychopharmacology*, **2**, 5–31.

Nair, N. P., Hariharasubramanian, N. & Pilapil, C. (1984). Circadian rhythm of plasma melatonin in endogenous depression. *Progress in Neuropsychopharmacolology and Biological Psychiatry*, **8**, 715–18.

Nasr, S. J., Pandey, G., Altman, E. G. et al. (1983). Symptom profile of patients with positive DST: a pilot study. *Biological Psychiatry*, **18**, 571–4.

Nemeroff, C. B., Widerlov, E., Bissett, G. et al. (1984). Elevated concentrations of CSF corticotropin-releasing factor-like immunoreactivity in depressed patients. *Science*, **226**, 1342–4.

Pepper, G. M. & Krieger, D. T. (1984). Hypothalamic–pituitary–adrenal abnormalities in depression: their possible relation to central mechanisms regulating ACTH release. *Neurobiology of Mood Disorders*, **16**, 245–70.

Pfeffer, C., Stokes, P. & Shindledecker, R. (1991). Suicidal behaviour and hypothalamic–pituitary–adrenocortical axis indices in child psychiatric inpatients. *Biological Psychiatry*, **29**, 909–17.

Post, R. M. & Weiss, S. R. (1997). Emergent properties of neural systems: how focal molecular neurobiological alterations can affect behavior. *Developments in Psychopathology*, **9**, 907–29.

Post, R., Rubinow, D. & Ballenger, J. (1986). Conditioning and sensitisation in the longitudinal course of affective illness. *British Journal of Psychiatry*, **149**, 191–201.

Puig-Antich, J., Goetz, R., Davies, M. et al. (1984a). Growth hormone secretion in prepubertal major depressive children. II. Sleep related plasma concentrations during a depressive episode. *Archives of General Psychiatry*, **41**, 463–6.

Puig-Antich, J., Novacenko, H., Davies, M. et al. (1984b). Growth hormone secretion in prepubertal children with major depression. III. Response to insulin-induced hypoglycemia after recovery from a depressive episode and in a drug-free state. *Archives of General Psychiatry*, **41**, 471–5.

Puig-Antich, J., Novancenko, H., Davies, M. et al. (1984c). Growth hormone secretion in prepubertal major depressive children: I. *Archives of General Psychiatry*, **41**, 455–60.

Puig-Antich, J., Dahl R. E., Ryan, N. D. et al. (1989). Cortisol secretion in prepubertal children with major depressive disorder. Episode and recovery. *Archives of General Psychiatry*, **41**, 455–60.

Reichlin, S. (1992) Neuroendocrinology. In *Williams Textbook of Endocrinology*, 8th edn, ed. J. D. Wilson & D. W. Foster, pp. 135–220. Philadelphia: W. B. Saunders Company.

Reiter, R. J. (1989). The pineal and its indole products: basic aspects and clinical applications. In *The Brain as an Endocrine Organ*, ed. M. P. Cohen & P. P. Foa, pp. 96–149. New York: Springer-Verlag.

Riddle, M. A., Anderson, G. M. & McIntosh, S. (1986). Cerebrospinal fluid monoamine precursor and metabolitic levels in children treated for leukemia: age and sex effects and individual variability. *Biological Psychiatry*, **21**, 69–72.

Risch, S. C., Ehlers, C. & Janowsky, D. S. (1988). Human growth hormone releasing factor infusion effects on plasma growth hormone in affective disorder patients and normal controls. *Peptides*, **9**, 45–8.

Rivier, C. & Plotsky, P. M. (1986). Mediation by corticotropin releasing factor (CRF) or adenohypophysial hormone secretion. *Annual Review of Physiology*, **48**, 475.

Robbins, D. & Alessi, N. (1985). Suicide and the dexamethasone suppression test in adolescence. *Biological Psychiatry*, **20**, 107–10.

Robbins, D., Alessi, N., Yanchyshyn, G. & Colfer, M. (1982). Preliminary report on the dexamethasone suppression test in adolescents. *American Journal of Psychiatry*, **22**, 467–9.

Robbins, D., Alessi, N., Yanchyshyn, G. & Colfer, M. (1983). The dexamethasone suppression test in psychiatrically hospitalized adolescents. *Journal of the American Academy of Child and Adolescent Psychiatry*, **22**, 467–9.

Rogeness, G. A., Mitchell, E. L., Custer, G. J. & Harris, W. R. (1985). Comparison of whole blood serotonin and platelet MAO in children with schizophrenia and major depressive disorder. *Biological Psychiatry*, **20**, 270–5.

Rubin, R. T., Poland, R. E., Lesser, I. M. et al. (1987) Neuroendocrine aspects of primary endogenous depression. *Archives of General Psychiatry*, **44**, 328–36.

Rubin, R., Poland, R. & Lesser, I. (1990). Neuroendocrine aspects of primary endogenous depression X serum growth hormone measures in patients and matched control subjects. *Biological Psychiatry*, **27**, 1065–82.

Rubin, R. T., Heist, E. K., McGeoy, S. S. et al. (1992). Neuroendocrine aspects of primary endogenous depression. XI. Serum melatonin measures in patients and matched control subjects. *Archives of General Psychiatry*, **49**, 558–67.

Rubinow, D. R., Gold, P. W. & Post, R. M. (1983). CSF somatostatin in affective illness. *Archives of General Psychiatry*, **40**, 403–12.

Ryan, N. D., Puig-Antich, J. & Rabinovich, H. (1988). Growth hormone response to desmethylimipramine in depressed and suicidal adolescents. *Journal of Affective Disorders*, **15**, 323–37.

Ryan, N. D., Birmaher, B. & Perez, J. et al. (1992). Neuroendocrine response to L-5hydroxytryptophan challenge in prepubertal major depression. *Archives of General Psychiatry*, **49**, 843–51.

Ryan, N. D., Dahl, R. E., Birmaher, B. et al. (1994). Stimulatory tests of growth hormone secretion in prepubertal major depression: depressed versus normal children. *Journal of the American Academy of Child and Adolescent Psychiatry*, **33**, 824–33.

Sachar, E. J., Finkelstein, J. & Hellman, L. (1971). Growth hormone responses in depressive illness. I. Response to insulin tolerance test. *Archives of General Psychiatry*, **25**, 263–9.

Sachar, E. J., Hellman, L., Roffwarg, H. P. et al. (1973). Disrupted 24-hour patterns of cortisol secretion in psychiatric depression. *Archives of General Psychiatry*, **28**, 19–24.

Scanlon, M. R. (1991). Neuroendocrine control of thyrotropin secretion. In *Werner and Ingbar's The Thyroid: a fundamental and clinical text*, 6th edn, ed. L. E. Braverman & R. D. Utiger, pp. 230–56. Philadelphia: J. B. Lippincott.

Schilkrut, R., Chandra, D. & Oswald, M. (1975). Growth hormone release during sleep and with thermal stimulation in depressed patients. *Neuropsychobiology*, **1**, 70–4.

Shafii, M., Foster, M. B., Greenberg, R. A. et al. (1990). The pineal gland and depressive disorders in children and adolescents. In *Biological Rhythms, Mood Disorders, Light Therapy, and the Pineal Gland*, ed. M. Shafii & S. L. Shafii, pp. 97–116. Washington, DC: American Psychiatric Press.

Shafii, M., MacMillan, D. R., Key, M. P. et al. (1996). Nocturnal serum melatonin profile in major depression in children and adolescents. *Archives of General Psychiatry*, **53**, 1009–13.

Siever, L. & Davis, K. (1985). Overview: towards a dysregulation hypothesis of depression. *American Journal of Psychiatry*, **142**, 1017–31.

Siever, L. J. & Uhde, T. W. (1984). New studies and perspectives on the noradrenergic receptor system in depression: effects of the alpha-adrenergic agonist clonidine. *Biological Psychiatry*, **19**, 131–56.

Siever, L. J., Uhde, T. W., Silberman, L. K. et al. (1982). Growth hormone response to clonidine as a probe of noradrenergic receptor responsiveness in affective disorder patients and controls. *Psychiatry Research*, **6**, 171–83.

Sitaram, N., Dube, S., Keshavan, M. et al. (1987). The association of supersensitive cholinergic REM-induction and affective illness within pedigrees. *Journal of Psychiatric Research*, **21**, 487–97.

Sokolov, S. T. H., Kutcher, S. P. & Joffe, R. T. (1994). Baseline thyroid indices in adolescent depression and bipolar disorder. *Journal of the American Academy of Child and Adolescent Psychiatry*, **33**, 469–75.

Sokolov, S. T. H., Kutcher, S. P. & Joffe, R. T. (1996). Changes with thyroid hormone levels associated with desipramine response in adolescent depression. *Progress in Neuropsychopharmacology and Biological Psychiatry*, **20**, 1053–63.

Souetre, E., Salvati, E., Belugou, J. L. et al. (1989) Circadian rhythms in depression and recovery: evidence for blunted amplitude as the main chronobiological abnormality. *Psychiatry Research*, **3**, 263–78.

Stokes, P. E. & Sikes, C. R. (1987). Hypothalamic–pituitary–adrenal axis in affective disorders. In *Psychopharmacology, The Third Generation of Progress*, vol. 59, ed. H. M. Melter, pp. 589–607. New York: Raven Press.

Stokes, P. E., Stoll, P. M., Koslow, S. H. et al. (1984). Pretreatment DST and hypothalamic–pituitary–adrenocortical function in depressed patients and comparison groups. *Archives of General Psychiatry*, **41**, 257–67.

Styra, R., Joffe, R. & Singer, W. (1991). Hyperthyroxinemia in major affective disorders. *Acta Psychiatrica Scandinavica*, **83**, 61–3.

Targum, S. & Capodanno, A. (1983). The dexamethasone suppression test in adolescent psychiatric inpatients. *American Journal of Psychiatry*, **140**, 589–91.

Thomas, E. B., Levine, S. & Arnold, W. J. (1968). Effects of maternal deprivation and incubator rearing on adrenocortical activity in the adult rat. *Developmental Psychobiology*, **1**, 21–3.

Thomas, R., Beer, R., Harris, B. et al. (1989). GH responses to growth hormone releasing factor in depression. *Journal of Affective Disorders*, **16**, 133–7.

Thompson, C., Mezey, G., Corn, T. et al. (1985). The effect of desipramine upon melatonin and cortisol secretion in depressed and normal subjects. *British Journal of Psychiatry*, **147**, 389–93.

Thompson, C., Franey, C., Arendt, J. & Checkley, S. A. (1988). A comparison of melatonin secretion in depressed patients and normal subjects. *British Journal of Psychiatry*, **152**, 260–5.

Traskman, L., Tybring, G., Asberg, M. et al. (1980). Cortisol in the CSF of depressed and suicidal patients. *Archives of General Psychiatry*, **37**, 761–7.

Troiani, M. E., Oaknin, S., Reiter, R. J. et al. (1987). Depression in rat pineal *N*-acetyltransferase activity and melatonin content produced by a hind leg saline injection is time and darkness dependent. *Journal of Pineal Research*, **4**, 185–95.

Troiani, M. E., Reiter, R. J., Vaughan, M. K. et al. (1998). The depression in rat pineal melatonin production after saline injection at night may be elicited by corticosterone. *Brain Research*, **450**, 18–24.

von Bardeleben, U. & Holsboer. F. (1991). Effect of age on the cortisol response to human CRH in depressed patients pretreated with dexamethasone. *Biological Psychiatry*, **29**, 1042–50.

Waterman, G. S., Ryan, N. D., Puig-Antich, J. et al. (1991). Hormonal responses to dextroamphetamine in depressed and normal adolescents. *Journal of the American Academy of Child and Adolescent Psychiatry*, **30**, 415–22.

Waterman, G., Ryan, N. & Percel, I. et al. (1992). Nocturnal urinary excretion of 6-hydroxy melatonin sulphate in prepubertal major depressive disorder. *Biological Psychiatry*, **31**, 582–90.

Weissman, M. & Klerman, G. (1992). Depression: current understanding and changing trends. *American Review of Public Health*, **13**, 319–39.

Wetterberg, L., Beck-Friis, J., Aperia, B. & Petterson, U. (1979). Melatonin/cortisol ratio in depression (letter). *Lancet*, **2**, 1361.

Wetterberg, L., Aperia, B., Beck-Friis, I. et al. (1982). Melatonin and cortisol levels in psychiatric illness (letter). *Lancet*, **2**, 100.

Wetterberg, L., Beck-Friis, J., Kjellman, B. F. & Ljunggren, J. G. (1984). Circadian rhythms in melatonin and cortisol secretion in depression. *Advances in Biochemical Psychopharmacology*, **39**, 197–205.

Whybrow, P. C., Coppen, A., Prange, A. I. Jr et al. (1972). Thyroid function and the response to liothyronine in depression. *Archives of General Psychiatry*, **26**, 242–5.

Wilson, B. W. (1988). Chronic exposure to ELF fields may induce depression. *Bioelectromagnetics*, **9**, 195–205.

Winokur, A., Caroff, S. N., Amsterdam, A. I & Maislin, G. (1984). Administration of thyrotropin-releasing hormone at weekly intervals in a diminished thyrotropin response. *Biological Psychiatry*, **19**, 695–702.

Wolkowitz, O. M., Reus, V. I., Keebler, A. et al. (1999). Double-blind treatment of major depression with dehydroepidandrosterone. *American Journal of Psychiatry*, **156**, 646–9.

Woodside, B., Brownstone, D. & Fisman, S. (1987). The dexamethasone suppression test and the children's depression inventory in psychiatric disorders in children. *Canadian Journal of Psychiatry*, **32**, 2–4.

Zadik, Z., Chalew, S. A., McCarter, R. et al. (1985). The influence of age on the 24-hour integrated concentration of growth hormone in normal individuals. *Journal of Clinical Endocrinology and Metabolism*, **60**, 513–16.

10

Suicidal behaviour in adolescents

Erik Jan de Wilde, Ineke C. W. M. Kienhorst and
René F. W. Diekstra

Introduction

Discussing the topic of suicidal behaviour without discussing the context of
depression is probably as precarious as is discussing depression without the
possible implication of suicidality. The two phenomena share aetiology and
epidemiology, and are overlapping but also distinct, since the majority of
depressed adolescents do not attempt or commit suicide, and not every suicidal
adolescent is depressed. Although in some other psychiatric disorders (e.g.
schizophrenia, anxiety disorders, personality disorders) there is certainly an
increased risk for suicide, depression clearly stands out in this respect. However, focusing on the commonalities between the aetiology and epidemiology
of suicidal phenomena and depression symptomatology is perhaps less interesting than focusing on their differences, studying depressed suicidal persons and
depressed nonsuicidal persons and learning from their differences. The fundamental question on which these results may shed a light is why some depressed
persons attempt or commit suicide and others do not. This chapter will discuss
studies that have used this approach, and other relevant studies. Before this, the
concept of suicide is described and some basic rates of the various suicidal
behaviours are given.

The words 'suicide' and 'suicidal' in everyday life are used to refer to
self-chosen behaviour that is intended to bring about one's own death. However, of all the behaviours and experiences to which these words are attached,
many are or might not be motivated by a wish to die or to do away with oneself
for good. Often they are not even meant to harm oneself, but only to express or
communicate complex emotions such as despair, hopelessness and anger.

'Suicide' refers to death that is the direct or indirect result of an act
accomplished by the victim him/herself which he or she knows or believes will
produce this result.

'Attempted suicide' covers behaviours that can vary from what is sometimes called suicidal gestures and manipulative attempts to serious but unsuccessful attempts to kill oneself. Sometimes a distinction is made between attempted suicide and 'parasuicide'; the first category is reserved for nonlethal attempts with none the less high suicidal intent, the latter for the other suicidal behaviours.

'Suicidal ideation' refers to cognitions that in research seem to vary from fleeting thoughts that life is not worth living, via very concrete well-thought-out plans for killing oneself to an intense delusional preoccupation with self-destruction (Goldney et al., 1989).

Epidemiology

Rates

Suicide statistics consist of official data only, which are known to be underestimates, therefore giving an incomplete estimate of the phenomenon (Jobes et al., 1986). Within the member states of the United Nations that reported mortality statistics, a considerable number of suicidal deaths – estimates vary from 30 to 200% – are not recorded as such. Suicide is underreported as a cause of death (Diekstra et al., 1995).

Although ranking as a major cause of death, completed suicide is still a rare event in young people, especially when compared to other age groups. Indeed, several authors state that one of the most basic facts about completed suicide is that its risk increases as a function of age (Diekstra, 1981). It is extremely rare in children under the age of 12 (Shaffer & Fisher, 1981; Brooksbank, 1985; Kienhorst et al., 1987). The highest European national suicide rates in the 15–24 year age group are found in Finland: 8 per 100 000 in females and 45 per 100 000 in young males (Hawton et al., 1998). The observation that completed suicide ranks as a major cause of death is mainly made because very few adolescents die from other causes, such as diseases.

Although national statistics are not yet adequately kept on the subject, the number of attempted suicides or parasuicidal acts is much higher than that of completed suicides. The data from the regional centres in the World Health Organization (WHO)/Euro Multicentre Study of Parasuicide suggest that in most centres the younger age groups (15–24 years) show the highest rates (Schmidtke et al., 1996). Futhermore, rates of completed suicide, attempted suicide or parasuicide are positively correlated (Hawton et al., 1998). Most rates of nonfatal suicidal behaviour are based on medical contacts such as hospital admissions or consultations with GPs. These data are therefore directly linked to the resultant medical seriousness of the suicidal act: adolescents who take too many paracetamol tablets with the expectation of dying, but who end up in the bathroom being sick because of it are unlikely to seek or get medical attention for this act of self-poisoning and will remain undetected. Similarly, adolescents who are on the verge of cutting themselves but do not do so because, for instance, they suddenly see someone arriving are unlikely to think that they need medical attention. These cases will not be included in the above-mentioned rates, but are none the less important to get a clear picture of the phenomenon under study. To make a more appropriate estimate of the rate of the behaviour in the general population, nationwide screenings may prove to be more accurate. Various studies have performed these screenings and arrived at percentages ranging from 2 to 8% year prevalence (Kienhorst et al., 1990a; Andrews & Lewinsohn, 1992; Garnefski et al., 1992; Meehan et al., 1992; Rossow & Wickstrom, 1994; Rey et al., 1997; E. J. De Wilde & C. W. M. Kienhorst, unpublished paper).

Although these rates should be interpreted carefully because of various problems with comparability and definition issues (De Wilde & Kienhorst, 1995), it is apparent that these self-reported self-harm rates are rather to be expressed in terms of percentages than in terms of rates per 100 000, which suggests that the number of self-reported yearly rates is likely to be about 100 times higher than the hospital admission rates.

Regarding suicidal ideation, it is evident that a significant proportion of adolescents report having thoughts about some sort of self-harm. Studies that use complete scales for suicidal ideation arrive at high percentages. Two studies (Schotte & Clum, 1982; Strang & Orlofsky, 1990) suggest that up to 61% of adolescents have 'some' recent suicidal ideation. Rudd (1989) reports that 43.7% of 737 university students experienced some suicidal ideation during the previous year. Smith & Crawford (1986) reported that 62.6% of high-school students experienced some degree of suicidal ideation or action during their lifetime. In the Netherlands Garnefski et al. (1992) report prevalence of 19% in the preceding year, and Kienhorst et al. (1990b) found that 3.5% of those adolescents reported recent suicidal thoughts, i.e. in the weeks preceding the administration. In a study of 4157 Mexican and Texan adolescents, 23% of the Texas youth and 12% of the Mexican youth admitted that they had thought about killing themselves during the past week (Swanson et al., 1992).

Correlates of suicide trends

Diekstra and co-workers, within the framework of the WHO programme on Preventive Strategies on Suicide (WHO, 1989), carried out an analysis of suicide rates among 15–29-year-olds in 18 European countries. They found that increases in suicides were related to increases in unemployment, the size of the population under 15, the number of women employed, the divorce rate, the homicide rate, alcohol use and decrease in church affiliation. In a multiple regression equation, this combination of variables showed a 0.84 correlation with the change in suicide rates.

From ideation to completion?

Suicidal ideation, attempted suicide and completed suicide are behaviours that are hierarchically related: suicidal thoughts generally precede suicidal acts, and many completed suicides were preceded by attempts. Although this may not apply for everyone, it is tempting to see these successive behaviours as part of a continuum of suicidality.

The studies that address this issue study the differences and similarities between groups that display these different behaviours. Brent et al. (1988) compare adolescent suicide victims ($n = 27$) with suicidal psychiatric inpatients, who had either seriously considered ($n = 18$) or actually attempted suicide ($n = 38$). There were no differences between rates of affective disorder and family history of affective disorder, antisocial disorder and suicide. However, four putative risk factors were more prevalent among the suicide victims: diagnosis of bipolar disorder; affective disorder with comorbidity; lack of previous mental health treatment and availability of firearms in the home. However, Kosky et al. (1990) were not able to differentiate adolescent suicide attempters ($n = 82$) from ideators ($n = 258$) with respect to clinical symptoms such as level of depression, anxiety, sleep disorders and irritability. Still, suicide attempts were more likely to be associated with chronic family discord and substance abuse. For boys, the odds of suicide attempts were substantially increased if the subject had experienced loss.

In a high-school sample ($n = 380$) Harkavy Friedman et al. (1987) suggested that suicidal ideators and suicide attempters represent overlapping groups. On the other hand, Carlson & Cantwell (1982), in a sample of 102 psychiatrically referred children and adolescents, concluded that 'suicide attempts did not reflect a continuum of suicidal ideation'. Also, attempters tend to be younger and more often women. Completers are more often male, older, and use more lethal methods for self-destruction (Blumenthal, 1990).

Correlates of suicidal behaviour

Concepts

The practice of describing risk factors or protective factors does not do justice to the complexity of the aetiology and idiosyncratic nature of suicidal phenomena. A single causal factor that can answer the question what provokes adolescents to attempt or commit suicide does not exist. Of course, clearly identifiable single events may precede a suicidal act, acting as a trigger for it. This may be a fight with a friend or even a lower grade than expected for an exam. However, the same trigger may provoke other kinds of morbidity; the effect of the event may be mediated by numerous psychological, social, or physiological circumstances, often preventing the behaviour occurring. These circumstances can also be interrelated. Isolation of these individual characteristics of the very complex prodromes of suicidal behaviour is only necessary for the purpose of clarity in description. A number of important descriptions of univariate correlates of suicidal behaviour have however been reported (Spirito et al., 1989; Blumenthal, 1990). A systematic description of univariate factors is a necessary first step in determining their interelationships with each other and their independent and/or combined effects for subsequent suicidal behaviour.

Determining the correlates of suicidal behaviour is, among other things, complicated by: (1) the lack of adequate widely accepted definitions; (2) the limitations of data collection (in most cases data can only be collected *ex post facto*, after the suicide or suicide attempt has taken place); and (3) the non-specificity of the correlates (De Wilde, 1992). Furthermore, no specific behavioural characteristics have been determined that delineate suicidal behaviour apart from the attempt itself.

As stated above, the typical suicidal adolescent does not exist, since the path to a suicide (attempt) is different for everyone. A complex conglomeration of factors precedes the behaviour and in specific individuals different combinations of elements may play a role. Nevertheless, adolescents who have to deal with a combination of problematic elements are more at risk. Mostly, these characteristics are identified by comparing adolescents who displayed suicidal behaviour with adolescents who did not. Although the interrelationship of some of the characteristics has been demonstrated (Kienhorst et al., 1990b, 1991), they have predominantly been described as separate correlates (Herjanic & Welner, 1980; Petzel & Riddle, 1981; Spirito et al., 1989; Blumenthal, 1990; Kienhorst et al., 1991; De Wilde et al., 1992). Here, a distinction is made between various categories: the environment, development, psychology and comorbid factors. Before doing so, characteristics of the suicide (attempt), such as method and intent, will be discussed, as well as the adolescents' own reasons.

Method, intent and reasons

The majority of suicide attempts by adolescents are by self-poisoning, such as drug overdose (Hawton & Goldacre, 1982; Hawton, 1986; Kienhorst et al.,

1991). Other methods include self-mutilation, hanging, jumping from a height and jumping in front of a moving vehicle.

It has often been conjectured that a suicide attempt by an adolescent is predominantly an effort to draw attention from others. The phrase 'a cry for help' reflects this opinion. There are, however, no differences between British and Dutch adolescents in the nature of suicidal intent of adolescent attempters or between adolescents and adults (Hawton et al., 1982; Kerkhof, 1985; Kienhorst et al., 1991). Apart from the fact that this would be a very dramatic way of focusing attention on oneself, which in our opinion should be heard at any time, some empirical evidence seems to contradict this. A few studies have focused on the attempters' own reported motivation for attempting suicide. Bancroft and colleagues (1976, 1979) formulated a number of reasons that describe why suicide was attempted. In two studies, one Dutch and one British, all frequently endorsed items by adolescent suicide attempters, referring to either stopping a certain state of mind or escape from a painful situation (Hawton et al., 1982; De Wilde, 1992), were rather congruent. All items concerning the appeal motive ('drawing attention'), and the revenge motive were only endorsed by a minority of adolescents. In our opinion, the phrase 'a cry of pain', suggested by Williams (1997), summarizes these adolescent motives much better. Interestingly, clinicians gave far more weight to the appeal items (Hawton et al., 1982).

Furthermore, there is evidence that the items 'I wanted to stop feeling pain', 'I wanted to die', 'I wanted to get relief from a terrible state of mind' are all verbalizations of the same construct: 'to die' also meant 'to stop an unbearable consciousness' (De Wilde, 1992). Possibly death, in this context, is the pathway to relief.

The direct environment

The study of environmental factors in relation to suicidal behaviour is extremely difficult, because of the impossibility of controlling for all other events and personal characteristics when studying a single factor. Nevertheless, a lot of effort has been put into demonstrating relations between suicidal behaviour and environmental factors. Comparison of suicidal groups with nonsuicidal 'normal' groups indicates that life events such as physical illness and previous accidents are associated with suicidal behaviour. The family seems to be a predominant source of influence here on the adolescent's suicidal behaviour (for an exhaustive review on this subject, see Wagner, 1997). In a Dutch cross-sectional study, suicide attempt reporters had more disturbed relationships with parents than adolescents who did not report attempted suicide

(Kienhorst et al., 1990a). These results may be related to the finding that self-reported suicide attempters also report much more physical and/or sexual abuse than nonreporters. This was securely established in a sample of 6637 Navaho youths (Grossman et al., 1991), 5730 Minnesota adolescents (Hernandez et al., 1993), 600 high-school students (Riggs et al., 1990) and 1050 students in grades 7–12 aged 11–17 (Wagner et al., 1995). In a Dutch sample ($n = 1490$), the report of attempted suicide in adolescents who also reported they had been sexually abused was five times higher in girls and 20 times higher in boys (Garnefski & Arends, 1998). Many of these differences are not apparent, however, when controlling for depression. Only some extreme and traumatic events or circumstances remain. Lewinsohn and colleagues (1994) followed a group of 1500 high-school students for 1 year and established that those adolescents who reported they had attempted suicide also showed a significantly lower level of family support, even after controlling for depression. Sexual and physical abuse were more common in the suicidal group as compared to a depressed nonsuicidal group (De Wilde et al., 1992). The suicide attempters in this study also reported knowing more significant others who attempted or committed suicide (see also the section on imitation, below).

Even accounting for problematic research designs (Wagner, 1997), the general image arises that attempters seem to grow up in families with more turmoil than other groups of adolescents do. These adolescents more often come from broken homes (by death or divorce), experience more changes in living situation, unemployment of father, psychopathology, drug addiction and suicidality of parents (Friedman et al., 1984; Kienhorst et al., 1990a). Many of these family problems are already present in childhood and do not stabilize in adolescence (De Wilde et al., 1992).

Besides the type of event, the accumulation of events is also of importance. Jacobs (1971) reports an escalation of stressful life events that occurred from the onset of puberty in the lives of adolescent suicide attempters more than it did in normal adolescents. The results were not only relevant, but also specific, as De Wilde and colleagues (1992) found similar results, even in the comparison with a depressed group. Especially during the year preceding the attempt, the differences were substantial, predominantly as concerns characteristics related to social isolation.

Adolescent suicide attempters reported less perceived support and understanding from their parents than depressed adolescents (Kienhorst et al., 1992), although this was not true for other persons in their social network, such as friends, other family members and peers. Accordingly, most of the adolescents who attempted suicide reported that problems in the relationship with their parents was the primary reason for attempting suicide. Mansmann & Schenck (1983) found that suicidal adolescents, in comparison with psychiatric and normal controls, rated their families as the least cohesive and most rigid. However, these perceptual differences did not occur after controlling for depression (De Wilde, 1992).

What is so suicidal about adolescence?

Why is it that, with adolescence, a period starts and ends in which suicidality, although nonfatal, takes such enormous proportions? A first answer to this question comes from taking into account the main developmental tasks specific for adolescence: achieving an adult (sexual) identity and learning new relationships to their age mates (including performing sex roles), achieving independence (from parents and economically), and an own system of values. Remschmidt (1975) comments on these tasks as follows:

When such tasks have to be accomplished by a person, who at the same time has to deal with profound physical changes, the realization of a balance between the 'sense of oneself', the 'sense of the other' and adaptation to social norms, is extremely difficult.

Looking more specifically at these tasks it becomes clear that they involve psychological abilities which still have to be obtained. For example, achieving independence from parents may involve the achievement of an adult, social and economic status which requires, for example, self-confidence. So, if in this process something falters it has a direct (negative) influence on the accomplishment of the other developmental tasks. Whereas most adolescents seem to accomplish these tasks rather well, an element of distress cannot be excluded. From a developmental point of view, this can be considered as an implicit request for help to achieve an adult identity and position, which will provide the desired – although sometimes feared – independence. This desire for independence may explain the relatively low number of suicides in comparison with the high numbers of suicide attempts. In spite of the risk, the suicide attempt has an adaptive developmental, rather than fatal, outcome.

A further explanation comes from the study of biological-developmental status. In the highly industrialized countries of Europe and North America a remarkable change has taken place in this respect over the course of the past 150 years. Around 1850 the average age of the menarche was 16 years, while today in most countries the average age is around 12.5 years. A similar trend seems to have taken place in boys (age of spermarche) but this is harder to document. A number of authors have tried to attribute the increases in secular changes in emotional disturbances in early adolescence to this change (Hamburg, 1989; E. Fombonne, unpublished paper). The assumption that physiological changes at puberty directly contribute to risk remains unclear (Angold & Rutter, 1992) and early-onset puberty does not automatically explain higher prevalence rates of depression or suicidal behaviour.

A more plausible explanation seems to be that the lowering of puberty has caused a disjunction of biological development on the one hand and psychological development and social development on the other hand. The brain still does not reach a fully adult state of development until the end of the teenage years (Hamburg, 1989) and social changes over two centuries and particularly during the last century have postponed the end of adolescence – and of social dependence – until much later. This phenomenon of biopsychosocial dysbalance is a distinctly human evolutionary novelty (Hamburg, 1989). This might pose stresses and strains on many youngsters that overtax their own coping repertoires as well as those of their families and other educators, at least for a number of years. Besides, in most countries the present average age of puberty coincides with another developmental task for the early adolescent – the transition from elementary to secondary or high school (Petersen et al., 1993).

Some researchers hypothesize (Fombonne, 1995) that these processes particularly affect girls. This hypothesis is supported by the fact that depressive disorders, suicidal ideation and parasuicide are more prevalent in girls than in boys. The rise in number of suicides is, however, greater among boys than among girls. In our opinion, the sex difference in adolescents (as well as in adults) may be understood from the perspective that many suicide attempts and helplessness and hopelessness accompanying depression can be considered as help-seeking behaviours. Girls, more than boys, are socialized to depend on the help of others in our society. Boys are more educated to be independent and to find their own solutions for their problems. Thus, boys may resort to less help-seeking behaviour than girls because they lack the socialized repertoire of behaviours to do so. This may help to explain the difference in suicide and suicide attempt rates between the sexes.

The psychology of adolescent suicidal behaviour

Focusing on external stressors or general developmental issues in relation to suicidal behaviour remains unsatisfactory from a psychological point of view. For why is it that many people (if not most) in similar circumstances who have to accomplish the same tasks do not develop suicidal ideas or behaviours? An explanation could be found in the psychological factors.

A central point of departure is that the development of suicidal behaviour is mediated or facilitated by certain thoughts or patterns of thoughts. These may reflect differences in the general normal cognitive style of dealing with social problems or difficult emotions, or they may be due to the presence of abnormal cognitive distortions.

Cognitive repertoire

Suicidal persons are reported as having a limited number of ways of dealing with problems. Schotte & Clum (1982) asked suicidal psychiatric patients and depressed nonsuicidal psychiatric patients to solve social problems described in a short story. They were given an introduction to the story and the final outcome, and had to fill in the steps in between. The suicidal group could think of fewer different steps, and fewer relevant steps. This was in line with similar research by Linehan et al. (1987), and also appeared to apply to younger people. Orbach et al. (1987) established that suicidal children could think of fewer alternative solutions in a predefined dilemma about life and death than children from a chronically ill and a normal group. Cohen-Sandler (1982) also observed the relative inability of suicidal children to generate alternative solutions to common interpersonal problems. This quantitative aspect of problem-solving is often referred to as inflexibility or rigidity. Suicidal adolescents (not different from suicidal adults), seem to be more unfortunate in this respect. For instance, Puskar et al. (1992) found that adolescent suicide attempters, in contrast to a nonsuicidal group, used only affect-oriented coping methods, whereas the others used problem-oriented methods as well. It is unclear if this characteristic is specific for suicidal persons or whether it is found in individuals with depression and/or psychiatric disorders. A recent study by Kingsbury and colleagues (1999), in which these differences disappeared after controlling for depression, suggests it is not. Schmidtke & Schaller (1992) concluded, in an adult sample, that cognitive rigidity is a common feature of persons in crisis and those with depressive states.

Apart from the quantity of cognitions, their quality is also open for debate. Hart et al. (1988) found that adolescent suicide attempters displayed more attributional errors compared to psychiatric controls. Kahn (1987) found that many suicidal adolescents, compared to nonsuicidal adolescents, experienced difficulties in coping with their emotions and could not think through the consequences of their actions. Topol & Reznikoff (1982) reported a significantly more external locus of control in hospitalized adolescent suicide attempters than control adolescents. De Wilde et al. (1993) confirmed these results but added that the locus of control was not more external than that of a comparable depressed group of adolescents.

Impulsivity

Apart from distortions or limitations of cognitive processes of suicidal persons, adolescents are said not to think at all about or plan a suicide attempt in most cases. In relation to suicidal behaviour, impulsiveness, as well as a lack of planning, has been conceptualized as a trait-like characteristic of personality. For example, Withers & Kaplan (1987) reported in a study of 173 adolescent suicide attempters that 54% of the male and 39% of the female subjects had an 'impulsive' personality characteristic. This suggests that, in this study, impulsivity failed to be present in a substantial proportion of suicidal adolescents.

Having no reflection implies a short time span between onset of the idea to attempt suicide and the actual behaviour. This is not a defect in planning. Planning refers to the ability to make decisions regarding the enacting of behaviour (for example, which method to use) and is preceded by reflection. A reflective adolescent may ruminate on suicidal ideation without immediately, or even in the near future, planning the act itself. Furthermore, as indicated from the Withers & Kaplan study, adolescents who are not impulsive, and therefore are reflective, are capable of suicidal behaviour.

An individual may appreciate for the first time that the potentiality to kill can be applied to oneself and crucially, in suicidal circumstances for some adolescents, be exercised almost immediately. For others, however, suicidal ideation may sometimes exist for years without provoking planned action. Suicidal ideation is, however, one of the most powerful predictors of future attempts, at any age. Overall the implication is that impulsivity, denoting a lack of reflection, is neither necessary nor a sufficient explanation of all forms of suicidal behaviour.

Despite these theoretical complexities, some authors have investigated the relation between impulsiveness and adolescent suicidal behaviour. Hawton & Catalan (1987) found that two-thirds of their subjects in two studies ($n = 48$; $n = 50$) only thought about attempting suicide within 1 hour of the attempt. They also report doubts about these findings by suggesting that at some time in the development of the crisis there must have been earlier thoughts about a suicide attempt. Stiffman (1989) concluded that 80% of the attempts (from 291 adolescent runaway youth) were not planned, not even a day in advance. Somewhat surprising are her contradictory reports that one in every five had thought of a suicide plan within the last 2 days, and one in every three had considered such a plan within the last week, whereas only 3% planned the attempt more than 1 week ahead of time. Hoberman & Garfinkel (1988) report that in their sample of 229 adolescent suicides it appeared that: 'in only 28% of the cases there was credible evidence of a plan to commit suicide and this typically appeared of brief duration'. As Spirito et al. (1989) also stated, given the frequent reference to teenage suicide attempts as impulsive, it is surprising how few studies have been conducted on the relation between impulsivity and adolescent development. Summarizing from the above findings, despite the common-sense idea that adolescent suicidal behaviour is impulsive, the operationalization of the concept seems quite diverse and the scientific verification of it is still unclear. Perhaps the frequent reference to the (supposed) relation between impulsivity and suicide attempts of adolescents serves as a belief that assumes that suicide attempts by adolescents are carried out without a rationale. As such, this belief may become a prejudice, which may inhibit reflections about the actual factors involved.

Imitation

Although no study has yet clearly demonstrated a causal relation between exposure to suicide and suicidal behaviour itself, there are various ways of comprehending this process: individuals can learn to react with suicidal acts under specific conditions. This can be done by direct learning (a person's own previous suicidal gestures or attempts) or by vicarious or observational learning (for example, observing a significant other attempting or committing suicide while being depressed or after a severe personal loss). Regarding this latter process, the role of media exposure has also been investigated.

In the field of observational learning, attention was focused on the direct environment of suicidal persons. Adolescent suicide attempters report more significant others who attempted or committed suicide than ideating, depressed or nonsuicidal adolescents (Jacobs, 1971; Smith & Crawford, 1986; Conrad, 1992; Kienhorst et al., 1992). There is however another explanation for this concurrence than that of learned behaviour: it is also possible that adolescent suicide attempters are situated in more difficult circumstances in their direct environment than the controls are, since they are living with more suicidal persons and have been more exposed to the mourning processes for a beloved person who committed suicide.

The imitation effect may also occur in a (high-school) community. Several studies (Robbins & Conroy, 1983; Gould & Shaffer, 1986; Philips & Carstensen, 1986; Brent et al., 1989; Davidson et al., 1989) describe clustering of teenage suicides or suicide attempts. Although Robbins & Conroy suggest 'contagion' as a possible cause for suicide attempts, Davidson et al. (1989) found that the adolescents who committed suicide ($n = 14$) were not more likely than the control subjects ($n = 42$) to have had direct exposure to suicide, as measured by their acquaintance with a person who committed suicide.

Even more indirect is learning of suicidal behaviour through media exposure. Kessler et al. (1988) could not find a direct relation between exposure to three fictional films and television newscasts about suicide and an increase in adolescent suicide afterwards. However, some studies do demonstrate an increase in this respect (Philips & Carstensen, 1986; Ostroff & Boyd, 1987). Not only an increase in adolescent suicides, but also an imitation of the exhibited method is observed (Ostroff & Boyd, 1987; Schmidtke & Häfner, 1988). Moreover, there is some evidence that adolescent suicides increase more than adult suicides (Schmidtke & Häfner, 1988), even if the model was not an adolescent (Philips & Carstensen, 1986).

Still, since these studies are purely correlational, an increase in suicides after media exposure of suicide does not demonstrate the existence of imitation. Imitation effects have to be established in controlled experiments. By exposing 116 high-school students to different video-simulated conditions, Steede & Range (1989) concluded that adolescents may not be influenced by news about suicide or may just deny such influence. In another experimental study, Range et al. (1988) reported that their 142 subjects acknowledged the existence of behavioural contagion after suicide is reported, and that they perceived themselves to be influenced by such information. Overall, the findings suggest that exposure to suicide increases current levels of personal distress but does not predict an inevitable increase in subsequent suicidal thinking. To conclude, the literature in this field is rather ambiguous. Therefore, important implications for preventive strategies are still unclear.

Hopelessness

Hopelessness is an attractive concept explaining the progression from depression to suicide. A depression may become unbearable when there is no expectation of getting less depressed. Thus, hopelessness is frequently investigated in relation to suicidal behaviour, also in adolescence. Earlier, the correlation between suicidal intent and depression appeared to be influenced by hopelessness among adults (Minkoff et al., 1973; Wetzel et al., 1980; Salter & Platt, 1990) and children (Kazdin et al., 1983), and hopelessness was a significant predictor of completed suicide in psychiatric adults (Beck et al., 1985). Unfortunately, for adolescents, the picture is less clear. On the one hand, Topol & Reznikoff (1982) found a significant difference in hopelessness between hospitalized suicidal adolescents and hospitalized nonsuicidal adolescents. On the other hand, Asarnow et al. (1987) saw the correlation between hopelessness and suicides diminish after controlling for depression in children and young adolescents. Rotherham-Borus & Trautman (1988) found no significant difference comparing minority adolescent female suicide attempters and a matched group of psychiatrically disturbed adolescents. De Wilde and colleagues (1993) found that the nonsuicidal depressed group was even more hopeless than the suicidal group, possibly explained by the relief present at the time of the interview, after the attempt. The relation between hopelessness and suicidal behaviour needs more clarification.

Entrapment: an integration through memory

Williams provides a fascinating theory linking the various cognitive correlates of suicidality with each other through their relation with memory deficits in suicidal patients. From experiments investigating the memory bias in mood-induced depressed people (who tend to retrieve positive events more slowly than nondepressed; Teasdale & Fogarty, 1979), Williams and colleagues replicated these findings for suicidal patients (Williams & Broadbent, 1986). Additionally, they discovered that depressed and suicidal persons tended to report more general memories (e.g. 'Being with John') and had more difficulties retrieving specific events ('When I went to see my daughter in her new house') as a reaction to emotional cue words (in this case, 'happy'). This difference may be caused by the experience of stressful events, which generates a defence against too specific and painful content. General memory may prevent a person from invoking the successful problem-solving skills: if you cannot recollect successful problem-solving strategies, you are less likely to generate successful alternatives for future problems (Evans et al., 1992). The nonspecificity of reported positive events that may occur in the future was correlated with hopelessness and was higher in overdose patients than other medical patients and controls (MacLeod et al., 1993). Williams (1997) summarizes his findings, describing this situation as a 'psychological entrapment': 'If life circumstances are the factors that put a person in a cage, it is memory that springs the door closed'.

Attitude

People who dismiss the idea of suicide, because of religious or other reasons, are less likely to engage in the behaviour as well. There is a significant relation between attitude and suicidal ideation (Stein et al., 1992). But what is the attitude towards suicide in adolescents? Domino & Takahashi (1991) addressed this question in a high-school sample of north American adolescents. His study showed that, in general, adolescents do not have a romanticized, idealistic view of the self-inflicted death. The adolescents were able to distinguish between mental illness in general and depression in particular as a significant precursor of suicide. A total of 89% were reported to agree with the statement that most people who attempt suicide are lonely or depressed. However, in Israeli students nearly half of the sample did not regard suicide as a shameful act, and approximately two-thirds considered it justifiable under certain conditions. There is also variation with age and gender: older students agree less with different reasons for suicide than younger students. Females sympathize more with reasons for suicide than males do (Stillion et al., 1984). The suicide attempters in the study of De Wilde and colleagues (1993) were more inclined towards approval of suicide in circumstances of social/relational loss and physical suffering than the normal control group. They were also making fewer moral judgements about it. However, they did not significantly differ from the depressed adolescents in attitude, although a trend was visible.

Comorbidity

Anxiety

Brady & Kendall (1992) reported that a substantial part of the group of children and adolescents that were identified as anxious or depressed had comorbid anxiety and depressive disorders. Given the comorbidity of anxiety and depression and the nondiscriminability of life events in this respect (e.g. Goodyer et al., 1990), it is surprising how little research is done on the relation between anxiety and suicidal behaviour in adolescents. A Finnish study (Marttunen et al., 1991) shows a relatively low occurrence of anxiety disorders in adolescents who died by suicide. In adults some studies indicate that suicidal persons have a higher level of anxiety than nonsuicidal controls (Diekstra, 1973, 1981; Kreitman, 1977). Schmidtke & Schaller (1992) were unable to find any difference on both state and trait anxiety between suicidal and nonsuicidal psychiatric patients, although differences on these dimensions were reported between their patient groups and normal controls. De Wilde et al. (1994) reported no difference in trait and state anxiety between the adolescent suicide attempters, and depressed adolescents who never attempted suicide. However, both these groups reported more state and trait anxiety than a group of 'normal' adolescents. Furthermore, state anxiety was higher than trait anxiety in the depressed as well as the suicidal adolescents. Only 7% and 3% of the suicidal subjects of the same study respectively reported feelings of anxiety in the last days and hours before the attempt (De Wilde, 1992).

Substance use

Use of drugs and alcohol ranks at the top of the most powerful predictive factors (Kienhorst et al., 1990b). Illustrative are those suicides or suicide attempts in which alcohol or drugs are used as part of the suicide or suicide attempt itself (Garfinkel et al., 1982). Many suicide victims and attempters frequently used alcohol or drugs in the days or hours before the attempt (Brent et al., 1987; De Wilde et al., 1994). In a Finnish psychological autopsy study, alcohol abuse or dependence was found in 26% of 53 adolescent suicide victims (Marttunen et al., 1991). Shafii and his colleagues (1985) matched the psychological autopsy results from a group of 20 adolescent suicide victims to those from a nonsuicidal control group. In the suicidal group 70% of the adolescents displayed a frequent use of nonprescribed drugs or alcohol – significantly more than the 29% found in the control group.

A study of Garnefski & De Wilde (1998) in a large self-report study of Dutch secondary-school students aged 16–19 years revealed an almost linear relationship between the number of reported addiction–risk behaviours and percentage of (nonfatal) suicide attempters. Although the prevalence of hard drugs was the lowest of all addiction–risk behaviours, there was a markedly high report of suicidal behaviours in youngsters who used these drugs: one out of each five boys and one out of each three girls. The most 'suicidal' combination of two addiction–risk behaviours reported by girls was that of sedatives and hard drugs: more than half of the girls who reported both these behaviours also reported a suicide attempt. In boys, 27% of those who reported sedatives and cigarettes also reported a suicide attempt. Drug addiction, whether of the person or of significant others, is also predictive of suicidal behaviour (McKenry et al., 1983). Most suicidal acts are performed by using poisoning substances and can be considered as a form of abuse of drugs. Once a person is accustomed to the use of drugs, the intake of an overdose (which is then often defined as a suicide attempt or a suicide) becomes more likely.

The same applies to alcohol abuse. Chronic and/or excessive alcohol use is associated with severe personal and social problems. Coping with these problems through the intake of a mind-changing chemical substance (i.e. alcohol) increases the risk of use of other chemical substances in high doses. There is some evidence that suicidal behaviour in adolescents is part of a general problematic reaction style (including the use of mind-changing chemical substances) towards problematic circumstances (Kienhorst, 1988; Kienhorst et al., 1992).

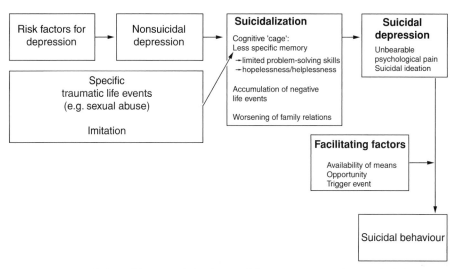

Figure 10.1. A psychological framework for the suicidalization process in depressed adolescents.

A conceptual framework

In an effort to integrate the above findings and coming back at the question raised in the introduction (Why do some depressed adolescents attempt or commit suicide and others do not?), Figure 10.1 shows a possible framework. It makes sense to distinguish between nonsuicidal depression and suicidal depression. The aetiology of nonsuicidal depression is described elsewhere in this book, and is simply summarized in the figure by 'depression risk factors'. The most predominant factors that contribute to the transformation of a non-suicidal depression into a suicidal depression are the cognitive entrapment – changes in the environment (worsening of family relations and accumulation of negative life events) and perhaps comorbid factors such as drug abuse. The act of the suicide (attempt) is then facilitated by the availability of means and imitation.

Prevention

Clearly one of the most effective strategies of dealing with suicidal behaviour is to prevent or treat depression. It occurs frequently and is an important precursor of suicidal thoughts, attempts, and completed suicides.

More specific, suicide-related primary prevention programmes, have been developed and were introduced, mainly in the USA during the 1980s (Garland et al., 1989). Briefly, the main goals are: (1) to raise awareness of the problem of adolescent suicide; (2) to train participants to identify adolescents who are at risk for suicide; and (3) to educate participants about community mental health resources and referral techniques. The programmes are presented by mental health professionals or educators and are most commonly directed to secondary-school students, their parents and educators. The mean duration of the programmes is approximately 2 hours.

Unfortunately, most suicide prevention programmes have fallen short on both of these requirements. Curriculum-based suicide prevention programmes have been operating since 1981 (Garland et al., 1989), but there are only a few published evaluation studies. The majority of these have no control group (Nelson, 1987; Ross, 1980), but two well-designed studies are worth noting. First, Spirito et al. (1988) evaluated a suicide awareness programme for ninth-graders (approximately 13 years old) and concluded that the programme was minimally effective in imparting knowledge, and ineffective in changing attitudes. Second, the New Jersey study of Shaffer et al. (1990) found few positive effects of three suicide prevention curriculum programmes and some possible negative effects. Further evaluation is clearly needed, with an emphasis on the assessment of behavioural variables, including suicidal behaviour and help-seeking behaviour.

Secondary prevention, or treatment strategies with depressed adolescents, was suggested by Kienhorst et al. (1992). The strategies should focus on three main areas: (1) attacking the suicidal adolescent's problematic life situation, which may include family therapy. Attention should be given to the conquering of possible traumatic experiences such as sexual and physical abuse; (2) changing a negative cognitive style with a special focus on hopelessness; and (3) changing the problem-solving and/or coping strategies, with special attention to replacing withdrawal reactions by more adequate strategies.

Concluding remarks

The field of adolescent suicide risk factors has been covered quite adequately during the past decades. However, the field of specific risk factors has not. This is mostly due to methodological shortcomings: retrospective research designs, small samples and, above all, inadequate control groups. The question why some depressed adolescents attempt suicide and others do not is still open for answering, although the scarce research is promising. Prospective research and, due to the cognitive nature of the promising variables, experimental approaches are to be recommended and supported.

Any suicidal thought or attempt increases the chance of eventual suicidal death. Any suicidal death causes a complicated distress in those people left behind. The burden of suicidal behaviour – emotionally, socially and financially – is therefore too big not to explore everything to prevent it. Understanding adolescent suicidal depression better should be a major target in this respect.

REFERENCES

Andrews, J. A. & Lewinsohn, P. M. (1992). Suicidal attempts among older adolescents: prevalence and co-occurrence with psychiatric disorders. *Journal of the American Academy of Child and Adolescent Psychiatry*, **31**, 655–62.

Angold, A. & Rutter, M. (1992). The effects of age and pubertal status on depression in a large clinical sample. *Development and Psychopathology*, **4**, 5–29.

Asarnow, J., Carlson, G. & Guthrie, D. (1987). Coping strategies, self-perceptions, hopelessness, and perceived family environments in depressed and suicidal children. *Journal of Consulting and Clinical Psychology*, **55**, 361–6.

Bancroft, J. H. J., Skrimshire, A. M. & Simkin, S. (1976). The reasons people give for taking overdoses. *British Journal of Psychiatry*, **128**, 538–48.

Bancroft, J., Hawton, K., Simkin, S. & Kingston, B. (1979). The reasons people give for taking overdoses: a further inquiry. *British Journal of Medical Psychiatry*, **52**, 353–65.

Beck, A., Steer, R., Kovacs, M. & Garrison, B. (1985). Hopelessness and eventual suicide: a 10-year prospective study of patients hospitalized with suicidal ideation. *American Journal of Psychiatry*, **142**, 559–63.

Blumenthal, S. J. (1990). Youth suicide: risk factors, assessment, and treatment of adolescent and young adult suicidal patients. Adolescence: psychopathology, normality, and creativity. *Psychiatric Clinics of North America*, **13**, 511–56.

Brady, E. U. & Kendall, P. C. (1992). Comorbidity of anxiety and depression in children and adolescents. *Psychological Bulletin*, **111**, 244–55.

Brent, D., Perper, J. & Allman, C. (1987). Alcohol, firearms, and suicide among youth: temporal trends in Allegheny county, Pennsylvania, 1960 to 1983. *Journal of the American Medical Association*, **257**, 3369–72.

Brent, D., Perper, J., Goldstein, C. et al. (1988). Risk factors for adolescent suicide. A comparison of adolescent suicide victims with suicidal inpatients. *Archives of General Psychiatry*, **45**, 581–8.

Brent, D. A., Kerr, M. M., Goldstein, C. et al. (1989). An outbreak of suicide and suicidal behavior in a high school. *Journal of the American Academy of Child and Adolescent Psychiatry*, **28**, 918–24.

Brooksbank, D. (1985). Suicide and parasuicide in childhood and early adolescence. *British Journal of Psychiatry*, **146**, 459–63.

Carlson, G. A. & Cantwell, D. P. (1982). Suicidal behavior and depression in children and adolescents. *Journal of the American Academy of Child Psychiatry*, **21**, 361–8.

Cohen-Sandler, R. (1982). Interpersonal problem-solving skills of suicidal and non-suicidal children: assessment and treatment. *Dissertation Abstracts International*, **43**, 17.

Conrad, N. (1992). Stress and knowledge of suicidal others as factors in suicidal behavior of high school adolescents. *Issues in Mental Health Nursing*, **13**, 95–104.

Davidson, L. E., Rosenberg, M. L., Mercy, J. A., Franklin, J. & Simmons, J. T. (1989). An epidemiologic study of risk factors in two teenage suicide clusters. *Journal of the American Medical Association*, **262**, 2687–92.

De Wilde, E. J. (1992). *Specific Characteristics of Adolescent Suicide Attempters*. Amsterdam: Thesis Publishers.

De Wilde, E. J. & Kienhorst, I. C. (1995). Suicide attempts in adolescence: 'self-report' and 'other-report'. *Crisis*, **16**, 59–62, 65.

De Wilde, E. J., Kienhorst, C. W. M., Diekstra, R. F. W. & Wolters, W. H. G. (1992). The relationship of life events in childhood and adolescence with adolescent suicidal behavior. *American Journal of Psychiatry*, **1**, 45–51.

De Wilde, E. J., Kienhorst, C. W. M., Diekstra, R. F. W. & Wolters, W. H. G. (1993). The specificity of psychological characteristics in adolescent suicide attempters. *Journal of the American Academy of Child and Adolescent Psychiatry*, **32**, 51–9.

De Wilde, E. J., Kienhorst, C. W. M., Diekstra, R. F. W. & Wolters, W. H. G. (1994). Social support, life events, and behavioral characteristics of psychologically distressed adolescents at high risk for attempting suicide. *Adolescence*, **29**, 49–59.

Diekstra, R. F. W. (1973). *Crisis en Gedragskeuze*. Amsterdam: Swets & Zeitlinger.

Diekstra, R. F. W. (1981). *Over Suïcide* (about suicide). Alphen aan den Rijn: Samsom.

Diekstra, R. F. W. (1989). Suicidal behavior and depressive disorders in adolescents and young adults. *Neuropsychobiology*, **22**, 194–207.

Diekstra, R. F. & Garnefski, N. (1995). On the nature, magnitude, and causality of suicidal behaviors: an international perspective. Special issue: suicide prevention: toward the year 2000. *Suicide and Life Threatening Behavior*, **25**, 36–57.

Diekstra, R. F. W., Kienhorst, C. W. M. & De Wilde, E. J. (1995). Suicide and suicidal behaviour among adolescents. In *Psychosocial Disorder in Young People. Time Trends and their Causes*, ed. M. Rutter & D. Smith, pp. 688–761. New York: Wiley.

Domino, G. & Takahashi, Y. (1991). Attitudes toward suicide in Japanese and American medical students. *Suicide Life Threatening Behavior*, **21**, 345–59.

Evans, J., Williams, J. M., O'Loughlin, S. & Howells, K. (1992). Autobiographical memory and problem-solving strategies of parasuicide patients. *Psychological Medicine*, **22**, 399–405.

Fombonne, E. (1992). Depressive disorders. Paper prepared for the Academia Study Group on Youth Problems.

Fombonne, E. (1995). Depressive disorders: time trends and possible explanatory mechanisms. In *Psychosocial Disorder in Young People. Time Trends and Their Causes*, ed. M. Rutter & D. Smith, pp. 544–615. New York: Wiley.

Friedman R. C., Corn, R., Hurt, S. W. et al. (1984). Family history of illness in the seriously suicidal adolescent. *American Journal of Orthopsychiatry*, **54**, 390–7.

Garfinkel, B. D., Froese, A. & Hood, J. (1982). Suicide attempts in children and adolescents. *American Journal of Psychiatry*, **139**, 1257–61.

Garland, A., Shaffer, D. & Whittle, B. (1989). A national survey of school-based, adolescent suicide prevention programs. *Journal of the American Academy of Child and Adolescent Psychiatry*, **28**, 931–4.

Garnefski, N. & Arends, E. (1998). Sexual abuse and adolescent maladjustment: differences between male and female victims. *Journal of Adolescence*, **21**, 99–107.

Garnefski, N. & De Wilde, E. J. (1998). Addiction-risk behaviours and suicide attempts in adolescents. *Journal of Adolescence*, **21**, 135–42.

Garnefski, N., Diekstra, R. F. & de Heus, P. (1992). A population-based survey of the characteristics of high school students with and without a history of suicidal behavior. *Acta Psychiatrica Scandinavica*, **86**, 189–96.

Goldney, R. D., Winefield, A. H., Tiggemann, M., Winefield, H. R. & Smith, S. (1989). Suicidal ideation in a young adult population. *Acta Psychiatrica Scandinavica*, **79**, 481–9.

Goodyer, I., Wright, C. & Altham, P. (1990). The friendships and recent life events of anxious and depressed school-aged children. *British Journal of Psychiatry*, **156**, 689–8.

Gould, M. & Shaffer, D. (1986). The impact of suicide in television movies. Evidence of imitation. *New England Journal of Medicine*, **315**, 690–4.

Grossman, D. C., Milligan, B. C. & Deyo, R. A. (1991). Risk factors for suicide attempts among Navajo adolescents. *America Journal of Public Health*, **81**, 870–4.

Hamburg, D. (1989). Preparing for life: the critical transition of adolescence. In *Preventive Interventions in Adolescence*, ed. R. F. W. Diekstra, pp. 4–15. Toronto: Hogrefe & Huber.

Harkavy Friedman, J. M., Asnis, G. M., Boeck, M. & DiFiore, J. (1987). Prevalence of specific suicidal behaviors in a high school sample. *American Journal of Psychiatry*, **144**, 1203–6.

Hart, E. E., Williams, C. L. & Davidson, J. A. (1988). Suicidal behavior, social networks and psychiatric diagnosis. *Social Psychiatry and Psychiatric Epidemiology*, **23**, 222–8.

Hawton, K. (1986). *Suicide and Attempted Suicide Among Children and Adolescents*. Beverly Hills: Sage Publications.

Hawton, K. & Catalan, J. (1987). *Attempted Suicide: a practical guide to its nature and management*. Oxford: Oxford University Press.

Hawton, K. & Goldacre, M. (1982). Hospital admissions for adverse effects of medicinal agents (mainly self-poisoning) among adolescents in the Oxford Region. *British Journal of Psychiatry*, **141**, 166–70.

Hawton, K., Cole, D., O'Grady, J. & Osborn, M. (1982). Motivational aspects of deliberate self-poisoning in adolescents. *British Journal of Psychiatry*, **141**, 286–91.

Hawton, K., Arensman, E., Wasserman, D. et al. (1998). Relation between attempted suicide and suicide rates among young people in Europe. *Journal of Epidemiology and Community Health*, **52**, 191–4.

Herjanic, B. & Welner, Z. (1980). Adolescent suicide. *Advances in Behavioral Pediatrics*, **1**, 195–223.

Hernandez, J., Lodico, M., & DiClemente, R. (1993). The effects of child abuse and race on risk-taking in male adolescents. *Journal of the National Medical Association*, **85**, 593–7.

Hoberman, H. & Garfinkel, B. (1988). Completed suicide in children and adolescents. *Journal of the American Academy of Child and Adolescent Psychiatry*, **27**, 689–95.

Jacobs, J. (1971). *Adolescent Suicide*. London: Wiley Interscience.

Jobes, D. A., Berman, A. L. & Josselsen, A. R. (1986). The impact of psychosocial autopsies on medical examiner's determination of manner of death. *Journal of Forensic Science*, **31**, 177–89.

Kahn, A. U. (1987). Heterogeneity of suicidal adolescents. *Journal of the American Academy of Child and Adolescent Psychiatry*, **1**, 92–6.

Kazdin, A., Esveldt, D. K., Unis, A. & Rancurello, M. (1983). Child and parent evaluations of depression and aggression in psychiatric inpatient children. *Journal of Abnormal Child Psychology*, **11**, 401–13.

Kerkhof, A. J. F. M. (1985). *Suicide en de Geestelijke Gezondheidszorg*. Amsterdam: Swets & Zeitlinger.

Kessler, R., Downey, G., Milavsky, J. & Stipp, H. (1988). Clustering of teenage suicides after television news stories about suicides: a reconsideration. *American Journal of Psychiatry*, **145**, 1379–83.

Kienhorst, C. W. M. (1988). *Suicidaal Gedrag bij Jongeren. Onderzoek naar Omvang en Kenmerken*. (Suicidal behaviour among adolescents. A study of the frequency and characteristics. Thesis.) Baarn: Ambo.

Kienhorst, C. W. M., Wolters, W. H. G., Diekstra, R. F. W. & Otte, E. (1987). A study of the frequency of suicidal behaviour in children aged 5 to 14. *Journal of Child Psychology and Psychiatry*, **28**, 153–65.

Kienhorst, C. W. M., De Wilde, E. J., Van den Bout, J. et al. (1990a). Self-reported suicidal behavior in Dutch secundary education students. *Suicide and Life-Threatening Behavior*, **20**, 101–12.

Kienhorst, C. W. M., De Wilde, E. J., Diekstra, R. F. W. & Wolters, W. H. G. (1990b). Characteristics of suicide attempters in a population-based sample of Dutch adolescents. *British Journal of Psychiatry*, **156**, 243–8.

Kienhorst, C. W. M., De Wilde, E. J., Diekstra, R. F. W. & Wolters, W. H. G. (1991). Construction of an index for predicting suicide attempts in depressed adolescents. *British Journal of Psychiatry*, **159**, 676–82.

Kienhorst, C. W. M., De Wilde, E. J., Diekstra, R. F. W. & Wolters, W. H. G. (1992). Differences between adolescent suicide attempters and depressed adolescents. *Acta Psychiatrica Scandinavica*, **85**, 222–8.

Kingsbury, S., Hawton, K., Steinhardt, K. & James, A. (1999). Do adolescents who take overdoses have specific psychological characteristics? *Journal of the American Academy of Child and Adolescent Psychiatry*, **38**, 1125–31.

Kosky, R., Silburn, S. & Zubrick, S. (1990). Are children and adolescents who have suicidal thoughts different from those who attempt suicide? *Journal of Nervous and Mental Disease*, **178**, 38–43.

Kreitman, N. (1977). *Parasuicide*. London: Wiley & Sons.

Lewinsohn, P. M., Rohde, P. & Seeley, J. R. (1994). Psychosocial risk factors for future adolescent suicide attempts. *Journal of Consulting and Clinical Psychology*, **62**, 297–305.

Linehan, M. M., Camper, P., Chiles, J. A., & Strosahl, K. (1987). Interpersonal problem solving and parasuicide. *Cognitive Therapy and Research*, **11**, 1–12.

MacLeod, A. K., Rose, G. S. & Williams, J. M. (1993). Components of hopelessness about the future in parasuicide. *Cognitive Therapy and Research*, **17**, 441–55.

Mansmann, V. & Schenck, K. (1983). Vordergrundige Motive und langfristige Tenden zen zum Suiczid bei Kindern und Jugendlichen. In *Suizid bei Kindern und Jugendlichen*, ed. I. Jochmus & E. Forster. Stuttgart: Enke.

Marttunen, M. J., Aro, H. M., Henriksson, M. M. & Lönnqvist, J. K. (1991). Mental disorders in adolescent suicide. *Archives of General Psychiatry*, **48**, 834–9.

McKenry, P. C., Tishler, C. L. & Kelley, C. (1982). Adolescent suicide – a comparison of attempters and nonattempters in an emergency room population. *Clinical Pediatrics*, **5**, 266–70.

McKenry, P. C., Tishler, C. L. & Kelley, C. (1983). The role of drugs in adolescent suicide attempts. *Suicide Life Threatening Behavior*, **13**, 166–75.

Meehan, P. J., Lamb, J. A., Saltzman, L. E. & O'Carroll, P. W. (1992). Attempted suicide among young adults: progress toward a meaningful estimate of prevalence. *American Journal of Psychiatry*, **149**, 41–4.

Minkoff, K., Bergman, E., Beck, A. T. & Beck, R. (1973). Hopelessness, depression and attempted suicide. *American Journal of Psychiatry*, **130**, 455–9.

Nelson, F. (1987). Evaluation of a youth suicide prevention school program. *Adolescence*, **22**, 813–25.

Orbach, I., Rosenheim, E. & Hary, E. (1987). Some aspects of cognitive functioning in suicidal children. *Journal of the American Academy of Child and Adolescent Psychiatry*, **26**, 181–5.

Ostroff, R. B. & Boyd, H. (1987). Television and suicide. *New England Journal of Medicine*, **316**, 877–9.

Petersen, A. C., Compas, B. E., Brooks-Gunn, J. & Stemmler, M. (1993). Depression in adolescence. Special issue: adolescence. *American Psychologist*, **48**, 155–68.

Petzel, S. V. & Riddle, M. (1981). Adolescent suicide: psychological and cognitive aspects. *Adolescent Psychiatry*, **9**, 343–98.

Philips, D. P. & Carstensen, L. L. (1986). Clustering of teenage suicides after television news. Stories about suicide. *New England Journal of Medicine*, **315**, 685–9.

Puskar, K., Hoover, C. & Miewald, C. (1992). Suicidal and nonsuicidal coping methods of adolescents. *Perspectives in Psychiatric Care*, **28**, 15–20.

Range, L., Goggin, W. & Steede, K. (1988). Perception of behavioral contagion of adolescent suicide. *Suicide and Life-Threatening Behavior*, **18**, 334–41.

Remschmidt, H. (1975). Psychologie und Psychopathologie der Adoleszenz. *Medischer Kinderheilkunde*, **123**, 316–23.

Rey, C., Michaud, P. A., Narring, F. & Ferron, C. (1997). Suicidal behavior in adolescents in Switzerland: role of physicians. *Archives of Pediatrics*, **4**, 784–92.

Riggs, S., Alario, A. J. & McHorney, C. (1990). Health risk behaviors and attempted suicide in adolescents who report prior maltreatment. *Journal of Pediatrics*, **116**, 815–21.

Robbins, D. & Conroy, R. C. (1983). A cluster of adolescent suicide attempts: is suicide contagious? *Journal of Adolescent Health Care*, **3**, 253–5.

Ross, C. P. (1980). Mobilizing schools for suicide prevention. *Suicide and Life Threatening Behavior*, **10**, 239–43.

Rossow, I. & Wichstrom, L. (1994). Parasuicide and use of intoxicants among Norwegian adolescents. *Suicide and Life Threatening Behavior*, **24**, 174–83.

Rotheram-Borus, M. & Trautman, P. (1988). Hopelessness, depression, and suicidal intent among adolescent suicide attempters. *Journal of the American Academy of Child and Adolescent Psychiatry*, **27**, 700–4.

Rudd, M. (1989). The prevalence of suicidal ideation among college students. *Suicide and Life-Threatening Behavior*, **19**, 173–83.

Salter, D. & Platt, S. (1990). Suicidal intent, hopelessness and depression in a parasuicide polpulation: the influence of social desirability and elapsed time. *British Journal of Clinical Child Psychology*, **29**, 361–71.

Schmidtke, A. & Häfner, H. (1988). The Werther effect after television films: new evidence for an old hypothesis. *Psychological Medicine*, **18**, 665–76.

Schmidtke, A. & Schaller, S. (1992). Covariation of cognitive styles and mood factors during crises. In *Suicidal Behavior in Europe*, ed. P. Crepet, G. Ferrari, S. Platt & M. Bellini, pp. 225–32. Rome: Wiley.

Schmidtke, A., Bille-Brahe, U., DeLeo, D. & Kerkhof, A. (1996). Attempted suicide in Europe: rates, trends and sociodemographic characteristics of suicide attempters during the period 1989–1992. Results of the WHO/EURO multicentre study on parasuicide. *Acta Psychiatrica Scandinavica*, **93**, 327–38.

Schotte, D. E. & Clum, G. A. (1982). Suicide ideation in a college population: a test of a model. *Journal of Consulting and Clinical Psychology*, **50**, 690–6.

Shaffer, D. & Fisher, P. (1981). The epidemiology of suicide in children and young adolescents. *Journal of the American Academy of Child Psychiatry*, **20**, 545–65.

Shaffer, D., Vieland, V., Garland, A. et al. (1990). Adolescent suicide attempters. Response to suicide-prevention programs. *Journal of the American Medical Association*, **264**, 3151–5.

Shafii, M., Carrigan, S., Whittinghill, J. R. & Derrick, A. (1985). Psychological autopsy of completed suicide in children and adolescents. *American Journal of Psychiatry*, **142**, 1061–4.

Smith, K. & Crawford, S. (1986). Suicidal behavior among 'normal' high school students. *Suicide and Life-Threatening Behavior*, **16**, 313–25.

Spirito, A., Overholser, J., Ashworth, S., Morgan, J. & Benedict, D. C. (1988). Evaluation of a suicide awareness curriculum for high school students. *Journal of the American Academy of Child and Adolescent Psychiatry*, **27**, 705–11.

Spirito, A., Brown, L., Overholser, J. & Fritz, G. (1989). Attempted suicide in adolescence: a review and critique of the literature. *Clinical Psychology Review*, **9**, 335–63.

Steede, K. K. & Range, L. K. (1989). Does television induce suicidal contagion with adolescents? *Journal of Community Psychology*, **17**, 166–72.

Stein, D., Witztum, E., Brom, D., DeNour, A. K. & Elizur, A. (1992). The association between adolescents' attitudes toward suicide and their psychosocial background and suicidal tendencies. *Adolescence*, **27**, 949–59.

Stiffman, A. (1989). Suicide attempts in runaway youths. *Suicide and Life-Threatening Behavior*, **19**, 147–59.

Stillion, J. M., McDowell, E. E. & May, J. H. (1984). Developmental trends and sex differences in adolescent attitudes toward suicide. *Death Education*, **8**, 81–90.

Strang, S. & Orlofsky, J. (1990). Factors underlying suicidal ideation among college students: a test of Teicher and Jacobs' model. *Journal of Adolescence*, **13**, 39–52.

Swanson, J. W., Linskey, A. O., Quintero-Salinas, R., Pumariega, A. J. & Holzer, C. E. (1992). A binational school survey of depressive symptoms, drug use, and suicidal ideation. *Journal of the American Academy of Child and Adolescent Psychiatry*, **31**, 669–78.

Teasdale, J. D. & Fogarty, S. J. (1979). Differential effects of induced mood on retrieval of pleasant and unpleasant events from episodic memory. *Journal of Abnormal Psychology*, **88**, 248–57.

Topol, P. & Reznikoff, M. (1982). Perceived peer and family relationships, hopelessness and locus of control as factors in adolescent suicide attempts. *Suicide and Life-Threatening Behavior*, **12**, 141–50.

Wagner, B. M. (1997). Family risk factors for child and adolescent suicidal behavior. *Psychological Bulletin*, **121**, 246–98.

Wagner, B. M., Cole, R. E. & Schwartzman, P. (1995). Psychosocial correlates of suicide attempts among junior and senior high school youth. *Suicide and Life Threatening Behavior*, **25**, 358–72.

Wetzel, R. D., Margulies, T., Davies, R. & Karam, E. (1980). Hopelessness, depression, and suicide intent. *Journal of Clinical Psychiatry*, **41**, 159–67.

WHO (1989). *World Health Statistic Annual*. Geneva: WHO.

Williams, J. M. (1997). *Cry of Pain*. London: Penguin Books.

Williams, J. M. & Broadbent, K. (1986). Autobiographical memory in suicide attempters. *Journal of Abnormal Psychology*, **95**, 144–9.

Withers, L. E. & Kaplan, D. W. (1987). Adolescents who attempt suicide: a retrospective clinical chart review of hospitalized patients. *Professional Psychology: Research and Practice*, **18**, 391–3.

11

Psychopharmacology of depressive states in childhood and adolescence

Eberhard Schulz and Helmut Remschmidt

Introduction

Over the past 50 years there has been a controversial debate concerning the issue of depression in childhood and adolescence. According to Carlson & Garber (1986), five historical phases of thinking can be distinguished:

1. The first one was represented by psychoanalysts who doubted the existence of depressive syndromes in children because children were said not to have a fully developed and well-organized superego, which is regarded as a precondition for depressive symptomatology.

2. The second phase can be characterized as the phase of masked depression, meaning that children show behavioural equivalents rather than pronounced and observable depressive symptoms.

3. In the third phase the notion was put forward that childhood depression includes the core symptomatology of adult depression, combined with additional symptoms such as somatic complaints, social withdrawal, conduct disorders and aggression.

4. The fourth perspective states a complete isomorphism with adult depression according to *DSM-III* and *DSM-III-R* criteria (American Psychiatric Association, 1980, 1987).

5. Finally, the fifth phase states that isomorphism between childhood and adult depression must be unrealistic from a developmental point of view. This viewpoint suggests that the classification of childhood psychopathology should go beyond the simple categorization of symptoms and behaviours and should include the broader notions of patterns of adaptation and competence (Carlson & Garber, 1986).

Depressive disorders are common, chronic and recurrent, and are associated with comorbid psychiatric conditions and poor outcome that can be alleviated by early identification and treatment. Depressive disorders confer a high risk for substance abuse, physical illness, early pregnancy and poor vocational,

292

academic and psychosocial functioning. Psychosocial difficulties often persist long after the remission of a major depressive episode (Birmaher et al., 1998a,b). In addition, follow-up studies have shown that depressed adolescents are at very high risk for suicidal behaviour (Rao et al., 1993). In this regard, one study showed that the most common method of completing suicide was tricyclic antidepressant (TCA) overdose (Kovacs et al., 1993).

Data derived from several controlled studies demonstrate that children and adolescents diagnosed as depressed are at increased risk of subsequent episodes of depression (Harrington & Vostanis, 1995). In this regard, Kovacs et al. (1994) were able to show that childhood-onset dysthymic disorder can be looked upon as an early marker of recurrent affective illness. The longer an episode of major depressive disorder (MDD) in school-aged children or adolescents persists, the greater the risk for long-lasting impairment in school, social or family domain. These impairments in social and cognitive development of depressed young-sters can subsequently increase the risk for psychiatric disorders into adolescent and adult life (Kovacs et al., 1994; Harrington & Vostanis, 1995; Goodyer et al., 1997).

In childhood and adolescence the features of depression are similar to those found in adults. In contrast to adults, the presentation of MDD and the response to pharmacotherapy vary in children and adolescents. These differen-ces may suggest developmental influences on the nature and characteristics of depression in young people (Kolvin, 1995). With respect to depressive signs and symptoms (Table 11.1), young children have a more depressed appearance, more somatic complaints, more separation anxiety, phobias and hallucinations. In the study of Ryan et al. (1987), adolescents presented with more anhedonia, hypersomnia, hopelessness and weight change (Ryan et al., 1987; Rosenberg et al., 1992). Early treatment is required because these recurrent disorders are frequently accompanied by poor psychosocial outcome, comorbid conditions and a high risk of suicide and substance abuse. Early detection and intervention are effective in ameliorating the poor psychosocial outcome (Birmaher et al., 1998a,b).

Goodyer et al. (1997) pointed to the fact that determining the nature and type of comorbid conditions (e.g. attention deficit hyperactivity disorder (ADHD), conduct disorder, obsessive-compulsive disorder (OCD), anxiety disorders) is also important, as this should influence the treatment strategy (psychopharmacological and/or psychotherapeutic). It is also important to assess for symptom clusters to define the subtypes of depression (e.g. seasonal-ity, atypical symptoms, psychosis or hypomania) in order to develop appropri-ate treatment strategies. In this regard, psychotherapy is an appropriate treat-

Table 11.1. Clinical features of child vs. adolescent depression

Signs and symptoms	Children	Adolescents
Anhedonia	Less	More
Hopelessness	Less	More
Sleep	Less	More
Weight	Little change	Often changes
Suicide	Decreased lethality	Increased lethality
Appearance	More depressed	Less depressed
Somatic complaints	More	Less
Fears and worries	More	Less

According to Ryan et al. (1987) and Rosenberg et al. (1992, 1994).

ment for all children and adolescents with depressive disorders. Antidepressant medications seem indicated for children and adolescents with: nonrapid-cycling bipolar or psychotic depression; severe symptoms which prevent effective psychotherapy; those symptoms failing to respond to an adequate trial of psychotherapy; and chronic or recurrent depression (Birmaher et al., 1998a,b). Therefore it is important to state that different treatment strategies in combination are required for the therapy of depressive states in children and adolescents. For patients requiring pharmacotherapy, selective serotonin reuptake inhibitors (SSRIs) are the initial antidepressants of choice, although the presence of comorbidities may require alternative initial agents.

Comparable with other fields of child psychopharmacology, the treatment of children and adolescents with MDD is characterized by the paucity of empirical studies evaluating the efficacy and safety of applied drugs. If we look at mood states and depressive syndromes in children and adolescents from a psychopharmacological point of view, we find remarkable differences, but also similarities between childhood/adolescence and adulthood. They are included in this chapter, giving an overview of the present state of pharmacological treatment of depressive syndromes in young people.

Psychopharmacological treatment strategies

In 1957, the antidepressive properties of imipramine were first described by Kuhn. Table 11.2 summarizes the time course and the development of an antidepressive mode of action in the past 40 years according to Möller & Volz (1996).

For simplicity, a general scheme (Table 11.3) can be used to describe the

Table 11.2. Antidepressive treatment strategies in the past 40 years

Time	Antidepressive mode of action and examples
1957–1979	Tricyclic antidepressants (TCAs): imipramine, clomipramine, amitriptyline
1960–1965	Monoamine oxidase inhibitors (MAOIs): phenelzine, pargyline, tranylcypromine
1970–1980	Newer-generation TCAs: lofepramine
1970–1980	Noradrenaline (norepinephrine) reuptake inhibitors (NARIs): maprotiline, levoprotiline
1970–1980	Atypical antidepressants: mianserin, trazodone
1980–1990	Selective serotonin reuptake inhibitors (SSRIs): fluoxetine, fluvoxamine, sertraline, paroxetine, citalopram
1980–1995	Reversible and selective inhibitors of monoamine oxidase type A (RIMAs): moclobemide, brofaromine
1975–2000	Noradrenergic and specific serotonergic antidepressant (NASSA): mirtazapine
1985–2000	Serotonin and noradrenaline reuptake inhibitors (SNRIs): venlafaxine

Table 11.3. Four basic steps of neurotransmission

1. Synthesis of transmitter substance
2. Storage and release of transmitter substance
3. Postsynaptic receptor–transmitter interaction
4. Reuptake of the transmitter from the synaptic cleft

basic steps of chemical transmission. The storage and release of neurotransmitters are mediated by synaptic vesicles which accumulate transmitter and release it at the synapse by exocytosis. In the nerve terminal, these vesicles are called synaptic vesicles. In the other regions of the neuron, the vesicles storing transmitter substances are called transmitter storage granules (Schwartz, 1985). If released into cytoplasm, neurotransmitters would be subject to intracellular degradative enzymes such as the monoamine oxidases, which are situated in the outer membrane of mitochondria.

The first support for the involvement of biogenic amines in depressive syndromes came from a series of observations in the early 1950s, which suggested that reserpine – a Rauwolfia alkaloid used in the treatment of hypertension – caused depressive states in some of the patients treated.

In the following years, animal studies demonstrated that reserpine inactivates aminergic storage granules, thus depleting the brain primarily of serotonin and noradrenaline. Released transmitters are unprotected within the cytoplasm and consequently become vulnerable as substrates to the degradation by monoamine oxidase. Iproniazid, an inhibitor of monoamine oxidase, initially developed to treat tuberculosis, was later found to be an effective antidepressant drug because of its mood-elevating action, as observed in tuberculosis patients. From a historical point of view, monoamine oxidase inhibitors (MAOIs) may be labelled as the first true antidepressants. The following section describes some of the basic biochemical actions of monoamine oxidase and the neurotransmitter systems involved.

Psychopharmacological aspects of monoamine oxidase inhibition

Neurochemical research has revealed that monoamine oxidase occurs in two subforms, MAO-A and MAO-B, with distinct distribution and different primary structures, each of which is coded by separate genes. The genes for the two enzyme forms are both located on the short arm of the human X chromosome. MAO-A and MAO-B genes are closely linked and have been assigned to the Xp11.23 and Xp22.1 regions respectively (for a review, see Cesura & Pletscher, 1992). MAO-A and MAO-B are distributed in most tissues found in both the central nervous system and in peripheral organs. MAO-A and MAO-B are distributed in distinct functional neurotransmitter systems and occur within glial cells. MAO-A deaminates serotonin, noradrenaline (norepinephrine) and normetanephrine. MAO-B deaminates dopamine and phenylethylamine. MAOIs prevent the metabolism and deactivation of these neurotransmitters. The effect of these actions is basically sympathomimetic.

MAOIs can be classified according to their relative specificity for the two subtypes of the enzyme, and by the reversibility or irreversibility of their actions (Table 11.4). Only the MAO-A inhibitors have been shown to have an antidepressant effect.

Irreversible MAO inhibitors are recognised by the enzyme as substrates and interact during the first phase of the reaction in a competitive fashion through noncovalent bonds. Thereafter the drug will be converted into reactive intermediates forming a stable covalent and therefore an irreversible complex in the following reactions (Dostert et al., 1989). After formation of such an irreversible complex, consisting of a stable covalent adduct, the recovery of catalytic activity depends on the synthesis of a new enzyme. For clinical purposes this irreversible blockade of the enzyme implicates that new MAO enzyme has to be resynthesized, thus accounting for the long duration of MAO inhibition, with a time span of up to 2 weeks after discontinuation of drug treatment.

Tranylcypromine, a nonselective MAOI, is chemically similar to amphetamine. This drug potentiates the blood pressure effect of tyramine and shows

Table 11.4. Classification of monoamine oxidase (MAO) inhibitors according to specificity

Nonselective MAO inhibitors	MAO-A selective inhibitors
Iproniazid (I)	Brofaromine (R)
Isocarboxazid (I)	Toloxatone (R)
Phenelzine (I)	Cimoxatone (R)
Tranylcypromine (I)	Amiflamine (R)
Clorgyline (I)	
Moclobemide (R)	MAO-B selective inhibitors
	Pargyline (I)
	L-Deprenyl (I)

I, Irreversible mode of action; R, reversible mode of action.

Table 11.5. The most common adverse effects of irreversible monoamine oxidase inhibitors

Orthostatic hypotension	Urinary retention
Hypertensive crisis precipitated by food amines	Constipation
Flushing and chills	Weight gain
Insomnia	Sexual dysfunction
Hypomania/mania	Oedema
Sedation	Headache
Blurred vision	Myoclonic jerking

indirect sympathomimetic effects. Phenelzine belongs to the hydrazine derivatives, with iproniazid as prototype. This class of irreversible inhibitors was mostly discredited because of adverse side-effects, such as increasing blood pressure due to strong interactions with food amines (e.g. tyramine), and the induction of liver damage (for reviews, see Larsen, 1988; Remick et al., 1989). Table 11.5 summarizes the most common adverse side-effects observed in studies with irreversible MAOI, predominantly involving phenelzine and tranylcypromine.

Moclobemide, a substituted benzamide, has been shown to be a reversible inhibitor of MAO-A under different experimental conditions. Reversible MAOIs appear to have fundamental advantages over irreversible ones. Table 11.6 demonstrates some of the major advantages of moclobemide in comparison with the first generation of MAOIs.

The study led by Frommer (1967) was the first controlled double-blind study with crossover design of antidepressant medication in prepubertal depression to be conducted. In a 2-week trial the author compared the irreversible nonselective MAOI phenelzine in combination with chlordiazepoxide to phenobarbitone. Out of 32 depressed children, 25 (78%) improved on the new

Table 11.6. Clinical profile of moclobemide

Reduced degree of tyramine potentiation and absence of cumulative effects
Short duration of action (half-life approximately 12 hours)
Side-effects less pronounced or comparable to tricyclic antidepressants
Co-administration with tricyclic antidepressants so far well tolerated by patients
Superiority over placebo and marked effectiveness in depressive syndromes in several adult clinical trials

For reviews, see Angst & Stahl (1992) and Cesura & Pletscher (1992).

combination of medications. It is difficult to interpret those results because of the treatment combination and the short duration of the trial period – a time span far below the latency of MAOIs to obtain antidepressive response. Interestingly, the relatively incomplete body of data dealing with the application of MAOIs in child and adolescent psychiatry came primarily from clinical trials with hyperkinetic children. Because of the suspected involvement of MAO in both externalizing symptoms and in ADHD (Young et al., 1980; Shekim et al., 1982; Browden et al., 1988; Stoff et al., 1989), a few clinical trials with MAOIs were conducted: Zametkin and co-workers, after observing a group of 14 children with ADHD under treatment with clorgyline ($n = 6$) and tranylcypromine ($n = 8$), found similar response patterns to those resulting from the dextroamphetamine-treated group (Zametkin et al., 1985). Trott et al. (1991, 1992) demonstrated the safe and efficient use of the 'new-generation' MAOI moclobemide, exhibiting short-lasting and reversible effects in 17 hyperkinetic children aged 6–12 years old. With respect to depressive disorder, a retrospective chart review, including 23 adolescent patients, was conducted (Ryan et al., 1988). Ryan's study assessed the outcome from 11 males and 12 females, aged 11–18 years (mean age 15 ± 2 years) with major depression who showed minimal or only partial response to TCAs. Because of nonresponse, those patients were thereafter treated with MAOIs tranylcypromine and phenelzine, as single treatment and in combination with TCAs. From this group, 74% of the adolescents, regardless of dietary compliance, showed fair or good clinical improvement, but 57% who also showed fair or good improvement had good dietary compliance. Except for dietary noncompliance, the side-effects resulting from usage of the two irreversible MAOIs were similar in intensity and frequency in comparison to TCAs.

Nutt & Glue (1989) labelled MAOIs as the 'Cinderella drugs of psychopharmacy'. In adult psychiatry the reevaluation of monoamine oxidase inhibition as a treatment strategy for treatment-resistant depression is still ongoing. As mentioned above, there are only anecdotal reports that MAOIs may be useful in the treatment of depressed children and adolescents who do not respond to typical antidepressant drugs. Therefore, caution should be taken in prescribing these medications and they should be used sparingly and only when other antidepressants have failed to respond (Viesselman, 1999).

MAOIs must not be used with serotonergic antidepressants (clomipramine, fluoxetine, fluvoxamine, paroxetine, sertraline, venlafaxine) or adrenergic agents. A serotonin syndrome can occur if serotonin-elevating agents are taken together with MAOIs. When administering a MAOI with a TCA, the TCA should always be administered before the MAOI (Viesselman, 1999).

In the presence of the new generation of reversible MAOIs it must be proven by careful clinical monitoring that these substances will be suitable for safe and practical usage in the age group of depressed prepubertal and adolescent patients.

The evaluation of tricyclic antidepressants

Over the years, TCAs have been an important class of medication in the treatment of child and adolescent psychiatric disorders. This class of antidepressants has been prescribed for a variety of disorders, including ADHD, enuresis, tic disorders, OCD, anxiety disorders and major depression (Green, 1995a).

In light of investigations performed during the last decade, early enthusiasm for the efficacy of TCAs has waned. None of the double-blind studies of TCAs in prepubertal or adolescent MDD found these drugs to be superior to placebo. Ambrosini (1987) published a review of the collective results from past placebo controlled studies (namely, those of Kramer & Feiguine, 1981; Petti & Law, 1982; Preskorn et al., 1982; Kashani et al., 1984; Puig-Antich et al., 1987). In prepuberty, of 52 children on tricyclic medication, 62% showed improvement, whereas a surprising 55% of 29 children reacted positively to placebo. Overall, approximately 60% of prepubertal depressives improved within 4–6 weeks regardless of the medication received. Of 44 adolescents on medication, 52% recovered, whereas 60% of 10 adolescents improved after having received treatment with placebo only. Similar to the prepubertal group, 55% of adolescent depressives responded within 4–6 weeks regardless of their medication regimen. Recently performed controlled trials with nortriptyline in prepubertal (Geller et al., 1989) and adolescent major depression (Geller et al., 1990), as well as in an uncontrolled study of imipramine in adolescents (Strober et al., 1990), confirmed these previous conflicting results.

Table 11.7. Metaanalysis data to calculate differences between tricyclic antidepressants (TCA) and placebo response rates during the treatment of depressive states in children and adolescents

Author	Year	Population	TCA	Dropout rate (*n*)	TCA response (*n*)	Placebo response (*n*)
Kashani et al.	1984	Children	Amitriptyline	0	7/9	5/9
Preskorn et al.	1987	Children	Imipramine	0	8/10	2/12
Puig-Antich et al.	1987	Children	Imipramine	Not noted	9/16	15/22
Geller et al.	1989	Children	Nortriptyline	10	8/13	4/29
Kramer & Feiguine	1981	Adolescents	Amitriptyline	0	5/10	1/10
Geller et al.	1990	Adolescents	Nortriptyline	4	1/14	4/21
Boulos et al.	1991	Adolescents	Desipramine	13	11/22	7/21
Total					48/132 (36%)	47/154 (31%)

According to P. J. Perry et al. (unpublished paper).

Boulos et al. (1991) evaluated the effectiveness of desipramine in the treatment of adolescents with MDD. Using an intent-to-treat analysis, 11 of the 22 (50%) adolescents randomized to desipramine responded, while 33% (7/21) of the placebo-treated group responded. This was not a significant difference. More recently, Kutcher et al. (1994) also evaluated the efficacy of desipramine in adolescents with MDD. Sixty subjects were randomized to desipramine 200 mg/day or placebo for 6 weeks. Eighteen adolescents dropped out. Forty-two subjects completed the trial and there was no significant difference in response between desipramine and placebo. A summary of these studies is presented in Table 11.7. According to these data, controlled studies have failed to demonstrate that TCAs are superior to placebo in the treatment of childhood and adolescent depression. Newer drugs have replaced TCAs as first-line treatment. These drugs have equal or greater efficacy and fewer serious side-effects.

It is crucial to determine whether the fact that TCAs failed to show superiority over placebo is due to problems in the methodology of these studies or due to developmental features of MDD and/or developmental aspects of drug metabolism in young people. Besides pharmacokinetic particularities, there are also possible pharmacodynamic influences, resulting from hormonal

Table 11.8. Tricyclic antidepressant pharmacotherapy of depression in different age groups

Age group	Effectiveness
Child	Ineffective
Adolescent	Ineffective
Middle-aged	Very effective
Elderly	Appears to be effective

According to Rosenberg et al. (1994).

status and other potential biological variables within the age group of young depressives (see below), which are regarded as being responsible for the relatively unsuccessful outcome of patients who have been treated with TCAs (Ryan et al., 1986).

Supposed factors associated with tricyclic nonresponse in children and adolescents with MDD are:

1. Heterogeneity in the age group of young depressives, although meeting research diagnostic criteria for major depression.
2. Depressed children and adolescents may represent a patient population that is more severely ill and more likely to be treatment-refractory.
3. Developmental and functional characteristics with special features in neuro-transmitter–receptor status are different from the adult brain.
4. Strong inter- and intraindividual variability in tricyclic drug metabolism and plasma level status with little knowledge about age-dependent influence on pharmacokinetics and pharmacodynamics.
5. Neuroendocrine factors with possibly different neuromodulator function in transmitter–receptor interaction as compared with adult brain.
6. Sample size and selectivity in the recruitment of young depressives for TCA clinical trials.

According to Rosenberg et al. (1994), TCA treatment of depression in different age groups raises the question of whether first, there is an age shift and second, at what age young adults begin to respond to TCAs (Table 11.8)?

Dosage regimens and plasma level monitoring of tricyclic antidepressant drugs

Notably, the plasma levels of TCAs show age-dependent variations (Nies et al., 1977; Ryan et al., 1986; Wilens et al., 1992). This is partially due to pharmacokinetic and pharmacodynamic special characteristics of childhood to the end of adolescence. In general, the child has an increased hepatic surface area and body weight. Additionally, antidepressants were found to be less highly protein-bound in children as compared with adults (for review, see Ereshefsky et al., 1988).

In childhood, many drugs, including tricyclics, are eliminated via hepatic metabolism at greater rates than in adults. In this regard, it is well known that prepubertal children may require higher dosing of psychotropics (including antidepressants), metabolized by the liver at higher doses than adults. Wilens and co-workers (1992) reported findings about developmental changes in serum concentrations of desipramine and its major metabolite between three main age groupings; the study involved 40 children (6–12 years), 36 adolescents (13–18 years) and 27 adult (19–67 years) patients. One of the study's main findings was that serum concentrations of desipramine, the metabolite 2-hydroxydesipramine, and the sum of the two concentrations were all found to be lowest in children, moderate in adolescents and highest in adults. Against expectation, children appeared to be more efficient in clearing both the parent drug and its metabolite than adult patients. Developmental aspects of cyto-chrome P450 isoenzymes are supposed to be of special relevance for the observed age-related differences in serum concentrations and drug metabolism (Oesterheld, 1998).

Preskorn and colleagues (1988b, 1989) demonstrated the interindividual variability of a fixed dose of 75 mg imipramine in 68 children. On this dosage, 78% of the children were outside the recommended therapeutic range (125–250 ng/ml). Of the 78% group, 66% were below the recommended range, and 12% were above. The authors recommend that, based on their plasma level data, the dosage should be adjusted using the formula: new dose = (initial dose/initial level) × desired level. If this dosage recommendation is followed properly, more recent results indicate that 84% of patients will stay within the desired therapeutic range. The remaining 16% with plasma levels below the recommended range will then simply require an additional increase in dosage (Preskorn et al., 1989). Central nervous system toxicity exhibits a strong correlation with the plasma level (even with fixed doses within recommended dosage range), and therefore, regular measurements and management of concentration levels appear to be a safe and predictable strategy to avoid iatrogenic damage of patients treated (Preskorn et al., 1988b). Table 11.9 shows the recommended combined dosage and plasma level range for most common tricyclic and tetracyclic antidepressants in child and adolescent psychiatry.

To date, studies of TCAs in prepubertal and adolescent depressives have shown inconsistent correlations between plasma drug concentrations and

Table 11.9. Dosage and plasma level recommendations for selected tricyclic and tetracyclic antidepressants used with young depressives

Drug	Daily dosage < 14 years (usual range)	Daily dosage > 14 years (usual range)	Plasma level range
Amitriptyline (range 1–5 mg/kg)[a]	50–75 mg	75–150 mg	100–250 ng/ml (amitriptyline + nortriptyline)
Imipramine (range 1–5 mg/kg)[a]	75 mg	75–150 mg	125–300 ng/ml (imipramine + desipramine)
Desipramine (range 1–5 mg/kg)[a]	50–75 mg	75–100 mg	100–300 ng/ml
Clomipramine (range 2–3 mg/kg)[a]	50–75 mg	75–100 mg	70–200 ng/ml (clomipramine + desmethylclomipramine)
Maprotiline	50–100 mg	75–150 mg	75–200 ng/ml

[a]According to Viesselman (1999).

responder versus nonresponder status. In this connection, Puig-Antich and co-workers (1987) described a linear relationship between imipramine plasma level and clinical response in prepubertal depressives. In support of this finding, two independent groups of investigators (Preskorn et al., 1982; Geller et al., 1986) showed that plasma level monitoring is a better predictor of response than dosage regimens of the tricyclic drug alone. Other studies have failed to find a positive correlation between plasma levels and clinical improvement (Ryan et al., 1986; Geller et al., 1992).

Despite the controversial connections between plasma level and response patterns, drug level monitoring is still considered to be a useful tool in drug safety management. Plasma level measurement enables the physician to cope with potential differences in drug metabolism (e.g. genetic polymorphisms), to avoid toxicity by means of dosage-dependent side-effects, and to adapt dosage regimens to the individual needs of the patient (for a review, see Preskorn et al., 1988a). Much of the interindividual variability in drug response and serum levels can be explained by differences in absorption, distribution, excretion and, in particular, biotransformation (for review, see Paxton & Dragunow, 1999). Hereditary differences in the amount or structure of key metabolizing enzymes (e.g. cytochrome P450 isoenzymes) may result in remarkable variations in the rate of drug biotransformation. With regard to biotransformation, an important polymorphism is that of the cytochrome P4502D6 isoenzyme involved in the metabolism of a number of drugs, including antidepressants such as imipramine, desipramine, amitriptyline, nortriptyline, fluoxetine, paroxetine and venlafaxine (Glue & Banfield, 1996; Nemeroff et al., 1996; Paxton & Dragunow, 1999). Between 5% and 10% of Caucasians have a genetic variation that results in decreased activity of the isoenzyme P4502D6. This polymorphism is known to be present in children presumably from its earliest genetic expression (Oesterheld, 1998). Nearly 8% of white children and 2% of Afro-American children under 18 years of age were poor metabolizers (Relling et al., 1991; Oesterheld, 1998). The child data are consistent with the known adult rates of this polymorphism. Individuals who are poor metabolizers will exhibit greater bioavailability, greater plasma levels and prolonged elimination half-lives as compared with normal metabolizers. Several investigators have found that poor metabolizers have two to four times higher serum levels than expected (Potter et al., 1982; Geller et al., 1985; Wilens et al., 1992). Therefore they may develop toxic serum levels at therapeutic TCA doses. In addition, pharmacogenetic studies demonstrated that a small proportion of the population can be identified as ultrarapid metabolizers with extremely high CYP2D6 activity. These subjects failed to respond to treatment due to excessively low serum concentrations of the applied drug (Paxton & Dragunow, 1999).

Due to high individual variability between TCA dose and resultant serum level, the TCA serum level is the critical parameter. Responsible treatment with TCAs includes monitoring of drug and metabolite serum levels. Commonly accepted therapeutic serum levels are: imipramine 125–300 ng/ml; desipramine 100–300 ng/ml; amitriptyline 100–250 ng/ml; and nortriptyline 50–150 ng/ml. Steady-state serum levels should be checked when the electrocardiogram is repeated. High serum levels are significantly correlated with cardiotoxicity. However, serum levels are poorly correlated with dose (Puig-Antich et al., 1987; Biederman et al., 1989a; Preskorn et al., 1989).

Side-effects of tricyclic antidepressants

The most common side-effects of TCAs result from their blockade at different receptor systems (for review, see Richelson, 1991). Cardiovascular toxicity of TCAs has attracted most attention because of sudden death in children receiving imipramine or desipramine (Saraf et al., 1974; Biederman, 1991; Riddle et al., 1991, 1994; Popper & Ziminitzky, 1995; Wilens et al., 1996; Varley &

McClellan, 1997). TCA-related cardiotoxicity can be divided into five categories (Warrington, 1988):

1. Arrhythmias or atrioventricular extrasystoles
2. Sudden death
3. Reduced left ventricular performance
4. Orthostatic (postural) hypotension
5. Accidental or deliberate overdose with intractable arrhythmia or hypotension

According to Warrington (1988), classical TCAs could be expected to cause sudden deaths on rare occasions because their quinidine-like activity might provoke a lethal arrhythmia. Electrocardiographic abnormalities, tachycardia, orthostatic hypotension, T-wave abnormalities, ventricular extrasystoles and bundle-branch block are potential risks described in clinical trials with children and adolescents using tricyclic medication (Gittelman-Klein & Klein, 1971; Hayes et al., 1975; Winsberg et al., 1975; Saraf et al., 1978; Ryan et al., 1986).

Additionally, it should be noted that, under careful clinical monitoring most clinical investigators found only few or minor changes in cardiovascular function (Biederman et al., 1989a; Schroeder et al., 1989; Bartels et al., 1991). Wilens et al. (1996) reviewed literature involving cardiovascular effects of TCAs in children or adolescents. They found that these studies yielded results which were consistent with mild changes in these parameters. PR interval changes or atrioventricular block appeared infrequently. Onset of incomplete intraventricular conduction block was common, and reported in up to 25% of paediatric patients treated with TCAs. This was predominantly a right bundle-branch block. Rarely, a complete bundle-branch block developed. Mild repolarization delays were also reported, with an increase in QT intervals. There was some evidence that higher doses or serum levels led to more pronounced electrocardiogram effects. This is a particularly important finding, especially in the group of patients who are slow hydroxylators and therefore have relatively higher serum levels at a given dose.

Other potential risks with TCAs result from a possible seizure induction (Petti & Campbell, 1975), which necessitates baseline and follow-up electroencephalogram monitoring. Blockade of histaminergic and muscarinic receptors is a common side-effect of tricyclic compounds. In a dose-dependent manner this receptor antagonism may provoke side-effects such as sedation, drowsiness, blurred vision, dry mouth, constipation, urinary retention and impaired cognitive function. Additionally, weight loss and growth deficits in children treated with tricyclic compounds such as desipramine and imipramine have been reported (Biederman et al., 1989b; Spencer et al., 1992). Table 11.10 shows

Table 11.10. Side-effects of tricyclic antidepressants in children and adolescents

Cardiac	Confusion	Incoordination
Anticholinergic	Insomnia	Anxiety
Psychosis	Nightmares	Sexual dysfunction
Mania	Rash	Photosensitization
Seizures	Tics	
Hypertension	Tremor	

some of the most common adverse effects of TCAs in children and adolescents.

For TCAs, electrocardiogram, resting blood pressure, pulse (supine or sitting, standing) and weight should be monitored regularly.

Comparing risks and benefits, however, TCAs remain viable second-line or third-line medications. Despite the fact that no double-blind placebo-controlled study found TCAs to be superior to placebo, several open studies, however, reported clinical effectiveness (Ambrosini et al., 1993). According to Green (1995b), there are some common reasons for using a second-line agent such as a TCA:

1. Unsatisfactory amelioration of symptoms with first-line agents
2. Inability to tolerate adverse effects (e.g. insomnia or exacerbation of self-destructive phenomena with SSRIs)
3. Inability to tolerate the pharmacokinetic properties of the first-line agent

Many have proposed guidelines for the use of TCAs in children and adolescents (Elliot & Popper, 1991; Rosenberg et al., 1994; Wilens et al., 1996; Birmaher et al., 1998a,b). In clinical practice, TCAs remain an important alternative treatment for ADHD, OCD (clomipramine only), tic disorders and enuresis, and possibly depressive and anxiety disorders (Flament et al., 1985; Leonard et al., 1989, 1991; Green, 1995a,b; Wilens et al., 1996; Popper, 1997). Because of the increased risk of death following an overdose, TCAs should be avoided as a first-line treatment for suicidal patients (Birmaher et al., 1998a,b).

Alternative treatment strategies with serotonin-specific drugs

Recent developments in molecular biology offer new insights into the heterogeneity of the serotonin (5-HT) receptor family and its functional equivalents. Serotonin is synthesized within neurons by two enzymatic steps: first, the amino acid tryptophan is converted to 5-hydroxytryptophan (5-HTP) by the enzyme tryptophan hydroxylase, and subsequently it is decarboxylated to 5-hydroxytryptamine (serotonin) by aromatic acid decarboxylase. Released

Table 11.11. Drug interactions with tricyclic antidepressants

May increase effect of:	May decrease effects of:
Central nervous system stimulants	Clonidine
Central nervous system depressants	Guanethidine
Monoamine oxidase inhibitors	
Sympathomimetics (i.e. ephedrine)	*Effects may be increased by:*
Alcohol	Phenothiazines
Antipsychotics	Methylphenidate
Benzodiazepines	Oral contraceptives (oestrogen)
Barbiturates	Marijuana (tachycardia)
Anticholinergic agents	*Effects may be decreased by:*
Thyroid medications (cardiac effects)	Lithium
Seizure-potentiating drugs	Barbiturates
Phenytoin	Chloral hydrate
	Smoking

serotonin is primarily inactivated through reuptake via the serotonin transporter (a sodium-dependent transmembrane carrier). Within neurons or glial cells this transmitter is metabolized by MAO-A and aldehyde reductase to the major metabolite 5-hydroxyindole acetic acid (5-HIAA; Hamon et al., 1974; Boadle-Biber, 1982; Youdim & Ashkenazi, 1982). In the serotonergic system there are presynaptic autoreceptors regulating activity in a negative feedback fashion by inhibiting the activity of serotonergic neurons in somatic regions, and thus inhibiting release of the transmitter into terminal regions. At the postsynaptic site, one finds an integral element in chemical signal transduction called the 5-HT receptors. Results from recent studies in molecular genetics have led to a reclassification of these receptors based on receptor structural homologies in DNA and amino acid sequences, rather than receptor affinity for ligands. All monoamine receptor subtypes identified to date fall into either of two gene superfamilies: the G protein-coupled receptor superfamily or the ligand-gated ion channel superfamily.

Fluoxetine belongs to a class of drugs characterized by selective *in vivo* and *in vitro* inhibition of serotonin uptake. Figure 11.1 illustrates the primary mechanisms by which antidepressants are supposed to interact with serotonergic transmission. SSRIs like fluoxetine do not directly affect the postsynaptic 5-HT receptor complex but facilitate 5-HT transmission via the serotonin transporter and at 5-HT$_1$ receptors by presynaptic disinhibition. Presynaptic 5-HT$_1$ receptors decrease the amount of serotonin released per action potential. Fluoxetine acts by blocking presynaptic 5-HT inhibition of 5-HT release. The 5-HT$_{1A}$

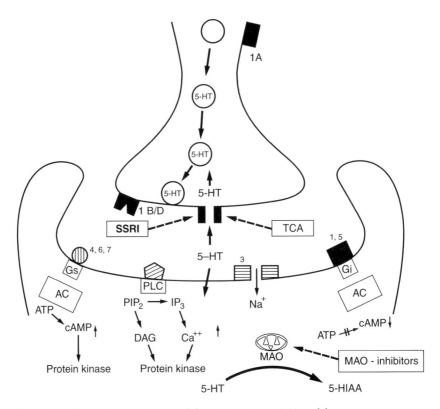

Figure 11.1. Synaptic transmission and drug interaction: 5-HT model.

receptors are autoreceptors in the cell body region and regulate activity of 5-HT neurons, and are also located postsynaptically. Regulation of postsynaptic activity involves the linkage of the activated receptor with its transmembrane second messenger system. The second messengers include adenylate cyclase and phosphoinositate and the activity of phosphorylated kinases which phosphorylate membrane proteins, thus altering membrane potentials and therefore facilitating or inhibiting neuronal activity. According to Figure 11.1, the 5-HT$_{1A}$ linked second messenger system decreases cyclic adenosine monophosphate (cAMP), the 5-HT$_2$ receptor is coupled to phosphatidyl inositol hydrolysis, whereas 5-HT$_2$ receptors are supposed to increase cAMP.

TCAs are typical reuptake blockers of different biogenic amines. TCAs like imipramine, amitriptyline and mianserin are also antagonists of 5-HT$_2$ receptors. In general, antidepressant treatment increases the amount of transmitter substance, thereby altering the balance between neurotransmitter levels and their receptors. The specific transmitter receptors are able to change their conformational state by regulation of affinity and/or maximal number of binding sites through interaction with the transmitter molecules. Linkage of the receptor complex to postsynaptic second messenger systems decides whether receptor binding results in facilitation or inhibition of the activated systems.

Within the spectrum of 5-HT-specific uptake inhibitors, fluoxetine, fluvoxamine, sertraline and paroxetine have been described as antidepressants with fewer antiadrenergic, anticholinergic and antihistaminergic side-effects compared to TCA drugs.

It has been suggested that childhood and adolescent depression are linked to alterations of central nervous serotonergic neurotransmission and therefore SSRIs may be more appropriate for pharmacological treatment in this age group. Indirect evidence for the involvement of serotonin in depressive states in young people originates from challenge tests. After L-5-hydroxytryptophan stimulation, depressed children ($n = 37$) who met the diagnostic criteria (Research Diagnostic Criteria) MDD secreted significantly less cortisol compared to a control group (Ryan et al., 1992). The blunted cortisol response after serotonergic stimulation is supposed to be linked with a dysregulation of central serotonergic function in childhood major depression. Interestingly, two open clinical trials found fluoxetine to be effective in TCA treatment-refractory young patients (Joshi et al., 1989). Apter et al. (1994) treated six TCA-refractory adolescents with fluvoxamine (100–300 mg/day) for 8 weeks, with significant improvements.

In total, there have been seven uncontrolled studies (Boulus et al., 1992; Jain et al., 1992; Colle et al., 1994; Ghaziuddin et al., 1995; Sallee et al., 1995; Tierney et al., 1995; McConville et al., 1996) and two controlled trials (Simeon et al., 1990; Emslie et al., 1997) evaluating the effectiveness of SSRIs in children and adolescents with depressive states. The open studies have shown improvements in depressed children and adolescents with different SSRIs, although one earlier placebo-controlled study showed only a slight superiority of fluoxetine over placebo (Simeon et al., 1990). Recently, Emslie et al. (1997) reported on the first double-blind placebo-controlled study of fluoxetine in depressed children and adolescents. Fifty-six per cent of patients on fluoxetine were rated as much or very much improved, compared to only 33% on placebo. Table 11.12 shows current dosage recommendations for SSRIs.

Since clinical improvement with SSRIs may take 4–6 weeks, patients should be treated with adequate and tolerable doses for at least 4 weeks. If, after 4 weeks, patients have not even shown minimal improvement, treatment should be modified (e.g. by increasing the dosage, changing the drugs). If the patient shows improvement after 4 weeks, the same dosage should be continued for at

Table 11.12. Selective serotonin reuptake inhibitor (SSRI) dosages for the treatment of major depressive disorder in school-aged children

Drug	Typical SSRI dosages (mg/day)
Fluoxetine	5–20
Fluvoxamine	50–150
Paroxetine	20
Sertraline	50

least 6 weeks (Birmaher et al., 1998a,b).

The SSRIs have a relatively flat dose–response curve, suggesting that maximal clinical response may be achieved at minimum effective doses. The SSRIs differ in elimination half-life, drug interactions and antidepressant activity of metabolites.

Abrupt discontinuation of SSRIs with shorter half-lives (Table 11.13), such as paroxetine, may induce withdrawal symptoms mimicking a relapse or recurrence of a depressive episode. Withdrawal symptoms can appear after only 6–8 weeks on SSRI.

The risk-to-benefit ratio in prescribing 5-HT-specific uptake inhibitors like fluoxetine to children is still under debate since exacerbation of self-destructive behaviour, mania or suicidality as potential risks have been reported (King et al., 1991; Power & Cowen, 1992; Venkataraman et al., 1992). Data so far available demonstrate that side-effects of all SSRIs are similar and dose-dependent. Most of them subside with time. However, it is evident that SSRIs may provoke behavioural activation, in which patients become impulsive, silly, agitated and daring. In this regard further investigations should be performed to decide whether these compounds (due to their lower toxicity) should preferably be administered in cases with suicidal and/or impulsive tendencies or not. Other side-effects include gastrointestinal symptoms, restlessness, diaphoresis, headaches, akathisia, bruising, and changes in appetite, sleep and sexual functioning. SSRIs inhibit to varying degrees the metabolism of several drugs (Tables 11.14 and 11.15) which depend on the cytochrome P450 isoenzymes (Birmaher et al., 1998a,b).

The most common psychotropic drug interactions (Table 11.15) with SSRIs can be summarized as follows:

1. SSRI may increase levels of TCAs and trazodone
2. Increased half-life of some benzodiazepines (monitor sedation)
3. Increased half-life of carbamazepine (monitor carbamazepine levels)

Table 11.13. Half-lives of selective serotonin reuptake inhibitors (SSRIs)

SSRI	Half-life (range: hours)	Average half-life (hours)	Steady state (days)
Fluoxetine	24–216	72	28–35
Fluvoxamine		20	7
Paroxetine	7–37	20 (highly variable)	7–14
Sertraline	26	26	7–12

According to Viesselman (1999).

Table 11.14. Selective serotonin reuptake inhibitor (SSRI) inhibition of cytochrome P450 isoenzymes

SSRI/metabolites	3A4	2D6	1A2	2C9
Fluoxetine	+	+++	+	++
Norfluoxetine	++/+++	+++	+	++
Sertaline	++	+	+	+
Desmethylsertaline	++	+	+	+
Paroxetine	+	+++	+	+
Fluvoxamine	++	+	+++	++
Nefazodone	+++	+	–	–
Venlafaxine	–	+	–	–

+ Mild; ++ moderate; +++ strong; – none.

4. Increased levels of SSRI by cimetidine
5. SSRIs increase clozapine effects and toxicity
6. Increased half-life of haloperidol
7. Decreased levels of SSRI by phenobarbitone
8. Decreased levels of SSRI by phenytoin
9. Decreased effect of buspirone
10. MAOIs are contraindicated because of potentially fatal serotonin syndrome

Bipolar disorder

In bipolar disorder the clinician should consider initiating a prophylactic mood-stabilizing agent, such as lithium carbonate, valproate or carbamazepine (Table

Table 11.15. Effects of selective serotonin reuptake inhibitors (SSRIs) on cytochromes and drug interactions

	Cytochrome	Polymorphism inhibitors	Potential interactions
IA 2	Possible	Fluvoxamine	Haloperidol
		Phenytoin	
		Theophylline	
		Caffeine	
		Clozapine	
IIC 9	Yes: 2–3% of whites;	Fluoxetine	Phenytoin
	15–25% of Asians	Fluvoxamine	Diazepam
		Sertraline	Tolbutamide
IID 6	Yes: 5–8% of whites;	Fluoxetine	Tricyclic antidepressants
	lower in Asians and	Fluvoxamine	Haloperidol
	African-Americans	Paroxetine	Perphenazine
		Sertraline	Thioridazine
		Clozapine	
		Risperidone	
		β-Blockers	
		Type IC	
		antiarrhythmics	
IIIA 4	Possible	Fluoxetine	Tricyclic antidepressants
		Fluvoxamine	Carbamazepine
		Sertraline	Alprazolam
		Triazolam	
		Astemizole	

11.16). For patients who do not respond to mood stabilizers alone, an antidepressant should be added to the treatment. In patients with psychotic depression, recovery appears to be more rapid when antidepressants (TCAs or SSRIs) are combined with an antipsychotic agent. Neuroleptics confer the risk of tardive dyskinesia and therefore should be tapered after remission of the depression. Newer antipsychotic drugs, including risperidone, olanzapine and clozapine, may be useful alternatives to typical neuroleptics (Birmaher et al., 1998a,b).

The indications, side-effects and pharmacological data of lithium are given in Tables 11.16–11.20.

Side-effects of valproic acid include nausea, gastrointestinal discomfort and

Table 11.16. Standard and alternative agents for the treatment of acute manic and depressive states

Standard prophylaxis	Acute treatment of depression[a]	Acute treatment of mania[a]
Lithium	SSRIs	Valproic acid
	MAOIs	Carbamazepine
	TCAs	Antipsychotics (Benzodiazepines)
Carbamazepine	TCAs	Valproic acid
	MAOIs	Lithium
	SSRIs	Antipsychotics (Benzodiazepines)
Lithium		
Starting dosage	30 mg/kg per day in divided doses	
Maintenance dosage	15–40 mg/kg per day	
Valproate		
Starting dosage	15 mg/kg per day in divided doses	
Maintenance dosage	15–60 mg/kg per day	
Carbamazepine		
Starting dosage	100 mg/day	
Maintenance dosage	400–800 mg/day	

[a]These drugs are to be added to the prophylactic treatment when possible.
SSRIs, Selective serotonin reuptake inhibitors; MAOIs, monoamine oxidase inhibitors; TCAs, tricyclic antidepressants.

sedation. Monitoring of carbamazepine involves the assessment of potential neurological side-effects and induction of manic states.

Conclusions

Antidepressant medication in childhood and adolescence is indicated in cases of severe depressive symptomatology which are unresponsive to psycho-therapeutic interventions. In particular, the persistence of functional impair-

Table 11.17. Pharmacokinetic properties of lithium

Absorption	Peak serum levels (hours)	Serum half-life (hours)	Principal route of excretion
Gastrointestinal	2–4	20–24	Renal

Table 11.18. Lithium carbonate dosage guide for prepubertal children

Weight (kg)	Dosage (mg)			Total daily dose (mg)
	8 a.m.	12 p.m.	6 p.m.	
< 25	150	150	300	600
25–40	300	300	300	900
40–50	300	300	600	1200
50–60	600	300	600	1500

Table 11.19. Indications for lithium carbonate in children and adolescents with mood disorders

FDA established	Bipolar disorder: acute mania in patients > 12 years
	Prophylaxis for bipolar disorder in patients > 12 years
Possible indications	Bipolar disorder: acute mania in children < 12 years
	Bipolar disorder: acute depression
	Unipolar depression
	Augmentation of tricyclic-refractory depression
	Prophylaxis for unipolar depression
	Cyclothymia

FDA, Food and Drug Administration.

ments in school, social or family domain and/or the continuing risk of suicidal behaviour are clinical indicators for pharmacological interventions (Remschmidt, 1992; Ambrosini et al., 1993).

Antidepressant medications seem indicated for children and adolescents: with nonrapid-cycling bipolar or psychotic depression; with severe symptoms preventing effective psychotherapy; whose symptoms fail to respond to an adequate trial of psychotherapy; and with chronic or recurrent depression (Birmaher et al., 1998a,b). For patients requiring pharmacotherapy, SSRIs are the initial antidepressants of choice, although the presence of comorbidities may require alternative initial agents.

Table 11.20. Side-effects of lithium carbonate

More frequent	Less frequent
Gastrointestinal (nausea/vomiting, diarrhoea)	Renal (polydipsia/polyuria)
Tremor	Ocular irritation/stomatitis
Leukocytosis	Hypothyroidism/nontoxic goitre
Malaise	Dermatological
	Cardiovascular
	Weight gain/oedema
	Encephalopathic syndrome
	Diabetes
	Hair loss
	Growth and development

Given the high rate of relapse and recurrence of depression, maintenance therapy is recommended for all patients for at least 6 months. If the patient is taking antidepressants, psychotherapy helps to foster medication compliance. Antidepressants must be continued at the same dose used to attain remission of acute symptoms. At the end of the continuation phase, for patients who do not require maintenance treatment, drugs should be discontinued gradually over 6 weeks or longer. Clinicians should consider maintenance therapy for patients with multiple or severe episodes of depression and those at high risk for recurrence. Youth with two or more episodes of depression should receive maintenance treatment for at least 1–3 years (Birmaher et al., 1998a,b).

The most likely reasons for treatment failure include inadequate drug dosage, pharmacogenetic abnormalities, inadequate length of drug trial, lack of compliance with treatment, comorbidity with other psychiatric disorders, comorbid medical illness, bipolar depression and exposure to chronic or severe life events that may require different modalities of therapy.

Several psychopharmacological strategies have been recommended for adults: optimization (extending the initial medication trial and/or adjusting the dose), augmentation or combination (e.g. lithium) and switching to the same or a different class of medications (Birmaher et al., 1998a,b). In this regard, Strober and colleagues (1992), in a 3-week open trial involving 24 adolescents (mean 15.4 years), assessed usage results of lithium carbonate in co-medication with imipramine. All had previously remained highly depressive after a 6-week treatment of imipramine alone while receiving a mean daily dose of 229 mg of the drug. Through drug monitoring, a mean steady-state concentration of 251 ng imipramine/ml plus desipramine plasma level was found. After addition of lithium, two patients had a dramatically positive response and eight other patients showed partial improvement. The study suggests the beneficial use of lithium carbonate adjunct to tricyclic medication in primary nonresponding adolescents, in spite of the fact that the co-medication treatment strategy appears less efficacious overall in this age group than in similar studies done on adults.

One major advantage over tricyclic and related antidepressants came from a constant line of evidence suggesting that SSRIs may be low-toxicity antidepressants. According to the consensus statement of the American College of Neuropsychopharmacology (Mann et al., 1993), there is to date no evidence that serotonin reuptake inhibitors such as fluoxetine may trigger emergent suicidal ideation above rates associated with other antidepressants or the underlying depressive illness. Therefore, SSRIs are the initial antidepressants of choice, although the presence of comorbidities may require alternative initial agents. SSRIs show some promise in treating depressive states in young patients. However, studies are still few and there is only one well-designed study indicating effectiveness in depression.

Main contraindications for the administration of TCAs are the following: cardiac conduction abnormalities, known hypersensitivity to TCAs and manifest seizure disorders. Prior to the initiation of TCA treatment the following routine assessments should be performed (Schulz & Remschmidt, 1988; Green, 1991): 1. careful physical examination; 2. baseline electrocardiogram; 3. baseline electroencephalogram; and 4. laboratory tests including full blood count, differential and haematocrit; serum electrolyte levels, blood urea nitrogen level, bilirubin and the basic liver function tests (aspartate aminotransferase, serum glutamic oxaloacetic transaminase, alanine aminotransferase, serum glutamic pyruvate transaminase, alkaline phosphatase and lactate dehydrogenase). In addition, thyroid function tests (thyroxine, triiodothyrosine resin uptake and thyroid-stimulating hormone are recommended. Abnormal thyroid function can aggravate abnormal cardiac function (Green, 1991). With respect to lithium carbonate administration, thyroid function tests and kidney function tests (baseline serum creatinine and urinalysis) are generally recommended. Lithium carbonate is known to cause hypothyroidism and to alter kidney function.

Derived from a prospective study of the electrocardiographic effects of imipramine in children (Fletcher et al., 1993) the following recommendations are given: a resting corrected QT interval greater than 450 ms or a bundle-branch heart block should be considered as contraindications to starting or continuing therapy with a tricyclic drug. The authors recommend that patients with a family history of sudden death, a baseline PR interval greater than the 90th percentile for age, or any degree of intraventricular conduction delay, should undergo further careful monitoring.

During TCA medication, plasma levels in children and adolescents show strong interindividual variabilities with a potential risk of toxic concentrations. A therapeutic plasma/serum level monitoring of the applied drug is still recommended. In addition to the well-known variabilities in plasma level concentrations, genetic polymorphisms in the hepatic enzyme cytochrome P4502D6 may play a causal role in clinical nonresponse and untoward effects owing to inadequate dosage regimens. Both TCAs and the specific serotonin reuptake inhibitors are substrates for this enzyme (Crewe et al., 1992; Van Harten, 1993). For practical purposes, therapeutic drug monitoring of anti-depressant drugs should be performed according to the following recommendations (Riederer & Laux, 1992): blood samples (serum collected in polypropylene tubes) should generally be taken prior to the morning dose, about 12 hours after the last administration. Blood sampling should be performed under strict steady-state conditions, i.e. when four or five half-life intervals have elapsed. As a result of recent knowledge gained from plasma level monitoring, recommendations for antidepressant drug dosage should be based on the measurement of the applied drugs and their major metabolites. According to Ambrosini et al. (1993), oral tricyclic dosing should provide plasma levels in the 200 ng/ml range, although for nortriptyline somewhat lower plasma levels of approximately 100 ng/ml are recommended. In cases of nonresponse and sufficient plasma levels of the tricyclic drug, lithium augmentation should be performed as a safe alternative.

There appears to be a consensus that the first-line drug treatment in MDD in an adolescent would be an SSRI, primarily because of a putative broader range of action, limited side-effect profile and safety in overdose. However, continued research is needed about the effectiveness and safety of treatment with SSRIs, specifically in children and adolescents.

REFERENCES

Ambrosini, P. J. (1987). Pharmacotherapy in child and adolescent major depressive disorder. In *Psychopharmacology. The third generation of progress*, ed. H. Y. Meltzer, pp. 1247–54. Raven Press, New York.

Ambrosini, P. J., Bianchi, M. D., Rabinovich, H. & Eha, J. (1993). Antidepressant treatments in children and adolescents. I. Affective disorders. *Journal of the American Academy of Child and*

Adolescent Psychiatry, **32**, 1–6.

American Psychiatric Association (1980). *Diagnostic and Statistical Manual of Mental Disorders*, 3rd edn (DSM-III). American Psychiatric Association, Washington, DC.

American Psychiatric Association (1987). *Diagnostic and Statistical Manual of Mental Disorders*, 3rd edn revised (DSM-III-R). American Psychiatric Association, Washington, DC.

Angst, J. & Stahl, M. (1992). Efficacy of moclobemide in different patient groups: a meta analysis of studies. *Psychopharmacology*, **106** (Suppl.), 109–13.

Apter, A., Ratzoni, G., King, R. A. et al. (1994). Fluvoxamine open-label treatment of adolescent inpatients with obsessive-compulsive disorder or depression. *Journal of the American Academy of Child and Adolescent Psychiatry*, **33**, 342–8.

Bartels, M. G., Varley, C. K., Mitchell, J. et al. (1991). Pediatric cardiovascular effects of imipramine and desipramine. *Journal of the American Academy of Child and Adolescent Psychiatry*, **30**, 100–3.

Biederman, J. (1991). Sudden death in children treated with a tricyclic antidepressant. *Journal of the American Academy of Child and Adolescent Psychiatry*, **30**, 495–8.

Biederman, J., Baldessarini, R. J., Wright, V. et al. (1989a). A double-blind/placebo-controlled study of desipramine in the treatment of ADD, II: serum drug levels and cardiovascular findings. *Journal of the American Academy of Child and Adolescent Psychiatry*, **28**, 903–11.

Biederman, J., Baldessarini, R. J., Wright, V. et al. (1989b). A double-blind placebo controlled study of desipramine in the treatment of ADD: 1. Efficacy. *Journal of the American Academy of Child and Adolescent Psychiatry*, **28**, 777–84.

Birmaher, B., Brent, D. A. and the Work Group on Quality Issues (1998a). Practice parameters for the assessment and treatment of children and adolescents with depressive disorders. *Journal of the American Academy of Child and Adolescent Psychiatry*, **37** (Suppl.), 63–83.

Birmaher, B., Brent, D. A., Benson R. S. and the Work Group on Quality Issues (1998b). Summary of the practice parameters for the assessment and treatment of children and adolescents with depressive disorders. *Journal of the American Academy of Child and Adolescent Psychiatry*, **37**, 1234–8.

Boadle-Biber, M. C. (1982). Biosynthesis of serotonin. In *Biology of Serotonergic Transmission*, ed. N. N. Osborne, pp. 63–94. New York: Wiley.

Boulos, C., Kutcher, S. & Marton, P. (1991). Response to desipramine treatment in adolescent major depression. *Psychopharmacology Bulletin*, **27**, 59–65.

Boulos, C., Kutcher, S., Gardner, D. & Young, E. (1992). An open naturalistic trial of fluoxetine in adolescents and young adults with treatment-resistant depression. *Journal of Child and Adolescent Psychopharmacology*, **2**, 103–11.

Browden, C. L., Deutsch, C. K. & Swanson, J. M. (1988). Plasma dopamine-betahydroxylase and platelet monoamine oxidase in attention deficit disorder and conduct disorder. *Journal of the American Academy of Child and Adolescent Psychiatry*, **27**, 171–4.

Carlson, G. A. & Garber, J. (1986). Developmental issues in the classification of depression in children. In *Depression in Young People. Developmental and clinical perspectives*, ed. M. Rutter, C. E. Izard & P. E. Read. New York: Guilford Press.

Cesura, A. M. & Pletscher, A. (1992). The new generation of monoamine oxidase inhibitors.

Progress in Drug Research, **38**, 171–297.

Colle, L. M., Belair, J., DiFeo, M. et al. (1994). Extended open-label fluoxetine treatment of adolescents with major depression. *Journal of Child and Adolescent Psychopharmacology*, **4**, 225–32.

Crewe, H. K., Lennard, M. S., Tucker, G. T. et al. (1992). The effect of selective serotonin re-uptake inhibitors on cytochrome P4502D6 (CYP2D6) activity in human liver microsomes. *British Journal of Clinical Pharmacology*, **34**, 262–5.

Dostert, P., Strolin Benedetti, M. & Tipton, K. F. (1989). Interactions of monoainine oxidase with substrates and inhibitors. *Medicinal Research Reviews*, **9**, 45–89.

Elliot, G. R. & Popper, C. W. (1991). Tricyclic antidepressants: the QT interval and other cardiovascular parameters. *Journal of Child and Adolescent Psychopharmacology*, **1**, 187–9.

Emslie, G., Rush, A. J., Weinberg, W. A. et al. (1997). Double-blind, randomized placebo-controlled trial of fluoxetine in depressed children and adolescents. *Archives of General Psychiatry*, **54**, 1031–7.

Ereshefsky, L., Tran-Johnson, T., Davis, C. M. & LeRoy, A. (1988). Pharmacokinetic factors affecting antidepressant drug clearance and clinical effect: evaluation of doxepin and imipramine – new data and review. *Clinical Chemistry*, **34**, 863–80.

Flament, M. F., Rapoport, J. L., Berg, C. J. et al. (1985). Clomipramine treatment of childhood obsessive-compulsive disorder: a double-blind controlled study. *Archives of General Psychiatry*, **42**, 977–83.

Fletcher, S. E., Case, C. L., Sallee, F. R. et al. (1993). Prospective study of the electrocardiographic effects of imipramine in children. *Journal of Pediatrics*, **122**, 652–4.

Frommer, E. A. (1967). Treatment of childhood depression with antidepressant drugs. *British Medical Journal*, **1**, 729–32.

Geller, B., Cooper, T. B. & Chesnut, E. C. (1985). Serial monitoring and achievement of steady state nortriptyline plasma levels in depressed children and adolescents. *Journal of Clinical Psychopharmacology*, **5**, 213–16.

Geller, B., Cooper, T. B., Chesnut, E. C. et al. (1986). Preliminary data on the relationship between nortriptyline plasma level and response in depressed children. *American Journal of Psychiatry*, **143**, 1283–6.

Geller, G., Cooper, T. D., McCombs, H. G. et al. (1989). Double-blind placebo-controlled study of nortriptyline in depressed children using a 'fixed plasma level' design. *Psychopharmacology Bulletin*, **25**, 101–8.

Geller, B., Cooper, T. B., Graham, D. L. et al. (1990). Double-blind placebo-controlled study of nortriptyline in depressed adolescents using a 'fixed plasma level' design. *Psychopharmacology Bulletin*, **26**, 85–90.

Geller, B., Cooper, T. B., Graham, D. L. et al. (1992). Pharmacokinetically designed double-blind placebo-controlled study of nortriptyline in 6- to 12-year-olds with major depressive disorder. *Journal of the American Academy of Child and Adolescent Psychiatry*, **31**, 34–44.

Ghaziuddin, N., Naylor, M. W. & King, C. A. (1995). Fluoxetine in tricyclic refractory depression in adolescents. *Depression*, **2**, 278–91.

Gittelman-Klein, R. & Klein, D. F. (1971). Controlled imipramine treatment of school phobia.

Archives of General Psychiatry, **25**, 204–7.

Glue, P. & Banfield, C. (1996). Psychiatry, psychopharmacology and P450s. *Human Psychophar-macology*, **11**, 97–114.

Goodyer, I. M., Herbert, J., Secher, S. M. et al. (1997). Short-term outcome of major depression: I. Comorbidity and severity at presentation as predictors of persistent disorder. *Journal of the American Academy of Child and Adolescent Psychiatry*, **36**, 179–87.

Green, W. H. (1991). *Child and Adolescent Clinical Psychopharmacology*. Baltimore, MD: Williams & Wilkins.

Green, W. H. (1995a). *Child and Adolescent Clinical Psychopharmacology*. Baltimore, MD: Williams & Wilkins.

Green, W. H. (1995b). The treatment of attention-deficit hyperactivity disorder with non-stimulant medications. *Child and Adolescent Psychiatric Clinics of North America*, **4**, 169–95.

Hamon, M., Bourgoin, S., Morot-Gaudry, Y. et al. (1974). Role of active transport of tryptophan in the control of 5-hydroxytryptamine biosynthesis. *Advances in Biochemical Psychopharmacology*, **11**, 153–62.

Harrington, R. & Vostanis, P. (1995). Longitudinal perspectives and affective disorder in children and adolescents. In *The Depressed Child and Adolescent. Developmental and clinical perspectives*, ed. I. M. Goodyer, pp. 311–41. Cambridge: Cambridge University Press.

Hayes, T. A., Panitch, M. L. & Barker, E. (1975). Imipramine dosage in children: a comment on 'imipramine and electrocardiographic abnormalities in hyperactive children'. *American Journal of Psychiatry*, **132**, 546–7.

Jain, U., Birmaher, B., Garcia, M. et al. (1992). Fluoxetine in children and adolescents with with mood disorders: a chart review of efficacy and adverse effects. *Journal of Child and Adolescent Psychopharmacology*, **2**, 259–65.

Joshi, P. T., Walkup, J. T., Capozzoli, J. A., Detrinis, R. B. & Coyle, J. T. (1989). The use of fluoxetine in the treatment of major depressive disorder in children and adolescents. Paper presented at the 36th Annual Meeting of the American Academy of child and Adolescent Psychiatry, October 11–15, 1984, New York.

Kashani, J. H., Shekin, W. O. & Reid, J. C. (1984). Amitriptyline in children with major depressive disorder: a double-blind crossover pilot study. *Journal of the American Academy of Child Psychiatry*, **23**, 348–51.

King, R. A., Riddle, M. A., Chappell, P. B. et al. (1991). Emergence of self-destructive phenomena in children and adolescents during fluoxetine treatment. *Journal of the American Academy of Child and Adolescent Psychiatry*, **30**, 179–86.

Kolvin, I. (1995). Childhood depression: clinical phenomenology and classification. In *The Depressed Child and Adolescent. Developmental and clinical perspectives*, ed. I. M Goodyer, pp. 111–25. Cambridge: Cambridge University Press.

Kovacs, M., Goldston, D. & Gastonis, C. (1993). Suicidal behaviours and childhood-onset depressive disorders: a longitudinal investigation. *Journal of the American Academy of Child and Adolescent Psychiatry*, **32**, 8–20.

Kovacs, M., Akiskal, H. S., Gastonis, C. et al (1994). Childhood onset dysthymic disorder: clinical features and prospective naturalistic outcome. *Archives of General Psychiatry*, **51**, 365–74.

Kramer, A. D. & Feiguine, R. J. (1981). Clinical effects of amitriptyline in adolescent depression: a pilot study. *Journal of the American Academy of Child Psychiatry*, **20**, 636–44.

Kuhn, R. (1957). Über die Behandlung depressiver Zustäande mit einem Iminodibenzylderivat (Geigy 22355). *Schweizerische Medizinische Wochenschrift*, **87**, 1135–40.

Kutcher, S., Boulos, C., Ward, B. et al. (1994). Response to desipramine treatment in adolescent depression: a fixed-dose placebo-controlled trial. *Journal of the American Academy of Child Psychiatry*, **33**, 686–94.

Larsen, J. K. (1988). MAO inhibitors: pharmacodynamic aspects and clinical implications. *Acta Psychiatrica Scandinavica*, **345** (Suppl. 78), 74–80.

Leonard, H. L., Swedo, S. E., Rapoport, J. L. et al. (1989). Treatment of obsessive-compulsive disorder with clomipramine and desipramine in children and adolescents: a double-blind crossover comparison. *Archives of General Psychiatry*, **46**, 1088–92.

Leonard, H. L., Swedo, S. E., Lenane, M. C. et al. (1991). A double-blind desipramine substitution during long-term clomipramine treatment in children and adolescents with obsessive-compulsive disorder. *Archives of General Psychiatry*, **48**, 922–7.

Mann, J. J., Goodwin, F. K., O'Brien, C. P. & Robinson, D. S. (1993). Suicidal behavior and psychotropic medication. *Neuropsychopharmacology*, **8**, 177–83.

McConville, B. J., Minnery, K. L., Sorter, M. T. et al. (1996). An open study of the effects of sertraline on adolescent major depression. *Journal of Child and Adolescent Psychopharmacology*, **6**, 41–51.

Möller, H. J. & Volz, H. P. (1996). Drug treatment of depression in the 1990s. An overview of achievements and future possibilities. *Drugs*, **52**, 625–38.

Nemeroff, C. B., DeVane, C. L. & Pollock, B. G. (1996). Newer antidepressants and the cytochrome P450 system. *American Journal of Psychiatry*, **153**, 311–20.

Nies, A., Robinson, D. S. & Friedman, M. J. (1977). Relationship between age and tricyclic antidepressant plasma levels. *American Journal of Psychiatry*, **134**, 790–3.

Nutt, D. & Glue, P. (1989). Monoamine oxidase inhibitors: rehabilitation from recent research? *British Journal of Psychiatry*, **154**, 287–91.

Oesterheld, J. R. (1998). A review of developmental aspects of cytochrome P450. *Journal of Child and Adolescent Psychopharmacology*, **8**, 161–74.

Paxton, J. W. & Dragunow, M. (1999). Pharmacology. In *Practitioner's Guide to Psychoactive Drugs for Children and Adolescents*, ed. J. S. Werry & M. G. Aman, pp. 23–50. New York: Plenum.

Petti, T. A. & Campbell, M. (1975). Imipramine and seizures. *American Journal of Psychiatry*, **132**, 538–40.

Petti, T. A. & Law, W. (1982). Imipramine treatment of depressed children: a double-blind pilot study. *Journal of Clinical Psychopharmacology*, **2**, 107–10.

Popper, C. W. (1997). Antidepressants in the treatment of attention-deficit/hyperactivity disorder. *Journal of Clinical Psychiatry*, **14** (Suppl.), 14–29.

Popper, C. W. & Ziminitzky, B. (1995). Sudden death putatively related to desipramine treatment in youth: a fifth case and a review of speculative mechanisms. *Journal of Child and Adolescent Psychopharmacology*, **5**, 283–300.

Potter, W. Z., Calil, H. M., Sutfin, T. A. et al. (1982). Active metabolites of imipramine and desipramine in man. *Clinical Pharmacology and Therapeutics*, **31**, 393–401.

Power, A. C. & Cowen, P. J. (1992). Fluoxetine and suicidal behavior. Some clinical and theoretical aspects of a controversy. *British Journal of Psychiatry*, **161**, 735–41.

Preskorn, S. H., Weller, E. B. & Weller, R. A. (1982). Depression in children: relationship between plasma imipramine levels and response. *Journal of Clinical Psychiatry*, **43**, 450–3.

Preskorn, S. H., Weller, E. B., Hughes, C. W. et al. (1987). Depression in prepubertal children: dexamethasone nonsuppression predicts differential response to imipramine vs. placebo. *Psychopharmacology Bulletin*, **23**, 128–33.

Preskorn, S. H., Dorey, R. C. & Jerkovich, G. S. (1988a). Therapeutic drug monitoring of tricyclic antidepressants. *Clinical Chemistry*, **34**, 822–8.

Preskorn, S. H., Weller, E., Jerkovich, G. et al. (1988b). Depression in children: concentration-dependent CNS toxicity of tricyclic antidepressants. *Psychopharmacology Bulletin*, **24**, 140–2.

Preskorn, S. H., Bupp, S. J., Weller, E. B. & Weller, R. A. (1989). Plasma levels of imipramine and metabolites in 68 hospitalized children. *Journal of the American Academy of Child and Adolescent Psychiatry*, **28**, 373–5.

Puig-Antich, J., Perel, J. M., Lupatkin, W. et al. (1987). Imipramine in prepubertal major depressive disorders. *Archives of General Psychiatry*, **44**, 81–9.

Rao, U., Weissman, M. M., Martin, J. A. et al. (1993). Childhood depression and risk of suicide: a preliminary report of a longitudinal study. *Journal of the American Academy of Child and Adolescent Psychiatry*, **32**, 21–7.

Relling, M. V., Cherrie, J., Schell, M. J. et al. (1991). Lower prevalence of the debrisoquin oxidative poor metabolizer phenotype in American black versus white subjects. *Clinical Pharmacology and Therapeutics*, **50**, 308–13.

Remick, R. A., Froese, C. & Keller, F. D. (1989). Common side effects associated with mono-amine oxidase inhibitors. *Progress in Neuro-Psychopharmacology and Biological Psychiatry*, **13**, 497–504.

Remschmidt, H. (1992). *Psychiatrie der Adoleszenz*. Stuttgart: Thieme Verlag.

Richelson, E. (1991). Biological basis of depression and therapeutic relevance. *Journal of Clinical Psychiatry*, **52**, 4–10.

Riddle, M. A., Nelson, J. C., Kleininan, C. S. et al. (1991). Sudden death in children receiving Norpramin: a review of three reported cases and commentary. *Journal of the American Academy of Child and Adolescent Psychiatry*, **30**, 104–8.

Riddle, M. A., Geller, B. & Ryan, N. D. (1994). The safety of desipramine. *Journal of the American Academy of Child and Adolescent Psychiatry*, **33**, 588.

Riederer, P. & Laux, G. (1992). Therapeutic drug monitoring of psychotropics: report of a consensus conference. *Pharmacopsychiatry*, **25**, 271–2.

Robertson, D. W. & Fuller, R. W. (1991). Progress in antidepressant drugs. *Annual Reviews in Medicinal Chemistry*, **26**, 23–32.

Rosenberg, D. R., Wright, B. A. & Gershon, S. (1992). Depression in the elderly. *Dementia*, **3**, 157–73.

Rosenberg, D. R., Holttum, J. & Gershon, S. (1994). *Textbook of Pharmacotherapy for Child and Adolescent Psychiatric Disorders*. New York: Brunner & Mazel.

Ryan, N. D., Puig-Antich, J., Cooper, T. et al. (1986). Imipramine in adolescent major depression: plasma level and clinical response. *Acta Psychiatrica Scandinavica*, **73**, 275–88.

Ryan, N. D., Puig-Antich, J., Ambrosini, P. et al. (1987). The clinical picture of major depression in children and adolescents. *Archives of General Psychiatry*, **44**, 854–61.

Ryan, N. D., Puig-Antich, J., Rabinovich, H. et al. (1988). MAOIs in adolescent major depression unresponsive to tricyclic antidepressants. *Journal of the American Academy of Child and Adolescent Psychiatry*, **27**, 755–8.

Ryan, N. D., Birmaher, B., Perel, J. M. et al. (1992). Neuroendocrine response to L-5-hydroxytryptophan challenge in prepubertal major depression – depressed vs normal children. *Archives of General Psychiatry*, **49**, 843–51.

Sallee, F. R., Nesbitt, L., Dougherty, D. et al. (1995). Lymphocyte glucocorticoid receptor: predictor of sertraline response in adolescent major depressive disorder (MDD). *Psychopharmacology Bulletin*, **31**, 339–45.

Saraf, K. R., Klein, D. F., Gittelman-Klein, R. & Groff, S. (1974). Imipramine side effects in children. *Psychopharmacologia*, **37**, 265–74.

Saraf, K. R., Klein, D F., Gittelman-Klein, R. et al. (1978). EKG effects of imipramine treatment in children. *Journal of the American Academy of Child Psychiatry*, **17**, 60–9.

Schroeder, J. S., Mullin, A. V., Elliott, G. R. et al. (1989). Cardiovascular effects of desipramine in children. *Journal of the American Academy of Child and Adolescent Psychiatry*, **28**, 376–9.

Schulz, E. & Remschmidt, H. (1988). Pharmakotherapie depressiver Syndrome im Kindes- und Jugendalter. *Zeitschrift für Kinder- und Jugendpsychiatrie*, **16**, 142–54.

Schwartz, J. H. (1985). Molecular steps in synaptic transmission. In *Principles of Neural Science*, 2nd edn, ed. E. R. Kandel & J. H. Schwartz, pp. 167–75. New York: Elsevier.

Shekim, W. O., David, L. G., Bylund, D. R. et al. (1982). Platelet MAO in children with attention deficit disorder and hyperactivity. *American Journal of Psychiatry*, **139**, 936–8.

Simeon, J. E., Dinicola, V. F., Ferguson, J. B. et al. (1990). Adolescent depression: a placebo-controlled fluoxetine study and follow-up. *Progress in Neuropsychopharmacology and Biological Psychiatry*, **14**, 791–5.

Spencer, T., Biederman, J., Wright, V. & Danon, M. (1992). Growth deficits in children treated with desipramine: a controlled study. *Journal of the American Academy of Child and Adolescent Psychiatry*, **31**, 235–43.

Stoff, D. M., Friedman, E., Pollock, L. et al. (1989). Elevated platelet MAO is related to impulsivity in disruptive behavior disorders. *Journal of the American Academy of Child and Adolescent Psychiatry*, **28**, 754–60.

Strober, M., Freeman, R. & Rigali, J. (1990). The pharmacotherapy of depressive illness in adolescence. I. An open trial on imipramine. *Psychopharmacology Bulletin*, **26**, 80–4.

Strober, M., Freeman, R., Rigali, J. et al. (1992). The pharmacotherapy of depressive illness in adolescence: II. Effects of lithium augmentation in nonresponders to imipramine. *Journal of the American Academy of Child and Adolescent Psychiatry*, **31**, 16–20.

Tierney, E., Paramjit, J. T., Leinas, J. F. et al. (1995). Sertraline for major depression in children and adolescents: preliminary clinical experience. *Journal of Child and Adolescent Psychopharmacology*, **5**, 13–27.

Trott, G. E., Menzel, M., Friese, H. J. & Nissen, G. (1991). Wirksamkeit und Verträglichkeit des selektiven MAO-A-Inhibitors Moclobemid bei Kindern mit hyperkinetischem Syndrom. *Zeitschrift für Kinder- und Jugendpsychiatrie*, **19**, 248–53.

Trott, E., Friese, H. J., Menzel, M. & Nissen, G. (1992). The use of moclobemide in children with attention deficit hyperactive disorder. *Psychopharmacology*, **106** (Suppl.), 134–6.

Van Harten, J. (1993). Clinical pharmacokinetics of selective serotonin reuptake inhibitors. *Clinical Pharmacokinetics*, **24**, 203–20.

Varley, C. K. & McClellan, J. (1997). Case study: two additional sudden deaths with tricyclic antidepressants. *Journal of the American Academy of Child and Adolescent Psychiatry*, **36**, 390–4.

Venkataraman, S., Naylor, M. W. & King, C. A. (1992). Mania associated with fluoxetine treatment in adolescents. *Journal of the American Academy of Child and Adolescent Psychiatry*, **31**, 276–81.

Viesselman, J. O. (1999). Antidepresant and antimanic drugs. In *Practitioner's Guide to Psychoactive Drugs for Children and Adolescents*, ed. J. S. Werry & M. G. Aman, pp. 249–96. New York: Plenum.

Warrington, S. J. (1988). The cardiovascular toxicity of antidepressants. *International Clinical Psychopharmacology*, **3** (Suppl. 2), 63–70.

Wilens, T. E., Biederman, J., Baldessarini, R. J. et al. (1992). Developmental changes in serum concentrations of desipramine and 2-hydroxydesipramine during treatment with desipramine. *Journal of the American Academy of Child and Adolescent Psychiatry*, **31**, 691–8.

Wilens, T. E., Biederman, J., Baldessarini, R. J. et al. (1996). Cardiovascular effects of therapeutic doses of tricyclic antidepressants in children and adolescents. *Journal of the American Academy of Child and Adolescent Psychiatry*, **35**, 1491–501.

Winsberg, B. G., Goldstein, S., Yepes, L. E. & Perel, J. M. (1975). Imipramine and electrocardiographic abnormalities in hyperactive children. *American Journal of Psychiatry*, **132**, 542–5.

Youdim, M. B. H. & Ashkenazi, R. (1982). Regulation of 5-HT catabolism. In *Serotonin in Biological Psychiatry*, ed. B. T. Ho, J. C. Schoolar & E. Usdin, pp. 35–60. New York: Raven Press.

Young, J. G., Cohen, D. J., Waldo, M. C. et al. (1980). Platelet monoamine oxidase activity in children and adolescents with psychiatric disorders. *Schizophrenia Bulletin*, **6**, 324–33.

Zametkin, A., Rappoport, J. L., Murphy, D. L. et al. (1985). Treatment of hyperactive children with monoamine oxidase inhibitors. *Archives of General Psychiatry*, **42**, 962–6.

12

The psychotherapeutic management of major depressive and dysthymic disorders in childhood and adolescence: issues and prospects

Maria Kovacs and Joel T. Sherrill

Introduction

This chapter addresses the state of the art in the psychotherapeutic management of depressed children and adolescents. We are specifically concerned with the treatment of psychiatrically diagnosable major depressive and dysthymic disorders, but we examine the management of depressive syndromes as well. We begin by briefly discussing clinical features of depressive disorders that have implications for the design and implementation of therapeutic interventions with youths. Then we summarize peer-reviewed articles of randomized controlled trials with clinically depressed youths as well as studies with youths classified as depressed based on symptom rating scales. Finally, we discuss current issues in the psychotherapeutic management of depressed youngsters and identify topics that require further attention.

Characteristics of depressive disorders

Several clinical and contextual features of childhood and adolescent depression have particular relevance for the design and evaluation of psychotherapeutic interventions. Specifically, episodes of early-onset depressive disorders are often protracted and have high rates of recurrence; these features should inform treatment duration and length of follow-up. Depression in youngsters is also associated with concurrent (comorbid) psychiatric conditions which can complicate the course of treatment, and family dysfunction which can derail specific treatment goals for a given child.

Duration of depressive episodes

An episode of major depressive disorder (MDD) in clinically referred children lasts about 11 months, on average, with a median time to recovery of about 7–9 months (McCauley et al., 1993; Kovacs, et al., 1997b). Recovery is most likely within the first 3–12 months after the onset of the episode, but about 15% of young patients with MDD have a first episode that lasts longer than 18 months (Kovacs et al., 1984a; M. Kovacs, et al., unpublished paper). Certain clinical subpopulations may have even longer episodes (Geller et al., 1985). Findings regarding nonreferred youths are consistent with the foregoing information but, as would be expected, indicate higher rates of remission and earlier recovery as compared to clinical samples. For example, in a study of unreferred youths (Warner et al., 1992), average MDD duration was about 10 months (46 weeks), while the median duration was 2.7 months (12 weeks). In another sample of unreferred youngsters with major depression, median episode duration was reported as 16 weeks (Keller et al., 1988).

The type of depression that has been designated in the *DSM-III* (American Psychiatric Association (APA), 1980) as dysthymic disorder (DD) appears to be a chronic and complicated condition among clinically referred school-age youths. As documented by one study, the first episode of DD is characterized by early onset (in some children, as early as 5 years of age) and protracted course. The average episode lasts about 4 years and recovery is quite gradual. Overall, it takes 8 years from the onset of dysthymic disorder to reach a 98% recovery rate (Kovacs et al., 1994). In a small sample of nonreferred children ($n = 9$) dysthymia was also reported to be protracted with a median duration of 5 years (Keller et al., 1988).

Furthermore, while the child is still dysthymic, and probably during the first 2 years of dysthymia, he or she is highly likely to have a first episode of major depression (Kovacs et al., 1984b, 1994). The superimposition of major depression on chronic dysthymia, originally delineated in studies of adults and labelled 'double depression' (Keller & Shapiro, 1982), has now been documented in various samples of juveniles (Kashani et al., 1987; Keller et al., 1988; Mitchell et al., 1988; Lewinsohn et al., 1991).

The information on length of depressive episodes in youths thus indicates that, while rates of recovery are high, the episodes are protracted, particularly among clinically referred children and adolescents. Therefore, a brief course of treatment may not be adequate to ensure symptomatic remission in most cases. Furthermore, treatment outcome in a clinical trial should be interpreted in the context of naturalistically observed timing of recovery from MDD.

Risk posed by initial depressive episodes

Early-onset depressive disorder portends a subsequent chronic course of affective illness. This pattern is particularly evident among childhood-onset dysthymic patients; about 75% of them progress to repeated episodes of major depression and a sizeable minority also develop bipolar illness. Excepting the fact that the onset of their depression tends to be at a younger age, dysthymic children who develop MDD are subsequently indistinguishable from those youths whose affective disorder history commenced with MDD. In other words, either DD or MDD in childhood appears to be a marker for subsequent episodes of MDD, bipolarity and other forms of affective illness. These youths move in and out of episodes, spending approximately 30% of their late childhood and adolescent years in some form of affective disorder (Kovacs et al., 1994).

There is also evidence that, even after recovery from the index episode of depression, youngsters may experience significant difficulties. For example, clinic-referred youths whose depression had remitted continued to be impaired in their communication and relationship with their mothers (Puig-Antich et al., 1985b). Similarly, Rohde et al. (1994) found residual problems or psychosocial 'scars' following episodes of depression among community adolescents. The problems included internalizing behaviours, stressful life events, emotional dependence, cigarette smoking and depressive symptoms.

The foregoing information suggests that treatment protocols for depressed children should include plans for the postrecovery period. It may be particularly important to teach ways of managing future stressors to maximize functioning during well intervals and to lessen the likelihood of episode recurrence.

Comorbidity

Information on both community and clinical samples suggests that a sizeable portion of depressed children and adolescents have multiple psychiatric disorders, with anxiety and conduct or disruptive behaviour disorders as the most common co-occurring conditions. According to a recent review (Kovacs & Devlin, 1998), in clinical samples of depressed youths comorbid anxiety disorders are about two- to threefold more prevalent than is conduct disorder. More specifically, rates of comorbid anxiety disorder in clinically referred samples range from 23% to 51% (Mitchell et al., 1988; Kovacs et al., 1989; Shain et al., 1991; Ferro et al., 1994; Rao et al., 1995). In contrast, rates of conduct disorder among youths referred for depression range from 7% to 24% (Ryan et al., 1987; Kovacs et al., 1988; Mitchell et al., 1988; Biederman et al., 1995; Rao et al., 1995). Results of follow-up studies also suggest that the initial patterns of comorbidity detected in index episodes are consistent with the longer-term diagnostic outcomes of depressed youths (Kovacs & Devlin, 1998).

The outcome of treatment trials can be strongly affected by comorbidity in the study cases because, compared to those with a single diagnosis, children with comorbid diagnoses evidence more functional impairment (Asarnow et al., 1988). Comorbidity is also related to higher rates of mental health service utilization (Fergusson et al., 1993), possibly suggesting more severe psycho-pathology.

Family context of depression in youths

Finally, the course and outcome of childhood-onset depressive disorders are complicated by family psychopathology and strife (Kazdin, 1990; Kaslow et al., 1994). Elevated rates of psychopathology among parents of clinically referred depressed children and adolescents are well documented (Strober & Carlson, 1982; Mitchell et al., 1989; Puig-Antich et al., 1989; Todd et al., 1993; William-son et al., 1995; Kovacs et al., 1997a). In addition, compared to families of nondepressed children, families of depressed youths have higher levels of marital (Forehand et al., 1988) and parent–child conflict (Puig-Antich et al., 1985a, 1993). Low levels of family cohesion (Fendrich et al., 1990; Garrison et al., 1990; Cole & McPherson, 1993) and diminished overall social support (Armsden et al., 1990; Daniels & Moos, 1990) have also been found among families of depressed youths. The combination of lack of social support and negative life events has, in fact, been associated with the development and maintenance of depression in youths (Compas, 1987; Compas et al., 1993). These ingredients, alone and in combination, may well jeopardize youths' ability to participate in and benefit from treatment.

Empirical treatment outcome studies

Studies of psychosocial treatments of depression among youngsters have traditionally included subjects who were clinically diagnosed with a depressive disorder, or subjects classified as depressed based on cut-off scores on self-rated depressive symptom inventories. A more recent trend has involved studies seeking to prevent depression in youngsters 'at risk', as determined by elevated depressive symptom profiles or similar criteria. Since our prior review of the field (Kovacs & Bastiaens, 1995), there has been steady, although slow progress in treatment outcome research with depressed young people.

Clinically diagnosed samples

As of early 1999, we identified seven peer-reviewed articles on controlled psychotherapy trials of youths, including five studies that were conducted since our 1995 review. The subjects in these studies met operational diagnostic criteria for major depressive or dysthymic disorder based on the *DSM-III* (APA, 1980) or *DSM-III-R* (APA, 1987), or were diagnosed by Research Diagnostic Criteria (Spitzer et al., 1978) with intermittent or minor depressive disorder. In each study we reviewed, diagnoses were determined through standardized, structured or semistructured psychiatric interviews. Across the seven studies, clinically depressed 8–18-year-old subjects typically received short-term cognitive behavioural therapy (CBT) delivered in individual (Vostanis et al., 1996b; Wood et al., 1996) or group (Lewinsohn et al., 1990; Fine et al., 1991; Clarke et al., 1999) format. A recent study included both individual CBT and family-based interventions (Brent et al., 1997), and another examined CBT and interpersonal psychotherapy (Rosselló & Bernal, 1999). The experimental therapies were compared to supportive or nonspecific interventions (Fine et al., 1991; Vostanis et al., 1996b; Wood et al., 1996; Brent et al., 1997) or wait-list conditions (Lewinsohn et al., 1990; Clarke et al., 1999; Rosselló & Bernal, 1999). At end of treatment, 35–90% of the youths reportedly recovered, with generally higher rates of success for experimental therapies than control conditions.

In their landmark study, Lewinsohn et al. (1990) tested the effectiveness of their Coping with Depression (CWD; G. N. Clarke & P. M. Lewinsohn, unpublished paper) course with 14–18-year-old symptomatic volunteers who met diagnostic criteria for major depression or intermittent or minor depression. The design included 59 subjects, randomly assigned to the CWD course, the CWD course with a parent component, or wait-list control. The 7-week protocol involved 14 2-hour skills-focused sessions targeting relaxation, positive event scheduling, dysfunctional thoughts, and social skills. Based on the assumption that parent–child conflicts are a common difficulty during adolescence, a conflict resolution component focusing on communication and problem-solving skills was also included. The two active treatments were identical, except that parents of the subjects in the CWD-with-parent modality also met once weekly.

Close to 50% of the treated youths were remitted from their depression at end of treatment, as compared to only 5% of the wait-list controls. The treated groups also evidenced significant improvements according to scores on self- and parent-rated scales. However, according to parental ratings, there were few differences between the CWD and the CWD-with-parent groups. Participants in both groups continued to improve during the following 2 years, although only 50% of the sample was available for the 2-year follow-up assessment.

Recently, Lewinsohn's group (Clarke et al., 1999) reported on a new clinical trial with 123 adolescents meeting criteria for MDD or dysthymia. As in the earlier study, the acute treatment involved randomization to CWD group, CWD group plus separate parents' group or a wait-list condition. The CWD protocol was modified to include skills training throughout the treatment course rather than in discrete segments. The other modification involved random assignment to one of three 24-month follow-up conditions: assessments plus booster sessions every 4 months, assessments without booster sessions every 4 months, or two annual assessments without booster sessions.

Recovery rates were similar in the two CWD treatments (65% and 69% in the adolescent group, and adolescent group plus parent group, respectively), and both were superior to the wait-list condition (48%). Additionally, compared to the control condition, both forms of CWD were associated with significantly greater pre- to posttreatment reduction in self-rated depression severity and improvement in clinician-rated global functioning.

Among youths who remained depressed at end of treatment, rates of recovery at 12-month follow-up were higher among those who received booster sessions (100%) than assessment only (50%). At 24 months, however, differences in rates of recovery were no longer apparent (overall recovery rate > 90%). Moreover, rates of recurrence were similar in the booster, frequent assessment and annual assessment conditions at 12-month (27%, 0% and 14%, respectively) and 24-month (36%, 0% and 23%, respectively) follow-up. Thus, while booster sessions during follow-up accelerated the recovery of refractory cases, they did not prevent recurrence.

Fine et al. (1991) compared supportive therapy and social skills training in a sample of 66 13–17-year-old adolescent patients, who had *DSM-III* major depressive or dysthymic disorder. Supportive therapy involved an emphasis on improving self-concept, discussion of common concerns and provision of emotional support. Social skill training focused on skills related to recognition of feelings, assertiveness, problem-solving and conflict negotiation. Treatment was delivered in group format during a period of 12 weeks. Fifty per cent of those who received supportive therapy and 40% of the subjects in social skills training experienced significant improvement in mood and hedonic capacity. It should be noted, however, that 41% of the study sample was receiving concomitant psychotherapy or medication. Subjects continued to improve after treatment; approximately 70% evidenced improved mood at the 9-month follow-up. However, 19 subjects did not complete the treatment and seven others dropped out during follow-up.

More recently, Vostanis and colleagues (1996b) compared CBT with a nonfocused control intervention (NFI) in a study with 57 8–17-year-old children and adolescents meeting *DSM-III-R* criteria for MDD, minor depression or DD. Both therapies were delivered in up to nine individual sessions during a 3.5-month period, on average. CBT focused on emotion recognition, self-reinforcement, social problem-solving and cognitive restructuring. NFI involved a review of symptom status and social functioning. At end of treatment, 87% of those receiving CBT and 75% of those treated with the NFI were no longer clinically depressed. Subjects in both conditions also evidenced significant and similar improvement on parent and child self-reports of depression and anxiety symptoms and self-esteem. Furthermore, according to parent and child self-reports at a 9-month follow-up, youths in both treatment conditions maintained their gains in psychosocial functioning (Vostanis et al., 1996a). However, although only 29% of those who received CBT and 25% of those treated with NFI met criteria for a depressive disorder at the follow-up, 46% of the sample reported severe depressive symptoms during the intervening period.

Wood et al. (1996) compared their version of CBT and a relaxation training (RT) control condition in a group of 53 9–17-year-old youths who met criteria for *DSM-III-R* MDD, or RDC minor depression. Wood et al.'s CBT involved three components: a focus on negative attributions, social problem-solving and specific strategies for symptom relief (e.g. sleep hygiene). RT did not actively address core symptoms of depression. Both treatments included five to eight sessions of individual therapy.

Youths treated with CBT reported significantly lower rates of depressive symptoms and lower scores of negative self-image than those treated with RT. Children treated with CBT also had higher rates of clinical remission than those assigned to RT (54% vs. 21%, respectively) and were more likely to be rated as improved (92% vs. 63%, respectively). However, differences between groups were generally not maintained. Rates of clinical remission did not significantly differ for the CBT and RT conditions at 3-month (45% vs. 25%, respectively) or 6-month (54% vs. 38%, respectively) follow-up.

In another recent controlled trial, Brent et al. (1997) compared individual CBT, systemic behaviour family therapy (SBFT) and individual nondirective supportive therapy (NST) for 107 13–18-year-olds with MDD. CBT involved an adaptation of Beck et al.'s model (1979) and focused on psychoeducation, modification of depressogenic thoughts, affect regulation, problem-solving and social skills. The first phase of SBFT involved identification of dysfunctional family patterns and reframing of the family's difficulties and concerns for purposes of clarification and engagement; the second phase focused on communication and problem-solving. In the NST control condition, therapists provided empathic support but did not give advice or teach specific skills. All treatments were delivered in 12–16 weekly sessions.

CBT resulted in a higher rate of remission (64.7%) than SBFT (37.9%) or NST (39.4%), as defined by absence of MDD and at least three consecutive scores lower than 9 on the Beck Depression Inventory (Beck et al., 1988). Interview-rated symptom relief was also achieved more rapidly with CBT than SBFT or NST. Correlates of poor outcome included comorbid anxiety, study entry by clinical referral (vs. response to advertisement), higher level of cognitive distortion and hopelessness (Brent et al., 1998). The authors concluded that CBT was relatively more efficacious, even in the face of multiple adverse predictors and for more complex cases.

However, as Brent et al. (1999) reported, within 24 months of terminating acute treatment, more than half (53%) of the adolescents received additional services; the median time to open treatment was approximately 3 months following termination of acute treatment. Rates of receiving additional services and the timing of additional therapy did not differ across the three treatment conditions. Dysthymic youths and those with higher self-rated depression at the 6-week point were more likely to receive adjunctive interventions during acute treatment. Clinician-rated depression severity, comorbid disruptive disorder and greater self-rated family problems were associated with obtaining additional services during posttreatment.

In a study with depressed youths in Puerto Rico, Rosselló & Bernal (1999) adapted and tested the efficacy of CBT and interpersonal therapy (IPT) for adolescents (Moreau et al., 1991; Mufson et al., 1993). The sample of 71 13–18-year-olds, who were referred by local schools, met *DSM-III-R* criteria for MDD or MDD with dysthymia, and were randomly assigned to CBT, IPT or a wait-list condition. CBT was based on a previously developed group intervention for Hispanic adults and focused on dysfunctional cognitions, pleasant activities, social support systems and assertiveness. IPT targeted the problem areas of grief, interpersonal disputes, role transitions and interpersonal deficits. Both treatments were detailed in manuals and delivered in 12 weekly individual sessions.

Compared to the wait-list condition, both treatments resulted in significant reductions in self-rated depression. The improvements were evident in terms of pre–posttreatment differences in depression severity scores and the number of youths scoring in the dysfunctional range. Moderate effect sizes for both treatments suggested that, on average, 72% of treated subjects were functioning better at the end of treatment than those not treated. In addition, while youths treated with IPT had improved more in self-esteem and social adaptation than those in the control condition, the two active treatments (IPT and CBT) did not show a difference on any of the outcome measures.

The above studies are noteworthy because the investigators utilized structured clinical assessments, operational diagnostic criteria, random assignment to groups, operationalized or 'manualized' treatments and follow-up. Additionally, the results clearly indicate that active, goal-oriented interventions are superior to inactive or wait-list conditions for depressed youths. However, the success rates for active treatments are somewhat disappointing. For example, in some studies (Lewinsohn et al., 1990; Fine et al., 1991; Wood et al., 1996), half or more of the treated cases were still in the midst of a depressive episode at the end of the trials. Furthermore, many treated cases continue to experience marked posttreatment depressive symptoms with possibly up to about 45% having relapses or recurrences during a less than 1-year interval (Vostanis et al., 1996a).

Admittedly, several features of the treatment trials may have made it difficult to obtain a better response. For example, some studies included subjects with either major depression, dysthymia, or both (Lewinsohn et al., 1990; Fine et al., 1991; Vostanis et al., 1996b; Clarke et al., 1999). These two disorders entail somewhat different symptoms, are presumed to represent different levels of severity, and have different durations (as discussed earlier in this chapter). Hence, the mixture of subjects with MDD and DD could have obscured a better response rate possibly associated with one (but not the other) condition.

Additionally, as also noted by Harrington et al. (1998), most studies did not consider the effects of comorbid disorders on treatment outcome. Indeed, Brent et al. (1998) found that comorbid anxiety disorders among depressed youngsters were associated with poor treatment response. As mentioned earlier, presence of a comorbid condition may signal a more severe form of psychopathology (Newman et al., 1996). Alternatively, for example, a depressed youngster who has preexisting attentional or learning problems may simply be at a disadvantage in a therapy that incorporates considerable written material and homework assignments. A condition such as attention deficit hyperactivity disorder may also continue to play a role in the coping style and interpersonal functioning of the individual, possibly predisposing to relapse or recurrence of the depressive symptoms.

Treatment and follow-up durations were also short in these studies, considering the average length of a depressive episode in youths. Recall that recovery rates were 60–73% at the 9-month follow-up in two studies (Fine et al., 1991; Vostanis et al., 1996a) and above 80% at the 24-month follow-up in the

Lewinsohn et al. (1990) study. But, as previously noted, the median recovery (evidenced by 50% of a sample) for an episode of MDD in childhood is about 9 months in clinically referred youths. Therefore, even a seemingly encouraging end-of-treatment recovery rate of 70% may represent no more than a 20% 'gain' over the natural remission rate.

Furthermore, given the wide age ranges of patients in some studies (Vostanis et al., 1996b; Wood et al., 1996) there may have been considerable within-sample developmental variability in the ability to recognize emotions, identify problems and in perspective taking and metacognitive functioning (Digdon & Gotlib, 1985; Kovacs, 1986; Leahy, 1988; Shirk, 1988). In so far as treatment gains are mediated by developmental readiness in the foregoing domains, youths at less mature levels may have evidenced comparatively less improvement, and thus negatively affected overall response rates. Additionally, psychiatrically disturbed youths may already have had delays in cognitive developmental milestones (Szajnberg & Weiner, 1989) that could have interfered with therapeutic learning.

Finally, as suggested earlier, treatment response of youths may be adversely affected by contextual factors such as parental psychopathology and negative family circumstances, including physical or emotional abuse. However, with the exception of the Brent et al. (1997) study, the social context of the youths or the mental health of their parents was neither investigated nor targeted for change.

Nondiagnosed depressed or at-risk samples

Since our 1995 review, three new studies have been reported with symptomatically depressed children and adolescents, bringing it to a total of eight peer-reviewed studies. Two of the recent studies sought to prevent clinical depression by targeting youths with minimal or mild symptoms (or related risk factors). In the investigations we now describe, the subjects were identified in school settings. Students were primarily selected based on cut-off scores on self-rated or parent-rated scales and/or teacher reports. Clinical diagnostic evaluations were not used, with one exception (Clarke et al., 1995). Treatment response rates appeared to be more favourable in general than in the studies of clinically diagnosed youths we reviewed above.

Butler et al. (1980) conducted one of the first controlled studies of a school-based treatment for symptomatically depressed fifth- and sixth-grade students ($n = 56$) using two target interventions: role play (enactment of common problems focusing on recognition of emotions and social and problem-solving skills) and cognitive restructuring (recognizing and replacing dysfunctional thoughts, enhancing listening skills and recognizing the relation between thoughts and feelings). The results revealed that depressive symptoms decreased and self-esteem increased significantly for youths in the two target interventions, compared to attention control and placebo conditions. The positive changes were mirrored in the reports of teachers.

Several years later, Reynolds & Coats (1986) reported on the treatment of 30 symptomatically depressed high-school students (mean age 15.7 years) with either cognitive behaviour (self-monitoring, self-evaluation and self-reinforcement skills) or relaxation (progressive muscle relaxation) techniques. At endpoint, approximately 80% of subjects in both active treatments scored below the clinical cut-off for depression on a self-report scale, compared to none of the wait-list controls. Stark et al. (1987) compared self-control therapy (teaching self-monitoring and self-reinforcement skills) and behavioural problem-solving training (monitoring pleasant events and improving social and problem-solving skills) with 9–12-year-old middle-school students. Although most subjects improved (78% and 60%, respectively), there were few significant differences between the two treatments according to subjects' self-reports and parental ratings.

Kahn et al. (1990) compared cognitive behavioural (based largely on CWD; G. N. Clarke & P. M. Lewinsohn, unpublished paper), and relaxation therapies (education and training in progressive relaxation) and self-modelling (feedback from video-taped rehearsal of nondepressed behaviour) for 10–14-year-old middle-school students. Subjects in all three treatment groups evidenced similarly significant improvement, as compared to a wait-list control condition. However, at 1-month follow-up, more subjects who were in the self-modelling group (50%) again scored in the dysfunctional ranges on self-report scales, compared to subjects who were in the cognitive behavioural and relaxation groups. In a school-based study of 7–11-year-old children, selected using cut-off scores on a self-rated scale as well as a symptom-based interview, Liddle & Spence (1990) failed to find specific effects for treatment delivered during an 8-week period. Children who received group-based social competence training (involving cognitive restructuring, and social and interpersonal problem-solving skills), attention placebo, or were in a wait-list control group, evidenced similar declines in levels of depression at end of treatment and by a 2-month posttreatment follow-up.

In a school-based prevention study, 10–13-year-olds, who reported slightly elevated depressive symptoms or parental conflict, were assigned to one of three 12-week group treatments (cognitive, social problem-solving or a combination of both) or a no-treatment condition (Jaycox et al., 1994). The three treatments were similarly superior to the control condition in terms of pos-ttreatment reduction in depressive symptoms and improvement in classroom behaviour, although rates of children reporting moderate or severe depression scores did not significantly differ between the treatment (15%) and control (23%) conditions. Results from a subsequent 2-year follow-up indicated that the effects of the prevention programme increased over time (Gillham et al., 1995). Compared to controls, children who had received treatment continued to report lower levels of depressive symptoms on average, and were significantly less likely to have overall scores above a clinical threshold. Rates of children reporting moderate or severe depression at 2-year follow-up were 22% and 44% for the prevention and control groups, respectively.

To prevent future depressive disorder among at-risk adolescents, Clarke et al. (1995) used an adaptation of the Adolescent Coping with Depression Course (CWD; Clarke et al., 1990). Subjects were 150 ninth- and 10th-grade adolescents (mean age 15.3 years) who had elevated depressive symptoms by self-rating but did not have diagnosable depression. They were randomized to either a 15-session CWD group delivered during a 5-week period or a 'usual care' control condition. Compared to the controls, adolescents assigned to the prevention groups reported lower levels of depression and were rated higher on global functioning at end of treatment but these differences were not maintained during a 12-month follow-up. Based on clinical evaluations, how-ever, the cumulative rates of MDD or dysthymia during the same 12-month follow-up were significantly lower in the experimental (14.5%) as compared to the control (25.7%) condition.

More recently, Weisz et al. (1997) assigned 48 children in grades 3–6 with mild-to-moderate depressive symptoms to either an eight-session cognitive behavioural intervention called the Primary and Secondary Control Enhance-ment Training (PASCET) programme or a no-treatment condition. The PAS-CET programme targeted primary control (e.g. skills and strategies for chang-ing one's situation to maximize reinforcement) and secondary control (e.g. altering attributions or using relaxation when objective conditions cannot be modified). Compared to untreated children, those in the PASCET programme showed greater symptomatic improvement and were more likely to score in the nonclinical ranges on self- and interviewer ratings on depression. Specifi-cally, at posttreatment, 50% of the treated children vs. 16% of the control children had moved from above to within the normal range on self-rated depression severity. These differences were generally apparent at the end of treatment and at a 9-month follow-up.

Although the overall response rates in the above-noted school-based interventions with symptomatically depressed or at-risk youths appear to be higher than the rates in clinically diagnosed samples, the results have to be interpreted with caution. With the exception of the Clarke et al. (1995) study, the assessments did not include diagnostic evaluations. Thus, it is not clear whether the findings can be generalized to young patients in clinical settings. Furthermore, in at least two investigations (Stark et al., 1987; Kahn et al., 1990), the outcome of assessments by teachers and parents did not coincide with self-reports, raising some questions about the cross-situational generalizability of treatment effects. A similar lack of convergence of results has been found even with identical assessment methods. For example, in one study (Clarke et al., 1995), outcome for one clinician-based measure (diagnosis) failed to parallel two other clinical-based indices (symptom scores and global functioning). However, these studies are distinguished by the fact that the interventions were initiated in the schools, making it feasible to reach a larger segment of potentially 'needy' youths.

Current issues

Expanding the armamentarium of psychosocial treatments

Psychosocial treatment efforts for depressed children and adolescents are still constrained by the paucity of appropriate, operationalized and 'manualized' interventions, and available treatment manuals generally represent modifications of interventions that had been designed for depressed adults. However, developmental considerations have been minimally integrated into these modifications. For example, the manuals rarely acknowledge that the level of cognitive, emotional and social maturity of depressed children and adolescents represents realistic constraints on the delivery of psychotherapy (DiGiuseppe, 1981; Barbanel, 1982; Kazdin, 1990).

One example of an adaptation of an intervention for adolescents is the CBT used by Brent et al. (1997) in the trial that was described above. Modifications of CBT to make it more appropriate for adolescent patients include the use of concrete examples to illustrate points and an emphasis on issues of autonomy and trust. Similarly, IPT, developed by Klerman et al. (1984), has been modified to accommodate the adolescent age group. Revisions included the addition of adolescent-specific therapy topics (e.g. the problem of single-parent families), provisions for involving parents and schools in the treatment, and phone contacts in the event of missed sessions (Moreau et al., 1991; Mufson et al., 1993). The version for adolescents (IPT-A) has been tested in a 12-week open clinical trial to assess its feasibility and preliminary efficacy (Mufson et al., 1994).

The pilot study of 14 clinically depressed adolescents yielded encouraging results; there were significant pre- vs. posttreatment differences in self-rated depressive symptoms, psychological and physical distress, and social adjustment, as well as in clinician-rated depressive symptoms, global functioning and diagnostic status.

Finally, we have ourselves developed an intervention for depressed children and adolescents, called Contextual Psychotherapy (CP). CP is based on the assumption that depression in youngsters is the outcome of a confluence of factors and represents, in large part, the inability to regulate dysphoric emotional reactions to stresses or stressful events. The treatment is grounded in concepts of normal development and developmental psychopathology and focuses on dysregulated emotion as a risk factor for early-onset affective disorders. It is posited that such dysregulation reflects the combination of lack of age-appropriate regulatory mechanisms, inappropriate use of existing regulatory mechanisms and adverse contextual factors. Under certain circumstances of stress or limited compensatory resources, the individual's propensity to emotion dysregulation may maintain or exacerbate depressive symptoms and culminate in an overt disorder.

The focus of CP is twofold: first, to help children recover from their depression by using more adaptive regulatory strategies and resource utilization, and second, to teach or reinforce coping skills and their use (M. Kovacs et al., unpublished paper). The treatment is applied through graduated intensity, starting with twice-a-week sessions, tapering to once a month maintenance. One novel feature of CP is that it requires the participation of at least one parent who is taught to function as a co-therapist or assistant coach in the process of the child's recovery and emotional education. Multiple and developmentally appropriate symptom reduction and coping strategies are presented to parents and children. We are in the process of testing the feasibility of CP in two open clinical trials: one sample involves psychiatrically diagnosed 8–13-year-old children with dysthymia or chronic depression; the other sample entails 8–16-year-old children and adolescents with insulin-dependent diabetes mellitus who are suffering from MDD.

The paucity of treatment outcome data

In their critical review of psychosocial interventions for depressed children and adolescents, Kaslow & Thompson (1998) noted that none of the available therapies are well-established according to the criteria of the Task Force on Promotion and Dissemination of Psychological Procedures (1995). The criteria specify that an intervention be shown by more than one research group to be superior to placebo, or equal to an empirically established effective treatment, in a sample with adequate power. Although Brent et al. (1997) and Rosselló & Bernal (1999) recently demonstrated that adaptations of CBT are effective for depressed adolescents, independent replications of a particular intervention are generally lacking. In addition, only two groups have replicated their own studies. As noted earlier, Clarke et al. (1999) replicated earlier results on CWD group treatment for adolescents (Lewinsohn et al., 1990). Additionally, in a nonpeer-reviewed report, Stark et al. (1991) briefly described a partial constructive replication of their earlier intervention for symptomatic children (Stark et al., 1987). Kaslow & Thompson (1998) concluded that, on the basis of these replications, the therapies examined in the foregoing studies meet criteria for 'probably' efficacious interventions but fall short of being well-established procedures.

Identifying those in need of treatment, and optimal treatment settings

According to reports commissioned by federal agencies of the USA, the vast majority of children in need of mental health care do not receive it (Office of Technology Assessment, 1987; Institute of Medicine, 1989). Indeed, studies of depressed children and adolescents in community settings both in the UK and the USA have yielded similar findings; treatment rates range from 0% (Goodyer & Cooper, 1993) to 60% (Lewinsohn et al., 1998). Poor service utilization probably reflects a combination of factors, including lack of identification of those in need and lack of access to service providers.

The school is probably the best single location for the early identification and treatment of children and adolescents with depressive disorders. A combination of self-, teacher- and parent-rated scales can provide first-stage screening, followed by more intensive diagnostic evaluations. Cases identified as needing treatment may then be served within the school setting. The large-scale application of such an approach has been documented in the well-known project of Kolvin et al. (1981).

The advantage of providing treatment in school settings is that the majority of depressed youths could be reached. Thus, practical problems or other burdens that may prevent parents from bringing a child to a clinic would be overcome. Treatment teams could work closely with teachers and school counsellors to evaluate progress and reinforce new coping skills. Reynolds & Coats (1986) suggested, for example, that the improved academic self-concept of some of the treated students in their study might have reflected the effects of using the school as the treatment milieu. Additionally, to obtain help for their children, parents may prefer the familiar setting of the school as compared to a clinic or mental health centre.

Disadvantages of providing treatment in school settings may include potential stigmatization of the student and difficulties in maintaining privacy and confidentiality. Additionally, because school-based interventions usually take the form of group therapy, they may not be suitable for more severely disturbed youths. Suicidality, psychotic symptoms or multiple comorbid conditions would be indicators for referral to a mental health clinic.

Mental health centres or outpatient child psychiatry clinics will probably remain the settings in which much of psychotherapy is delivered. However, attempts have also been made to provide care in the community at large, using recreational or youth centres that already have established activities (Institute of Medicine, 1989). The use of such community centres could be ideal for cultural and ethnic groups that may be uncomfortable with or distrustful of mainstream institutional environments. Finally, partial hospitalization programmes and inpatient units continue to be necessary to provide care for youths with incapacitating depressive disorders.

The duration of treatment

As long ago as 1959, Levitt et al. posed the question as to what time period or number of hours should constitute 'a course of psychotherapy'. Based on their examination of the rates and predictors of obtaining services beyond those provided in their clinical trial, Brent et al. (1999) concluded that 'Subsequent clinical trials for early-onset depression must focus on the treatment of the entire episode, rather than on acute treatment alone . . .' It would therefore seem sensible that decisions about what constitutes a course of treatment be made empirically, with disorder duration as one variable guiding decisions about treatment length.

Because children are in the process of growth and maturation, the duration of therapy also takes on a degree of importance for which there is no precedence in the literature on adults. Thus, the extent of the depressed child's developmental stage (as opposed to chronological age alone) may be another variable that could guide treatment duration. Finally, the goals of most therapeutic systems embrace learning new ways of behaving, perceiving relationships and interpreting interpersonal and other events of relevance. In so far as learning requires rehearsal, repeated execution of the target behaviours across multiple settings and internationalization of the new rules, developmental-stage specific learning trajectories may provide additional guidance for selecting optimal treatment durations.

Topics that require further attention

The role of parents in treatment

The ambiguous role of parents in psychotherapy trials of depressed youngsters is a notable aspect of the literature, just as it is a problem in child psychotherapy research in general (Kovacs & Lohr, 1995). The omission of parents from most treatment trials may partly reflect the fact that many studies were carried out in school settings. However, the sparse attention paid to parents persists in several currently available psychotherapy treatment manuals and is remarkable in light of practical and clinical issues.

First, at a practical level, parental cooperation is critical to the treatment of their offspring. The political and social reality is that children and adolescents have limited legal rights and, in most instances, parents or care-taking adults are the 'gatekeepers' with respect to initial referral and financial coverage. Second, parental mental health is likely to be a significant moderator of children's response to and compliance with treatment. There exists considerable literature suggesting a relationship between parental and offspring psychopathology (Harder et al., 1980; Beardslee et al., 1983; Cantwell & Baker, 1984; Turner et al., 1987; Puig-Antich et al., 1989; Weissman et al., 1997). Therefore, treatment of the parents' own disorders should be seriously considered in tandem with the psychotherapy of a youngster. Indeed, in one of the recent trials with depressed adolescents, Brent et al. (1997, 1998) found that maternal depression was associated with a diminished response to CBT.

Third, assuming reasonable parental mental health, the omission of parents from treatment trials diminishes the educational and psychological roles they play in their children's lives. Treatment studies of conduct-disordered youths have documented that parents can be important agents of behaviour change in the home (Dadds et al., 1987; Kazdin et al., 1987). Furthermore, Harter (1990) has demonstrated that positive parental attitude is a powerful contributor to self-worth in childhood and adolescence. At the very least, therefore, including the parents in some aspect of their offspring's therapy may help parents to become more effective in the subsequent care of young patients.

Fourth, we believe that a major factor that contributes to the surprisingly long episodes of depression among clinically referred youths is the disruptive effect of the depression on the parent–child relationship and on the behaviour of the parent. Clinically, one of the notable features of depressed children and adolescents is the nonreciprocity of their interpersonal interactions, coupled with an unwillingness or inability to verbalize their affective experience. In return, the parents can be expected to withhold emotional support, guidance and expressions of affection, or to become inconsistent with their offspring in these regards. Such negative interactions have been identified among depressed adults (Coyne et al., 1991) and also have been detected between depressed children and their parents, particularly the alienation of the mothers (Puig-Antich et al., 1985a,b; Cole & Rehm, 1986).

Importantly, the negative effects of the child on the parent and the eventual recursive nature of these consequences may undermine the attachment relationship between them. From a developmental viewpoint, the attachment bond or relationship between parent and child remains an important crucible for maturation and the growth of the child's self-esteem and is an ongoing process (Cicchetti & Schneider-Rosen, 1986; Cummings & Cicchetti, 1990). Thus, inclusion of parents in their children's treatment may also help to preserve or improve the attachment relationship.

Finally, in actual clinical practice, most therapists who work with children and adolescents do involve the parents at some level as well (Fauber & Long, 1991), although the nature and scope of parental involvement have not been well documented. Empirical treatment studies of depressed youths may therefore contribute to clinical practice by providing explicit practical rules for parental participation and clear guidelines regarding the nature of their involvement in their children's treatment.

Yet, only two research groups have systematically studied parent involvement in controlled trials. Lewinsohn and colleagues (Lewinsohn et al., 1990; Clarke et al., 1999) found no beneficial effects of adding separate parent groups to their school-based group CWD therapy. In Brent et al.'s (1997) study of depressed adolescents, SBFT, which included parents of the young patients, was not superior to the other treatments. However, parental participation in these trials involved groups as an adjunct (Lewinsohn et al., 1990; Clarke et al., 1999) or the context of family therapy (Brent et al., 1997). Therefore, there have been no empirical studies involving parents with their children in sessions that explicitly focus on the depressed youth's needs and concerns.

Which interventions are likely to benefit which children?

As noted in recent reviews by Kaslow & Thompson (1998) and Kazdin & Weisz (1998), little attention has been devoted to questions regarding which interventions, or parts of an intervention, are likely to be effective with children depending on their individual characteristics. With few exceptions (Brent et al., 1998), sociodemographic and clinical characteristics (e.g., illness history variables, comorbid conditions) that might relate to treatment efficacy have not been studied. Kaslow & Thompson (1998) and Kazdin & Weisz (1998) also noted that researchers have typically studied multicomponent interventions, most often incorporating elements of cognitive restructuring as well as problem-solving and other skills training. Yet, none of these research teams has addressed which particular ingredient is instrumental in positive treatment response in general, or among children with specific characteristics. Furthermore, as Harrington et al. (1998) noted, although CBTs are the most well-studied interventions, it is not known whether cognitive behavioural processes correlate with treatment response or change with treatment.

In contrast, in the adult literature, various patient-related factors have been identified that are associated with treatment efficacy, including the presence of comorbid conditions or marital discord (Sotsky et al., 1991; Whisman, 1993). The relative importance of specific components of multifaceted treatments has also been addressed in component analysis or 'dismantling' studies with depressed adults (Jacobson et al., 1996). There is a need for similar empirical initiatives in studies of depressed youths. Such initiatives may eventually yield data to help with the task of choosing and implementing an intervention for a particular adolescent or child.

Populations with special needs

Populations with special needs or characteristics include children whose lives are complicated by extreme poverty and homelessness, parental substance abuse and human immunodeficiency virus infection, the increasing cohort of children with chronic medical disorders, as well as those representing cultural minorities. Depressed homeless children, for instance, are unlikely to have access to individual psychotherapy and family support systems for them may be nonexistent. Indeed, several empirical issues raised in the present chapter may be irrelevant in the face of the multiple deprivations such children have to endure, and the fact that their unstable environments probably negate any long-term interventions. For these youths, psychotherapeutic strategies would have to be part of a comprehensive social service 'module' that can be offered in the form of crisis intervention.

The needs of juveniles who have a chronic medical disorder also require attention. Increased understanding of the pathogenesis of various childhood-onset diseases, including insulin-dependent diabetes mellitus, asthma or cystic fibrosis, and concomitant advances in their medical management have led to reduced mortality and better prognosis. However, youngsters with medical problems and depression (or other emotional problems) have generally been ignored in child psychotherapy research and treatment development. Existing treatment approaches will need to be modified in order to take into account functional issues and psychological concerns that are specific to the chronically ill, and to facilitate these youngsters' medical management in tandem with their psychotherapy.

Similarly, since most treatment outcome research has failed to include ethnic minorities, very little is known regarding the ecological validity of empirically studied treatments outside of the majority culture (Bernal et al., 1995). Yet, minority groups constitute a sizeable portion of modern society. As noted by Rosselló & Bernal (1999), their successful extension of CBT and IPT to Puerto Rican adolescents suggests that the development and testing of culturally sensitive adaptations of empirically supported interventions may be fruitful.

Conclusions

During the juvenile years, episodes of major depression and dysthymia are more protracted than hitherto thought, they are associated with high rates of comorbid psychiatric disorders and impairment in various areas of functioning, and they appear to portend future bouts of affective illness. Thus, there is an obvious need for effective interventions. In this chapter, we summarized the available information regarding the treatment of depressed youngsters. Although there has been some progress in the field during the last 5 years, data are still scant in regard to what form of psychotherapy may be most appropriate to bring about symptomatic remission, prevent relapse and improve the functioning of young patients. We also raised several issues that have not received sufficient consideration in treatment outcome studies of depressed youths and remain to be addressed in current treatment development efforts.

Mental health professionals who treat depressed youths are faced with several challenges. These challenges include not only the relative lack of information about efficacious treatments, but also the fact that the pool of professionals is not sufficiently large to meet the mental health needs of our juvenile population. Under these circumstances, what is to be done? From a practical viewpoint, evidence about the treatment of depressed youths together with information on psychotherapies that have been documented as effective with depressed adults can provide some guidelines. Thus, for example, it appears that structured, goal-directed or problem-solving oriented interventions that focus on symptom reduction, enhancement of self-esteem and social/interpersonal skill development are appropriate for depressed juveniles. The best implementation of available strategies may, however, require a closer collaboration between clinicians and academically oriented developmental psychologists. Additionally, if the literature on the treatment of depressed adults is any indication, it would seem advisable to provide youths with some form of maintenance psychotherapy as well, in order to reinforce the skills they have learned, and to prevent relapse. Clarke et al.'s (1999) examination of maintenance or booster sessions represents a step in this direction. Possibly, the concomitant use of antidepressant pharmacotherapy could also be considered, although that form of intervention is beyond the scope of our chapter.

In the treatment of depressed youths, we would also argue for the systematic involvement of the parents or primary care-takers. This involvement should occur on at least two levels. First, parents should be assessed to determine if they themselves suffer from some form of emotional or mental disorder: those who are symptomatic should be treated. Second, parents should be engaged, whenever possible, as agents of change in the treatment of their own children. Such involvement may not only help to reestablish or strengthen attachment bonds, but may teach parents some skills to manage their offspring better in the future.

Finally, to meet the needs of the population of depressed children and adolescents, treatment goals may have to vary depending on the setting in which services can be delivered. As we discussed, although school settings or community-based centres may allow easier access to more youths, certain youngsters may not be adequately served in such places. Possibly, multistage screening coupled with alternative forms of intervention could be implemented in nonclinical settings. However, even as more effective therapies and forms of service delivery are developed and new theories of early-onset depression emerge, the best solution will require a better understanding of risk and predisposing factors in order to make primary prevention possible.

Acknowledgements

Preparation of this chapter was supported in part by grants MH33990 and MH56193 from the National Institute of Mental Health, Rockville, MD, USA.

REFERENCES

American Psychiatric Association (1980). *Diagnostic and Statistical Manual of Mental Disorders*, 3rd edn. Washington, DC: American Psychiatric Association.

American Psychiatric Association (1987). *Diagnostic and Statistical Manual of Mental Disorders*, 3rd edn revised. Washington, DC: American Psychiatric Association.

Armsden, G. C., McCauley, E., Greenberg, M. T., Burke, P. M. & Mitchell, J. R. (1990). Parent and peer attachment in early adolescent depression. *Journal of Abnormal Child Psychology*, **18**, 683–97.

Asarnow, J. R., Goldstein, M. J., Carlson, G. A. et al. (1988). Childhood-onset depressive disorders. A follow-up study of rates of rehospitalization and out-of-home placement among child psychiatric inpatients. *Journal of Affective Disorders*, **15**, 245–53.

Barbanel, L. (1982). Short-term dynamic therapies with children. In *The Handbook of School Psychology*, ed. C. R. Reynolds & T. B. Gutkin, pp. 554–69. New York: John Wiley and Sons.

Beardslee, W. R., Bemporad, J., Keller, M. B. & Klerman, G. L. (1983). Children of parents with major affective disorder: a review. *American Journal of Psychiatry*, **140**, 825–32.

Beck, A. T., Rush A. J., Shaw, B. F. & Emery, G. (1979). *Cognitive Therapy of Depression*. New York: Guilford Press.

Beck, A. T., Steer, R. A. & Garbin, M. G. (1988). Psychometric properties of the Beck Depression Inventory: twenty-five years of evaluation. *Clinical Psychology Review*, **8**, 77–100.

Bernal, G., Bonilla, J. & Bellido, C. (1995). Ecological validity and cultural sensitivity for outcome research: issues for the cultural adaptation and development of psychosocial treatments with Hispanics. *Journal of Abnormal Child Psychology*, **23**, 67–87.

Biederman, J., Faraone, S., Mick, E. & Lelon, E. (1995). Psychiatric comorbidity among referred juveniles with major depression: fact or artifact? *Journal of the American Academy of Child and Adolescent Psychiatry*, **34**, 579–90.

Brent, D. A., Holder, D., Kolko, D. J. et al. (1997). A clinical psychotherapy trial for adolescent depression comparing cognitive, family, and supportive therapy. *Archives of General Psychiatry*, **54**, 877–85.

Brent, D. A., Kolko, D. J., Birmaher, B. et al. (1998). Predictors of treatment efficacy in a clinical trial of three psychosocial treatments for adolescent depression. *Journal of the American Academy of Child and Adolescent Psychiatry*, **37**, 906–14.

Brent, D. A., Kolko, D. J., Birmaher, B., Baugher, M. & Bridge, J. (1999). A clinical trial for adolescent depression: predictors of additional treatment in the acute and follow-up phases of the trial. *Journal of the American Academy of Child and Adolescent Psychiatry*, **38**, 263–70.

Butler, L., Miezitis, S., Friedman, R. & Cole, E. (1980). The effect of two school-based intervention programs on depressive symptoms in pre-adolescents. *American Educational Research Journal*, **17**, 111–19.

Cantwell, D. P. & Baker, L. (1984). Parental mental illness and psychiatric disorders in 'at risk' children. *Journal of Clinical Psychiatry*, **45**, 503–7.

Cicchetti, D. & Schneider-Rosen, K. (1986). An organizational approach to childhood depression. In *Depression in Young People: developmental and clinical perspectives*, ed. M. Rutter, C. E. Izard & P. B. Read, pp. 71–134. New York: Guilford Press.

Clarke, G. N., Lewinsohn, P. M. & Hops, H. (1990). *Instructor's Manual for the Adolescent Coping with Depression Course*. Eugene, OR: Castalia Press.

Clarke, G. N., Hawkins, W., Murphy, M. et al. (1995). Targeted prevention of unipolar depressive disorder in an at-risk sample of high school adolescents: a randomized trial of a group cognitive intervention. *Journal of the American Academy of Child and Adolescent Psychiatry*, **34**, 312–21.

Clarke, G. N., Rohde, P., Lewinsohn, P. M., Hops, H. & Seeley, J. R. (1999). Cognitive-behavioral treatment of adolescent depression: efficacy of acute group treatment and booster sessions. *Journal of the American Academy of Child and Adolescent Psychiatry*, **38**, 272–9.

Cole, D. A. & McPherson, A. E. (1993). Relation of family subsystems to adolescent depression: implementing a new family assessment strategy. *Journal of Family Psychology*, **7**, 119–33.

Cole, D. A. & Rehm, L. P. (1986). Family interaction patterns and childhood depression. *Journal of Abnormal Child Psychology*, **14**, 297–314.

Compas, B. E. (1987). Stress and life events during childhood and adolescence. *Clinical Psychology Review*, **7**, 275–302.

Compas, B. E., Orosan, P. G. & Grant, K. E. (1993). Adolescent stress and coping: implications for psychopathology during adolescence. *Journal of Adolescence*, **16**, 331–49.

Coyne, J. C., Burchill, S. A. L. & Stiles, W. B. (1991). An interactional perspective on depression. In *Handbook of Social and Clinical Psychology: the health perspective*, ed. C. R. Snyder & D. R. Forsyth, pp. 327–49. New York: Pergamon Press.

Cummings, E. M. & Cicchetti, D. (1990). Toward a transactional model of relations between attachment and depression. In *Attachment in the Preschool Years. Theory, research, and intervention*, ed. M. T. Greenberg, D. Cicchetti & E. M. Cummings, pp. 339–72. Chicago: University of Chicago Press.

Dadds, M. R., Schwartz, S. & Sanders, M. R. (1987). Marital discord and treatment outcome in behavioral treatment of child conduct disorders. *Journal of Consulting and Clinical Psychology*, **55**, 396–403.

Daniels, D. & Moos, R. H. (1990). Assessing life stressors and social resources among adolescents: applications to depressed youth. *Journal of Adolescent Research*, **5**, 268–89.

Digdon, N. & Gotlib, I. H. (1985). Developmental considerations in the study of childhood depression. *Developmental Review*, **5**, 162–99.

DiGiuseppe, R. A. (1981). Cognitive therapy with children. In *New Directions in Cognitive Therapy*, ed. G. Emery, S. D. Hollon & R. C. Bedrosian, pp. 50–67. New York: Guilford Press.

Fauber, R. L. & Long, N. (1991). Children in context: the role of the family in child psychotherapy. *Journal of Consulting and Clinical Psychology*, **59**, 813–20.

Fendrich, M., Warner, V. & Weissman, M. M. (1990). Family risk factors, parental depression, and psychopathology in offspring. *Developmental Psychology*, **26**, 40–50.

Fergusson, D. M., Horwood, L. J. & Lynskey, M. T. (1993). Prevalence and comorbidity of DSM-III-R diagnoses in a birth cohort of 15-year-olds. *Journal of the American Academy of Child and Adolescent Psychiatry*, **32**, 1127–34.

Ferro, T., Carlson, G. A., Grayson, P. & Klein, D. N. (1994). Depressive disorders: distinctions in children. *Journal of the American Academy of Child and Adolescent Psychiatry*, **33**, 664–70.

Fine, S., Forth, A., Gilbert, M. & Haley, G. (1991). Group therapy for adolescent depressive disorder: a comparison of social skills and therapeutic support. *Journal of the American Academy of Child and Adolescent Psychiatry*, **30**, 79–85.

Forehand, R., Brody, G., Slotkin, J. et al. (1988). Young adolescents and maternal depression: assessment, interrelations, and family predictors. *Journal of Consulting and Clinical Psychology*, **56**, 422–6.

Garrison, C. Z., Jackson, K. L., Marstellar, F., McKeown, R. E. & Addy, C. (1990). A longitudinal study of depressive symptomatology in young adolescents. *Journal of the American Academy of Child and Adolescent Psychiatry*, **29**, 581–5.

Geller, B., Chestnut, E. C., Miller, M. D. et al. (1985). Preliminary data on DSM-III associated features of major depressive disorder in children and adolescents. *American Journal of Psychiatry*, **142**, 643–4.

Gillham, J., Reivich, K., Jaycox, L. & Seligman, M. (1995). Prevention of depressive symptoms in school children: two-year follow-up. *Psychological Science*, **6**, 343–51.

Goodyer, I. M. & Cooper, P.J. (1993). A community study of depression in adolescent girls II: The clinical features of identified disorder. *British Journal of Psychiatry*, **163**, 374–80.

Harder, D. W., Kokes, R. F., Fisher, L. & Strauss, J. S. (1980). Child competence and psychiatric risk. IV. Relationships of parent diagnostic classifications and parent psychopathology severity to child functioning. *Journal of Nervous and Mental Disease*, **168**, 343–7.

Harrington, R., Whittaker, J. & Shoebridge, P. (1998). Psychological treatment of depression in children and adolescents. A review of treatment research. *British Journal of Psychiatry*, **173**, 291–8.

Harter, S. (1990). Causes, correlates and the functional role of global self-worth: a life-span perspective. In *Competence Considered*, ed. R. J. Sternberg & J. Kolligian, pp. 67–97. New Haven, CT: Yale University Press.

Institute of Medicine (1989). *Research on Children and Adolescents with Mental, Behavioral and Developmental Disorders: mobilizing a national initiative*. Washington, DC: National Academy Press.

Jacobson, N. S., Dobson, K. S., Truax, P. A. et al. (1996). A component analysis of cognitive-behavioral treatment for depression. *Journal of Consulting and Clinical Psychology*, **64**, 295–304.

Jaycox, L. H., Reivich, K. J., Gillham, J. & Seligman, M. E. P. (1994). Prevention of depressive symptoms in school children. *Behavioral Research and Therapy*, **32**, 801–16.

Kahn, J. S., Kehle, T. J., Jenson, W. R. & Clark, E. (1990). Comparison of cognitive-behavioral, relaxation, and self-modeling interventions for depression among middle-school students. *School Psychology Review*, **19**, 196–211.

Kashani, J. H., Carlson, G. A., Beck, N. C. et al. (1987). Depression, depressive symptoms, and depressed mood among a community sample of adolescents. *American Journal of Psychiatry*, **144**, 931–4.

Kaslow, N. J. & Thompson, M. P. (1998). Applying the criteria for empirically supported treatments to studies of psychosocial interventions for child and adolescent depression. *Journal of Clinical Child Psychology*, **27**, 146–55.

Kaslow, N. J., Deering, C. G. & Racusin, G. R. (1994). Depressed children and their families. *Clinical Psychology Review*, **14**, 39–59.

Kazdin, A. E. (1990). Childhood depression. *Journal of Child Psychology and Psychiatry*, **31**, 121–60.

Kazdin, A. E. & Weisz, J. R. (1998). Identifying and developing empirically supported child and adolescent treatments. *Journal of Consulting and Clinical Psychology*, **66**, 19–36.

Kazdin, A. E., Esveldt-Dawson, K., French, N. H. & Unis. A. S. (1987). Effects of parent management training and problem-solving skills training combined in the treatment of antisocial child behavior. *Journal of the American Academy of Child and Adolescent Psychiatry*, **26**, 416–24.

Keller, M. B. & Shapiro, R. W. (1982). 'Double depression': superimposition of acute depressive episodes on chronic depressive disorders. *American Journal of Psychiatry*, **139**, 438–42.

Keller, M. B., Beardslee, W., Lavori, P. W. et al. (1988). Course of major depression in non-referred adolescents: a retrospective study. *Journal of Affective Disorders*, **15**, 235–43.

Klerman, G. L., Weissman, M. M., Rounsaville, B. J. & Chevron, E. S. (1984). *Interpersonal Psychotherapy of Depression*. New York: Basic Books.

Kolvin, I., Garside, R. F., Nicol, A. R. et al. (1981). *Help Starts Here. The maladjusted child in the ordinary school*. New York: Tavistock Publications.

Kovacs, M. (1986). A developmental perspective on methods and measures in the assessment of depressive disorders: the clinical interview. In *Depression in Young People*, ed. M. Rutter, C. E. Izard & P. B. Read, pp. 435–65. New York: Guilford Press.

Kovacs, M. & Bastiaens, L. J. (1995). The psychotherapeutic management of major depressive and dysthymic disorders in childhood and adolescence: issues and prospects. In *The Depressed Child and Adolescent: developmental and clinical perspectives*, ed. I. M. Goodyer, pp. 281–310. New York: Cambridge University Press.

Kovacs, M. & Devlin, B. (1998). Internalizing disorders in childhood. *Journal of Child Psychology and Psychiatry*, **39**, 47–63.

Kovacs, M. & Lohr, W. D. (1995). Research on psychotherapy with children and adolescents: an overview of evolving trends and current issues. *Journal of Abnormal Child Psychology*, **23**, 11–30.

Kovacs, M., Feinberg, T. L., Crouse-Novak, M. A. et al. (1984a). Depressive disorders in childhood. I. A longitudinal prospective study of characteristics and recovery. *Archives of General Psychiatry*, **41**, 229–37.

Kovacs, M., Feinberg, T. L., Crouse-Novak, M. et al. (1984b). Depressive disorders in childhood. II. A longitudinal study of the risk for a subsequent major depression. *Archives of General Psychiatry*, **41**, 643–9.

Kovacs, M., Paulauskas, S., Gatsonis, C. & Richards, C. (1988). Depressive disorders in childhood. III. A longitudinal study of comorbidity with and risk for conduct disorders. *Journal of Affective Disorders*, **15**, 205–17.

Kovacs, M., Gatsonis, C., Paulauskas, S. L. & Richards, C. (1989). Depressive disorders in childhood. IV. A longitudinal study of comorbidity with and risk for anxiety disorders. *Archives of General Psychiatry*, **46**, 776–82.

Kovacs, M., Akiskal, H. S., Gatsonis, C. & Parrone, P. L. (1994). Childhood-onset dysthymic disorder: clinical features and prospective naturalistic outcome. *Archives of General Psychiatry*, **51**, 365–74.

Kovacs, M., Devlin, B., Pollock, M., Richards, C. & Mukerji, P. (1997a). A controlled family history study of childhood-onset depressive disorder. *Archives of General Psychiatry*, **46**, 776–82.

Kovacs, M., Obrosky, D. S., Gatsonis, C. & Richards, C. (1997b). First episode major depressive and dysthymic disorder in childhood: clinical and sociodemographic factors in recovery. *Journal of the American Academy of Child and Adolescent Psychiatry*, **36**, 777–84.

Leahy, R. (1988). Cognitive therapy of childhood depression. In *Cognitive Development and Child*

Psychotherapy, ed. S. R. Shirk, pp. 187–202. New York: Plenum Press.

Levitt, E. E., Beiser, H. R. & Robertson, R. E. (1959). A follow-up evaluation of cases treated at community child guidance clinic. *American Journal of Orthopsychiatry*, **291**, 337–49.

Lewinsohn, P. M., Clarke, G. N., Hops, H. & Andrews, J. (1990). Cognitive-behavioral treatment for depressed adolescents. *Behavior Therapy*, **21**, 385–401.

Lewinsohn, P. M., Rohde, P., Seeley, J. R. & Hops, H. (1991). Comorbidity of unipolar depression: I. Major depression with dysthymia. *Journal of Abnormal Psychology*, **100**, 205–13.

Lewinsohn, P. M., Rohde, P. & Seeley, J. R. (1998). Treatment of adolescent depression: frequency of services and impact on functioning in young adulthood. *Depression and Anxiety*, 7, 47–52.

Liddle, B. & Spence, S. H. (1990). Cognitive-behavior therapy with depressed primary school children: a cautionary note. *Behavioral Psychotherapy*, **18**, 85–102.

McCauley, E., Myers, K., Mitchell, J. et al. (1993). Depression in young people: initial presentation and clinical course. *Journal of the American Academy of Child and Adolescent Psychiatry*, **32**, 714–22.

Mitchell, J., McCauley, E., Burke, P. M. & Moss, S. J. (1988). Phenomenology of depression in children and adolescents. *Journal of the American Academy of Child and Adolescent Psychiatry*, **27**, 12–20.

Mitchell, J., McCauley, E., Burke, P., Calderon, R. & Schloredt, K. (1989). Psychopathology in parents of depressed children and adolescents. *Journal of the American Academy of Child and Adolescent Psychiatry*, **28**, 352–7.

Moreau, D., Mufson, L., Weissman, M. M. & Klerman, G. L. (1991). Interpersonal psychotherapy for adolescent depression: description of modification and preliminary application. *Journal of the American Academy of Child and Adolescent Psychiatry*, **30**, 642–51.

Mufson, L. H., Moreau, D., Weissman, M. M. & Klerman, G. L. (1993). Interpersonal psychotherapy for adolescent depression. In *New Applications of Interpersonal Psychotherapy*, pp. 129–66, ed. G. L. Klerman & M. M. Weissman. Washington, DC: American Psychiatric Press.

Mufson, L., Moreau, D., Weissman, M. M. et al. (1994). Modification of interpersonal psychotherapy with depressed adolescents (IPT-A): phase I and II studies. *Journal of the American Academy of Child and Adolescent Psychiatry*, **33**, 695–705.

Newman, D. L., Moffitt, T. E., Caspi, A. et al. (1996). Psychiatric disorder in a birth cohort of young adults: prevalence, comorbidity, clinical significance, and new case incidence from ages 11 to 21. *Journal of Consulting and Clinical Psychology*, **64**, 552–62.

Office of Technology Assessment (1987). *Children's Mental Health. Problems and services*. Durham, NC: Duke University Press.

Puig-Antich, J., Lukens, E., Davies, M. et al. (1985a). Psychosocial functioning in prepubertal major depressive disorders. I. Interpersonal relationships during the depressive episode. *Archives of General Psychiatry*, **42**, 500–7.

Puig-Antich, J., Lukens, E., Davies, M. et al. (1985b). Psychosocial functioning in prepubertal major depressive disorders. II. Interpersonal relationships after sustained recovery from the affective episode. *Archives of General Psychiatry*, **42**, 511–17.

Puig-Antich, J., Goetz, D., Davies, M. et al. (1989). A controlled family history study of prepubertal major depressive disorder. *Archives of General Psychiatry*, **46**, 406–18.

Puig-Antich, J., Kaufman, J., Ryan, N. D. et al. (1993). The psychosocial functioning and family environment of depressed adolescents. *Journal of the American Academy of Child and Adolescent Psychiatry*, **32**, 244–53.

Rao, U., Ryan, N. D., Birmaher, B. et al. (1995). Unipolar depression in adolescents: clinical outcome in adulthood. *Journal of the American Academy of Child and Adolescent Psychiatry*, **34**, 566–78.

Reynolds, W. M. & Coats, K. I. (1986). A comparison of cognitive-behavioral therapy and relaxation training for the treatment of depression in adolescents. *Journal of Consulting and Clinical Psychology*, **54**, 653–60.

Rohde, P., Lewinsohn, P. M. & Seeley, J. R. (1994). Are adolescents changed by an episode of major depression? *Journal of the American Academy of Child and Adolescent Psychiatry*, **33**, 1289–98.

Rosselló, J. & Bernal, G. (1999). The efficacy of cognitive-behavioral and interpersonal treatments for depression in Puerto Rican adolescents. *Journal of Consulting and Clinical Psychology*, **67**, 734–45.

Ryan, N. D., Puig-Antich, J., Ambrosini, P. et al. (1987). The clinical picture of major depression in children and adolescents. *Archives of General Psychiatry*, **44**, 854–61.

Shain, B. N., King, C. A., Naylor, M. & Alessi, N. (1991). Chronic depression and hospital course in adolescents. *Journal of the American Academy of Child and Adolescent Psychiatry*, **30**, 428–33.

Shirk, S. (1988). Children's understanding of therapeutic interpretations. In *Cognitive Development and Child Psychotherapy*, ed. S. R. Shirk, pp. 53–87. New York: Plenum Press.

Sotsky, S., Glass, D. R., Shea, M. T. & Pilkonis, P. A. (1991). Patient predictors of response to psychotherapy and pharmacotherapy: findings in the NIMH treatment of depression collaborative research program. *American Journal of Psychiatry*, **148**, 997–1008.

Spitzer, R. L., Endicott, J. & Robins, E. (1978). Research diagnostic criteria: rationale and reliability. *Archives of General Psychiatry*, **35**, 773–82.

Stark, K. D., Reynolds, W. M. & Kaslow, N. J. (1987). A comparison of the relative efficacy of self-control therapy and a behavioral problem-solving therapy for depression in children. *Journal of Abnormal Child Psychology*, **15**, 91–113.

Stark, K., Rouse, L. & Livingston, R. (1991). Treatment of depression during childhood and adolescence: cognitive-behavioral procedures for the individual and family. In *Child and Adolescent Therapy*, ed. P. Kendall, pp. 165–206. New York: Guilford Press.

Strober, M. & Carlson, G. (1982). Bipolar illness in adolescents with major depression: clinical, genetic, and psychopharmacologic predictors in a three- to four-year prospective follow-up investigation. *Archives of General Psychiatry*, **39**, 549–55.

Szajnberg, N. M. & Weiner, A. (1989). Children's conceptualization of their own psychiatric illness and hospitalization. *Child Psychiatry and Human Development*, **20**, 87–97.

Task Force on Promotion and Dissemination of Psychological Procedures (1995). Training in and dissemination of empirically-validated psychological treatments: report and recommendations. *Clinical Psychologist*, **8**, 3–24.

Todd, R. D., Neuman, R., Geller, B., Fox, L. W. & Hickok, J. (1993). Genetic studies of affective disorders: should we be starting with childhood onset probands? *Journal of American Academy of Child and Adolescent Psychiatry*, **32**, 1164–71.

Turner, S. M., Beidel, D. C. & Costello, A. (1987). Psychopathology in the offspring of anxiety disorders patients. *Journal of Consulting and Clinical Psychology*, **55**, 229–35.

Vostanis, P., Feehan, C., Grattan, E. & Bickerton, W.-L. (1996a). A randomized controlled out-patient trial of cognitive-behavioural treatment for children and adolescents with depression: 9-month follow-up. *Journal of Affective Disorders*, **40**, 105–16.

Vostanis, P., Feehan, C., Grattan, E. & Bickerton, W.-L. (1996b). Treatment for children and adolescents with depression: lessons from a controlled trial. *Clinical Child Psychology and Psychiatry*, **1**, 199–212.

Warner, V., Weissman, M. M., Fendrich, M. et al. (1992). The course of major depression in the offspring of depressed parents. Incidence, recurrence, and recovery. *Archives of General Psychiatry*, **49**, 795–801.

Weissman, M. M., Warner, V., Wickramaratne, P., Moreau, D. & Olfson, M. (1997). Offspring of depressed parents. 10 years later. *Archives of General Psychiatry*, **54**, 932–40.

Weisz, J., Thurber, C., Sweeney, L., Proffitt, V. & LeGagnoux, G. (1997). Brief treatment of mild to moderate child depression using primary and secondary control enhancement training. *Journal of Consulting and Clinical Psychology*, **65**, 703–7.

Whisman, M. A. (1993). Mediators and moderators of change in cognitive therapy of depression. *Psychological Bulletin*, **114**, 248–65.

Williamson, D. E., Ryan, N. D., Birmaher, B. et al. (1995). A case-control family history study of depression in adolescents. *Journal of the American Academy of Child and Adolescent Psychiatry*, **34**, 1596–1607.

Wood, A., Harrington, R. & Moore, A. (1996). Controlled trial of a brief cognitive-behavioral intervention in adolescent patients with depressive disorders. *Journal of Child Psychology and Psychiatry*, **37**, 737–46.

13

Natural history of mood disorders in children and adolescents

Richard Harrington and Bernadka Dubicka

Knowledge of the natural history of an illness is critical to understanding its origins and to optimizing its management. Over the past 15 years or so, data have been accumulating steadily on the course and outcome of juvenile affective conditions. The main purpose of the present chapter is to review these studies. The chapter is divided into five parts. The first part is concerned with the risk of recurrence of juvenile depression and the second part with the mechanisms that might be involved. The third part describes the prospects for recovery. The fourth part reviews the natural history of other juvenile affective disorders, principally bipolar disorder. The chapter concludes with a discussion of some of the clinical implications of these research findings.

Continuity and recurrence of depression

Continuities in the short term

Many studies of clinical samples have reported that young people with a depressive disorder have a high risk of recurrence or persistence (King & Pittman, 1970; Kovacs et al., 1984a; Asarnow et al., 1988; Goodyer et al., 1991; McCauley et al., 1993; Emslie et al., 1997b). For example, Kovacs and colleagues (1984a) undertook a systematic follow-up of child patients with a major depressive disorder, a dysthymic disorder, an adjustment disorder with depressed mood, and some other psychiatric disorder. The development of subsequent episodes of depression was virtually confined to children with major depressive disorders and dysthymic disorders. Thus, within the first year at risk, 26% of children who had recovered from major depression had had another episode; by 2 years this figure had risen to 40%; and by 5 years the affected cohort ran a 72% risk of another episode. On long-term follow-up major depression and dysthymia were associated with similar rates of most outcomes (Kovacs et al., 1994).

Asarnow and co-workers (1988) found that children who had been hospitalized with major depression were at increased risk of rehospitalization because of suicidal behaviour or increasing depression. Within a little less than 2 years 45% were rehospitalized – a rate that was not significantly different from that found for children with schizophrenia spectrum disorders. McCauley et al. (1993) found that 54% of their sample of depressed children had a recurrence within 3 years.

Surveys of community samples have generally also found that depressive disorders among young people tend to be recurrent (McGee & Williams, 1988; McGee et al., 1992; Fleming et al., 1993; Lewinsohn et al., 1993, 1994a; Garrison et al., 1997). For instance, Lewinsohn et al. (1993, 1994a) found that the 1-year relapse rate for unipolar depression (18.4%) was much higher than the relapse rate found in most other disorders. Interestingly, among adolescents in that study who experienced two episodes of depression there was low concordance across episodes in the symptoms of depression (Roberts et al., 1995). Only one community study has failed to find significant continuity for depressive disorder (Cohen et al., 1993a,b).

Investigators of the short-term stability of questionnaire ratings of depressive symptoms in community samples of young people have also found significant correlations over time (Garrison et al., 1990; Larsson et al., 1991; Edlsohn et al., 1992; Stanger et al., 1992; Charman, 1994; Cole et al., 1998). Larsson et al. (1991) for instance, found that the correlation over a 4–6-week period on the Beck Depression Inventory was 0.66. Garrison et al. (1990) reported that the stability of adolescents' self-reports of depression was 0.53 at 1 year and 0.36 at 2 years after the initial assessment.

Continuities in the long term

It seems, then, that both depressive symptoms and depressive disorder show significant continuity over time. Do these continuities extend into adulthood? The available data suggest that they do. Harrington et al. (1990) followed up 63 depressed children and adolescents on average 18 years after their initial contact. The depressed group had a substantially greater risk of depression after the age of 17 years than a control group who had been matched on a large number of variables, including nondepressive symptoms and measures of social impairment. This increased risk was maintained well into adulthood and was associated with significantly increased rates of attending psychiatric services and of using medication as compared to the controls. Depressed children were no more likely than the control children to suffer nondepressive disorders in adulthood, suggesting that the risk for adult depression was specific and unrelated to comorbidity with other psychiatric problems. Rao et al. (1995) also found high rates of recurrence of major depression in a clinical sample of depressed adolescents who were followed up 7 years later.

Continuity from childhood into adult life has also been found in community surveys, such as the Dunedin Multidisciplinary Health and Development Study (DMHDS). In the DMHDS mental health data were gathered at ages 11, 13, 15, 18 and 21 years. Follow-back longitudinal analyses found that subjects with a mood disorder at age 21 years were much more likely to have a history of previous mood disorder than of nondepressive disorders earlier in life (Newman et al., 1996). Similarly, prospective longitudinal analyses from the Oregon Adolescent Depression Project (Lewinsohn et al., 1999) found significant continuity from late adolescence (age 17 years) into early adult life (age 24 years). Thus, major depression in young adulthood was significantly more common in subjects who had had major depression in late adolescence than subjects who had had nonaffective mental disorders or no psychiatric disorder (average annual rate 9.0%, 5.6% and 3.7% respectively). About 45% of adolescents with a history of major depression developed a new episode of depression between the ages of 19 and 24. In the New York longitudinal study (Cohen et al., 1993a,b) anxiety or depression in adolescence predicted anxiety or depression in early adult life (Pine et al., 1998). Most adult anxiety or depression was preceded by earlier anxiety or depression. The British birth cohort follow-up of individuals born in 1946 found that evidence of affective disturbance at ages 13 and 15 years was a strong predictor of major affective disorder in middle life (Os et al., 1997).

Depressive symptoms rated on questionnaires have also been shown to have significant long-term stability (Devine et al., 1994; Ferdinand & Verhulst, 1995). For instance, Ferdinand & Verhulst (1995) found that an anxious/depressed syndrome derived from the Child Behavior Checklist (Achenbach & Edelbrock, 1983) was a relatively strong predictor (odds ratio 3.0) of the same syndrome 8 years later. Nevertheless, a significant proportion of young people with high levels of depressive symptoms do not show persistent symptoms of internalizing disorders (Ollendick & King, 1994).

Subsequent social impairment

There are a number of reasons for thinking that early-onset depression might not only predict further depression, but also could be associated with effects on social and cognitive functioning. Thus, depression in young people is frequently accompanied by social withdrawal and irritability, and so depressed youngsters may find it more difficult to establish and maintain social relationships. In addition, symptoms such as loss of concentration and psychomotor retardation may interfere with the process of learning. This in turn might lead to low self-esteem and so on to further academic failure. Kovacs & Goldston (1991) pointed out that young people suffering from major depression are impaired for a significant proportion of the life span and they are handicapped at a time when learning takes place rapidly. Perhaps, then, they will eventually show cognitive as well as social delays.

Several studies have examined the social outcomes of depressed young people. In one of the first systematic studies, Puig-Antich and colleagues (1985a,b) found that impairment of peer relationships persisted several months after recovery from depression. In the longer term, Kandel & Davies (1986) reported that self-ratings of dysphoria in adolescence were associated with heavy cigarette smoking, greater involvement in delinquent activities and impairment of intimate relationships as young adults. Garber et al. (1988) found that depressed adolescent inpatients reported more marital and relationship problems when they were followed up 8 years after discharge than non-depressed psychiatric control subjects.

These findings have important theoretical as well as clinical implications since they suggest that the social isolation and lack of a supporting relationship that have been found in cross-sectional studies of adult depression (Brown & Harris, 1978) may reflect social selection as much as social causation. However, none of these studies excluded the effects that childhood conduct problems, which are commonly associated with adolescent depression, could have on these outcomes. Harrington et al. (1991) found that juvenile depression seemed to have little direct impact on social functioning in adulthood, whereas comorbid conduct disorder was a strong predictor of subsequent social maladjustment. Similar findings were reported by Renouf and colleagues (1997) in an intensive longitudinal study of depressed children and nondepressed psychiatric controls. Social dysfunction associated with comorbid depression and conduct disorder seemed to be mainly related to the effects of conduct disorder. Bardone et al. (1998) found that adolescent conduct disorder predicted more smoking, sexually transmitted diseases and early pregnancy in adult life. Adolescent depression only predicted tobacco dependence and more medical problems. The implication is that it is important to differentiate the course of depressive disorder from the course of other comorbid disorders.

Links with suicidal behaviour

Adolescents who are depressed and those who attempt suicide share many psychosocial risk factors (Lewinsohn et al., 1994c). Indeed, depressed young people very commonly have suicidal thoughts and some of them make suicidal attempts (Andrews & Lewinsohn, 1992). Ryan et al. (1987), for instance, found in a clinical sample that about 60% of children and adolescents with major depression had suicidal ideation. Mitchell et al. (1988) reported that 67% of depressed young people had suicidal thoughts, and nearly 40% had made a suicidal attempt.

Several community surveys have found that depressive disorder predicts subsequent suicidality. For example, Lewinsohn and colleagues (1994c) reported that depression was one of the strongest predictors of a subsequent suicidal attempt, even when the association with other risk factors was controlled. Conversely, it seems that suicidal children are at increased risk of depression. For example, Pfeffer et al. (1991) found that young people who had attempted suicide were 10 times more likely to have a mood disorder during the 6–8-year follow-up period than young people who had not made an attempt. Reinherz et al. (1995) found that suicidal ideation at age 15 years predicted major depression at age 18.

Myers et al. (1991) examined the risk factors for suicidality in the depressed sample studied by Mitchell et al. (1988). Three variables predicted later suicidality: severity of initial suicidality, anger and age. Kienhorst et al. (1991) also found that previous suicidality was a predictor of subsequent attempts, as were features of the initial depression, a broken home and feelings of hopelessness. In a review of the association of depression and suicidal behaviour, Pfeffer (1992) concluded that the risk indicators for suicidal attempts among depressed young people included previous suicidality, suicidal ideation, hopelessness, comorbid problems such as substance abuse and anger, easy access to the method and lack of social support. The importance of comorbidity with conduct disturbance and/or substance abuse is underlined by the findings of Kovacs and colleagues (1993). They reported that the presence of these problems more than doubled the risk of suicide attempts among depressed child patients.

Relatively little is known about the risk of completed suicide in depressed young people. In our follow-up of 80 depressed probands (Harrington et al., 1990) all three deaths in adulthood were due to 'unnatural causes', of which two were definite suicides. Although no statistical weight can be attached to these small numbers, they seem far in excess of those expected in the general population of young adults. Similarly, in a preliminary communication from a longitudinal study of the depressed children and adolescents initially studied by Puig-Antich and his group, Rao et al. (1993) reported that seven (4.4%) had committed suicide. There were no suicides in the psychiatric control group.

Another way of looking at the relationship between depression and suicide is through 'psychological autopsy' studies of young people who have killed

themselves. Such studies involve the interviewing of relatives and the collection of data from a variety of other sources in order to make a diagnostic
assessment on the suicide victim. Several psychological autopsy studies of
suicide in young people have found high rates of affective disorders (Brent et
al., 1988; Groholt et al., 1998; Marttunen et al., 1991; Shaffer et al., 1996). The
association between suicide and depression seems to be particularly strong in
females (Marttunen et al., 1995). It is, however, important to note that other
mental disorders may also be relevant in suicide. For instance, Marttunen et al.
(1991) found that nearly one-fifth of suicides aged between 13 and 19 years had
a conduct disorder or antisocial personality, and that a quarter abused alcohol
or drugs.

A high rate of comorbidity with behavioural problems and substance abuse
is also found in attempted suicide. Brent et al. (1990) reported that, among
those depressed patients who had attempted suicide, the degree of intent was
associated with conduct disorder and comorbid substance abuse. In a birth
cohort of 16-year-old New Zealanders, suicidal attempts were not only associated with depression but with many other forms of psychopathology (e.g.
conduct disorder) and with delinquency (Fergusson & Lynskey, 1995).

Perhaps, then, it is the combination of depression and certain personality
characteristics, such as aggression or the propensity to take risks, that is
especially likely to lead to suicidal behaviour in young people. Substance abuse
may also be important. Nevertheless, it is clear that juvenile depression poses a
substantial independent risk factor for suicidal behaviour.

Mechanisms involved in continuity and recurrence

Direct persistence of the initial depression

The review thus far suggests that depression in young people is associated with
a variety of adverse outcomes, particularly further episodes of depression and
suicidal behaviour. What processes could underpin these strong continuities
over time? The first point is that the strength and specificity of the continuities
clearly support the idea that in some cases there may be direct persistence of
the initial depression. At first sight, the finding that most cases of major
depression among the young remit within a year (see below) would seem to
suggest that direct persistence is uncommon. However, a detailed 12-year
prospective study of adults who had presented with major depression found
that, whilst only 15% had major depressive disorder level symptoms during the
follow-up, 43% had subthreshold depression (Judd et al., 1998). The same may
apply to depression in young people; major depression and dysthymia often

overlap and one can lead to the other (Kovacs et al., 1994). The symptomatic course of depression seems to be malleable, and symptoms of major depression, dysthymia and minor depression alternate over time in the same patients.

Scarring or sensitization

Another potential mechanism of continuity is that individuals are changed in one way or another by their first episode so that they become more likely to have subsequent ones. This notion, sometimes referred to as 'scarring' or sensitization, has attracted a good deal of attention from investigators of the neurobiological (Post, 1992) and psychological (Rohde et al., 1990) processes that may be involved in the relapsing and remitting course of depression in adults. Post (1992), for instance, has suggested that the first depressive episode may sensitize people to further episodes. He hypothesized that such sensitization may help to explain three characteristics of depression in adults: the tendency to recur, the decreasing length of interval between episodes and the greater role of psychosocial stress at the first episode. The idea is that the first episode of depression, which can often be linked to a psychosocial stressor, is associated with long-lasting changes in biology and responsivity to stressors. There may be biochemical and microstructural changes in the central nervous system that put the individual at risk of further episodes (Post et al., 1996).

The idea of scarring may also be relevant to depression in young people. Lewinsohn and colleagues (1994b) found in cross-sectional comparisons that formerly depressed individuals shared many psychosocial characteristics with depressed individuals. A subsequent prospective study by the same research group identified 45 adolescents who experienced and recovered from a first episode of depression between two assessment points (Rohde et al., 1994). Psychosocial scars (characteristics evident after but not before the episode) included stressful life events, excessive emotional reliance on others and subsyndromal depressive symptoms. This level of scarring was more severe than found in previous research by the same team with depressed adults.

Cognitive vulnerability

Scarring should be distinguished from the related concept of vulnerability, in which the predisposition to depression precedes the first episode.

Two types of cognitive problem are thought to make young people vulnerable to depression: general cognitive deficits such as reading retardation or low intelligence, and cognitive distortions, such as a negative attributional style, that are believed to be specific to depression.

There may be early neurodevelopmental precursors of affective illness in both childhood and adult life. In a retrospective study of hospital records, Sigurdsson et al. (1999) found that adolescents with severe affective disorders (bipolar, manic or psychotic depression) were significantly more likely to have experienced delayed language, social or motor development. Associations between childhood developmental problems (such as low cognitive ability) and affective disorder were studied prospectively in the British 1956 national birth cohort study (Os et al., 1997). Affective disorder was assessed at interview when subjects were aged 36 and 43 years. Teacher questionnaires at age 13 and 15 years also identified subjects with evidence of affective disturbance. Early cognitive ability independently predicted both adolescent affective disturbance and affective disorder in adult life. So, continuity could be due to an underlying neurodevelopmental problem that increases the liability to depression in both childhood and adult life.

The 'depressogenic' cognitive distortions that may make some individuals vulnerable to depression are dealt with in other parts of this book and so need not be considered in detail here (see Chapters 2 and 3 for discussions relating to normal and abnormal emotion and cognitive psychology and Chapter 12 for their application of these to current psychotherapeutic methods). For the purposes of this chapter, however, it is worth noting that negative cognitions such as self-criticism can be remarkably stable (Koestner et al., 1991). Several longitudinal studies have shown that they may precede depressive symptoms in young people (Seligman & Peterson, 1986; Reinherz et al., 1989; Nolen-Hoeksema et al., 1992; Cole et al., 1997). However, different results have been obtained when depressive disorders have been studied. Thus, in an investigation that included the offspring of women with affective disorders, Hammen et al. (1988) found that depression at follow-up was best predicted by initial symptoms and life events but not by negative attributions. Similarly, Asarnow & Bates (1988) found that inpatient children whose depressive disorder had remitted did not show negative attributional patterns. Dalgleish et al. (1998) reported that recovered depressed subjects did not differ from matched controls in their judgements about the likelihood that negative events would happen to themselves.

At first sight, these findings would seem to suggest that negative cognitive distortions may be a state-dependent symptom of depressive disorder rather than a trait-like predisposition. In interpreting these results, however, it must be borne in mind that much of the research published thus far has been based on pencil-and-paper questionnaire measures of cognition. There has been relatively little experimental research using mood induction techniques. Kelvin and colleagues (1999) found that adolescents at risk for depression because of high emotionality did not show negative cognitions until mild dysphoric mood was induced by listening to a sad piece of music. The implication is that cognitive vulnerability to depression may be latent, and not easily assessed by questionnaires.

Biological vulnerability

Evidence of biological indices has up to now been focused on the kinds of markers that have been studied in depressed adults, such as abnormalities of cortisol physiology (Casat et al, 1989), melatonin (Shafii et al., 1996), thyroid hormone levels (Kutcher et al., 1991; Dorn et al., 1996), sleep (Emslie et al., 1987) and brain imaging (Steingard et al., 1996).

Several studies have shown that, in comparison with nondepressed patients, depressed young people show less nonsuppression of cortisol secretion following administration of the exogenous corticosteroid dexamethasone (Casat et al., 1989), but are more likely to have sleep abnormalities (Lahmeyer et al., 1983; Cashman et al., 1986; Emslie et al., 1987; Appelboom-Fondu et al., 1988; Kutcher et al., 1992; Riemann & Schmidt, 1993).

There has been very little longitudinal research on most of these measures. There is, however, some evidence that cortisol levels predict subsequent depression. Goodyer and colleagues (1998) found that higher cortisol/dehydroepiandrosterone levels at night predicted both the persistence of major depression and subsequent disappointing life events. They hypothesized that adrenal steroids might be involved in abnormal cognitive or emotional processes associated with the continuation of disturbed interpersonal behaviour. Susman et al. (1997) reported that adolescents who showed increased cortisol levels in a challenging situation had higher levels of depressive symptoms a year later than adolescents whose cortisol did not change or decreased. (Further discussions on the role of cortisol and other neuroendocrine aspects of depression can be found in Chapters 4 and 9. Correlates between sex hormones and depression in females are described in Chapter 6.)

Family–genetic vulnerability

The offspring of depressed parents are at greatly increased risk of depression, especially in childhood and early adult life (Wickramaratne & Weissman, 1998). Many other forms of psychopathology are increased amongst these children (Wickramaratne & Weissman, 1998) and they are also at increased risk of medical problems (Kramer et al., 1998). Several prospective longitudinal studies have suggested that these increased risks extend for many years (Hammen, 1991; Beardslee et al., 1993; Weissman et al., 1997). For example, Weissman and colleagues (1997) evaluated the effects of parental depression on offspring over a 10-year period. High rates of depression, panic disorder and alcoholism were found among the children.

There is evidence that affective disorders in adults have a genetic component. Genetic influences seem strongest for bipolar disorders (McGuffin & Katz, 1986), but unipolar major depressions also show significant heritability (Kendler et al., 1993), as do seasonal affective disorders (Madden et al., 1996). There have thus far been no large systematic twin or adoption studies of depressive disorder in young people. There is however evidence from twin studies of modest genetic influences on depressive symptoms in late childhood and adolescence (Thapar & McGuffin, 1994; Eaves et al., 1997; Silberg et al, 1999), though this has not been replicated in adoption studies (Eley et al., 1998). Twin studies also suggest that some of the stability in depressive symptoms arises from genetic factors (O'Connor et al., 1998).

Family environment

It is likely, however, that family environment also plays an important role in continuities. Some kinds of family adversity, such as marital discord, can be highly persistent (Richman et al., 1982; Rutter & Quinton, 1984) and there is growing evidence of the relevance of these factors to continuities of depressive disorders in young people. For example, Hammen and colleagues (1991) found a close temporal relationship between episodes of depression in children and episodes of depression in the mother. Fergusson et al. (1995) reported that maternal depression was only associated with depressive symptoms in adolescent offspring in so far as maternal depression was associated with social disadvantage or family adversity. Depression in parents is associated with many problems that could lead to depression in offspring, including impaired child management practices, insecure attachment, poor marital functioning and hostility towards the child (Cummings & Davies, 1994). Indeed, Asarnow and colleagues reported (Asarnow et al., 1993) that relapse of depression after discharge from a psychiatric inpatient sample was virtually confined to children who returned to a home environment characterized by high expressed emotion and hostility. Goodyer et al. (1997c) found that family dysfunction and lack of a confiding relationship with the mother predicted persistent psychiatric disorder in a sample with major depression.

Other environments

Other kinds of adverse experience may also contribute to the persistence of depression. For example, events such as physical assault or sexual abuse are strongly associated with subsequent depressive symptoms, even when the association of both with previous symptoms and family relationships problems is controlled statistically (Boney-McCoy & Finkelhor, 1996). A history of childhood physical or sexual abuse may be associated with a particular pattern of reversed neurovegetative depressive symptoms, such as increased appetite and hypersomnia (Levitan et al., 1998). Poor peer relationships are also associated with persistence of depression (Goodyer et al., 1997c).

Role of comorbidity with nondepressive psychopathology

Several studies have reported that comorbidity with nondepressive disorders predicts a worse outcome for juvenile depressive disorder (Sandford et al., 1995; Goodyer et al., 1997a; Kovacs et al., 1997). For instance, Kovacs et al. (1997) found that comorbid externalizing disorder predicted a much more protracted recovery from dysthymic disorder. Goodyer et al. (1997a) reported that comorbid obsessive-compulsive disorder was associated with persistence of major depression at 36-week follow-up.

Combinations of risk factors

It seems, then, that the risk of further episodes of depression is predicted by many factors. It is likely that it is the combination of several of these risk factors that poses the greatest risk. Thus, for instance, Beardslee et al. (1996) examined risk factors for affective disorder within a random sample of 139 adolescents. Single risk factors such as parental major depression, parental nonaffective diagnosis or a previous child psychiatric diagnosis increased the risk of subsequent affective disorder from 7% to 18%. However, when all three risk factors were present the risk jumped to 50%!

It is not clear whether the factors that lead to continuity simply add up, or whether there is some kind of interaction such that some risk factors only operate in the presence of others. There is some evidence of such interactions in adult depression. For instance, studies of major depression in women suggest that genetic influences may alter the sensitivity of individuals to the depression-inducing effect of adverse life events (Kendler et al., 1995). In other cases, it seems as if people act in ways that increase their likelihood of adversity, which in turn increases their risk of depression. One of the best known examples of this phenomenon comes from the research of Brown et al. (1986) with young women in an inner city. They found that women who had experienced lack of care during childhood (e.g. abuse) were more likely to become pregnant while young. In turn, early pregnancy increased the risk of other forms of adversity, such as marrying an abusive partner. These later forms of adversity were strongly associated with depression.

Similar kinds of processes may occur in juvenile depression. Daley and colleagues (1998) conducted a community study of personality functioning in older adolescents, who were then followed up for 2 years. They found that certain personality disorder features seemed to generate chronic interpersonal stress, which increased vulnerability to depression. Goodyer & Altham (1991) reported that the families of depressed girls seemed to become 'life event prone' as a result of parental psychopathology. In their study it seemed that young people became depressed when depressed parents were no longer able to protect them from adversity.

Summary

In summary, if the available evidence is put together, it seems probable that early-onset depression is associated with subsequent depression through several different mechanisms, though knowledge on their relative importance is lacking. Clearly, the strength and specificity of the links point to a relatively uninterrupted form of continuity, as would occur in the direct persistence of the initial disorder. There appears to be a substantial self-perpetuating quality to juvenile depressive disorders. Nevertheless, environmental influences, particularly those that occur within families, also appear to be important. Probably there are circular processes in which the effects of social experiences change the child's views of him/herself and the world, which in turn leads to depression, which then alters the child's experiences of the environment.

Discontinuity and recovery

Developmental discontinuities

The findings thus far suggest that juvenile depressive disorders show substantial continuities over time. Nevertheless, the available data also suggest that many depressed young people will not go on to have another episode, and so it is important to consider the reasons for discontinuity. There is a surprising lack of knowledge on this issue, but some limited evidence is available.

The first point to make is that there may be developmental differences in the continuity of depressive disorders. Interest in the possibility of such differences has been increased by the finding of marked age differences in the prevalence of affective phenomena such as depression, suicide and attempted suicide (Harrington et al., 1996). Thus, for example, it seems that depressive disorders show an increase in frequency during early adolescence (Angold et al., 1998). The reasons for these age trends are still unclear but there is some evidence that they are accompanied by developmental differences in continuity. Thus, in our child-to-adult follow-up of depressed young people, continuity to major depression in adulthood was significantly stronger in pubescent/postpubertal depressed probands than in prepubertal depressed subjects (Harrington et al., 1990). All five cases of bipolar disorder in adulthood occurred in the postpubertal group. Similarly, Kovacs et al. (1989) reported that, among cases who had recovered from their index episode of major depression, older children would go into a new episode faster than younger ones. Other studies, too, have found that older age predicts greater persistence of depression (Sandford et al., 1995; Goodyer et al., 1997b).

What do these differences mean? Clearly, the association with age and/or puberty suggests that maturational factors could play an important part. For example, perhaps the relative cognitive immaturity of younger children protects them from the development of cognitive 'scars' arising from an episode of depression. Or it may be that the massive changes in sex hormone production that occur around the time of puberty are involved. There is evidence that the increase in rates of depression in girls at puberty is related to changes in androgen and oestrogen levels (Angold et al., 1999). However, it would be unwise to dismiss the effects of environment altogether. After all, puberty is associated not only with maturational changes but also with marked changes in social/family environment (Buchanan et al., 1992). Indeed, there is evidence that children who develop depression are more likely to come from families in which there is much discord and expressed emotion than depressed adolescents (Harrington et al., 1997). It could be that for depression to occur at a developmentally inappropriate period (i.e. early childhood), stressors need to be particularly severe.

Recovery from an episode of depression

It is important to distinguish between long-term continuities/discontinuities in the course of depressive disorders and the prognosis for the index attack. Indeed, the available data suggest that the majority of children with major depression will recover within 2 years. For example, Kovacs et al. (1984b) reported that the cumulative probability of recovery from major depression by 1 year after onset was 74% and by 2 years was 92%. The median time to recovery was about 28 weeks. This study included many subjects who had previous emotional-behavioural problems and some form of treatment, and might therefore have been biased towards the most severe cases. Very similar results were reported in a retrospective study of recovery from first episode of major depression in young people by Keller et al. (1988, 1991) who had mostly not received treatment, and by Warner et al. (1992) in a study of the children of depressed parents. In a community survey, Garrison et al. (1997) found that only one-fifth of those with major depression at baseline continued to have it at 1 year. The probability of recovery for adolescent inpatients with major depression also appears to be about 90% by 2 years (Strober, 1992), though those with long-standing depressions seem to recover less quickly than those whose presentation was acute (Shain et al., 1991).

How do young people recover from an episode of depression? The paucity of systematic studies among the young makes it impossible to draw firm conclusions about this issue. Indeed, even the adult literature is sparse and has for the most part been concerned with recovery in the context of treatment trials rather than with the process itself. It has provided, however, a number of pointers about the mechanisms that could be involved in young people. It may be, for instance, that environmental circumstances change. For example, perhaps there is a reduction in adversity. Alternatively, it could be that some kind of positive event needs to occur before depression will abate (Needles & Abramson, 1990; Brown et al., 1992).

There are also a number of biological explanations for the periodicity of affective disorders. It could be, for instance, that the physiological systems involved in recurrent affective conditions oscillate endogenously. The recovery phase occurs because homeostatic mechanisms come into force in order to correct underlying biochemical imbalances. Or, it might be that there is some kind of external photic or temperature-related seasonal cue that leads to cycling. Recovery occurs when the external biological cue has ceased.

Treatment may also influence recovery from depression. There is quite a lot of evidence that some psychological therapies, particularly cognitive-behavioural therapies, are effective in mild or moderately severe depression in this age group (Harrington et al., 1998b). Pharmacological treatments, too, may be effective (Emslie et al., 1997a).

Chronicity

Although these results clearly provide some grounds for optimism regarding the short-term outcome of early-onset major depressions, it is worth noting that the speed of recovery found in some studies appears to be slower than reported in comparable studies of depressed adults (Strober et al., 1995). Moreover, recovery from dysthymic disorder tends to be slower than recovery from major depression. Kovacs et al. (1997) reported that the median duration of dysthymic disorder was 3.9 years.

In addition, it seems that a significant proportion of cases will become chronic to the extent that recovery takes many months or even years. Thus, Shain et al. (1991) found that about 10% of severe cases of adolescent-onset depression became chronic to the extent that they had not recovered by 1 year. Ryan et al. (1987) estimated that nearly one-half of depressed children and adolescents in their clinical sample had been ill for over 2 years. Goodyer and colleagues (1997a) reported that, at 36-week follow-up, 50% of a clinical sample with major depression still had the disorder.

Course of other affective disorders

Adolescent bipolar disorder

Bipolar disorder in adults is usually recurrent, though there is marked individual variability in episode duration and cycle length (Goodwin & Jamison, 1984). The interval between attacks shows a tendency to shorten as the disorder progresses (Goodwin & Jamison, 1984) and in about 10% of cases rapid cycling (four or more affective episodes per year) occurs (Bauer & Whybrow, 1991). Even with aggressive pharmacological maintenance treatment, the risk of relapse into mania or depression is high (Gitlin et al., 1995).

It can be difficult to diagnose bipolar disorder in adolescents. Mild forms are easily confused with problems such as conduct disorder and attention deficit disorder (Kovacs & Pollock, 1995). Severe psychotic manic states are often diagnosed initially as schizophrenia (Carlson et al., 1994). Indeed, typical adult-like bipolar disorder appears to be uncommon in adolescence. For example, in the first two waves of the Oregon study, only two of the 1500 adolescents who were evaluated met full diagnostic criteria for bipolar disorder (Lewinsohn & Klein, 1995).

Nevertheless, the available data suggest that those bipolar disorders that do occur in adolescence often follow the remitting and relapsing course of adult cases. Strober et al. (1995) followed up 54 consecutive admissions of adolescents with bipolar illness to a university inpatient service. At the time of admission, 20 were manic and the remainder depressed or in mixed states. Time to remission was much quicker in manic subjects (median 9 weeks) than in depressed subjects (median 26 weeks). Nearly 50% of the sample had a relapse during the 5-year follow-up. However, the prognosis of early-onset bipolar disorder is probably better than of early-onset schizophrenia (Werry et al., 1991).

It has been suggested that juvenile-onset depressions often presage bipolar disorder in adulthood (Akiskal, 1995). Long-interval follow-ups do not at present support this hypothesis (Harrington et al., 1990). Nevertheless, a proportion of adolescent patients who present with depression will go on to develop mania. Strober et al. (1992) found that five out of 58 adolescents with major depression developed manic or hypomanic episodes during the 24-month follow-up period. In line with the findings from adult follow-up studies (Akiskal et al., 1983) many of these cases had psychotic features during their depressive episode. Other predictors of outcome include premorbid personality (Werry & McClellan, 1992) and family history. Duffy and colleagues (1998) found that a family history of bipolar disorder that responded to lithium was associated with a relapsing and remitting course of affective disorder in offspring. Psychiatrically ill children of lithium-nonresponsive parents, however, had high rates of comorbid illness and experienced nonremitting affective disorders.

There has recently been interest in milder forms of bipolar disorder in adolescents, such as bipolar II disorder (episodes of major depression and hypomania) and cyclothymia (chronic mild states characterized by symptoms such as irritability, decreased need for sleep, and so on). These problems show moderate short-term stability (Lewinsohn & Klein, 1995) and may be a manifestation of a temperamental vulnerability to typical manic depression (Akiskal, 1995). However, at present they are of uncertain nosological validity.

Childhood bipolar disorder

Although childhood mania is regarded by many clinicians as extremely rare, some researchers have identified cases with mania-like symptoms suggestive of child-onset bipolar disorder. For example, Wozniak et al. (1995) found 43 children 12 years or younger who met *DSM* criteria for mania (American Psychiatric Association, 1994). Geller et al. (1994) found that bipolarity developed in 25 of 79 children with major depression, the majority of whom were prepubertal.

Little is known about the course of childhood mania, but in the study of Wozniak and colleagues the course seemed chronic, without the relapses and remissions that characterize mania in adults. Geller & Luby (1997) hypothesized that, in comparison with older adolescent and adult bipolar disorder, prepubertal bipolar disorder has the following distinguishing features. First, it is more likely to present with major depression. Second, it is typically rapid-cycling, without the discrete onset and offsets that characterize the adult forms of the condition. Third, episodes last for longer. Fourth, there is less recovery between episodes.

Seasonal affective disorder

Seasonal affective disorder (SAD) is characterized by depressions that occur at certain times of the year. Most often, the episodes begin in autumn or winter and remit in spring. Prominent symptoms include loss of energy, sleep disturbance and craving for carbohydrates. Carskadon & Acebo (1993) estimated a 3–5% prevalence for seasonal depression among children. Giedd and colleagues (1998) followed up six children (aged 6–17 years) with a diagnosis of SAD. Subjects were followed for 7 years and outcomes were assessed using standardized methods. All subjects had persistent seasonal symptoms, which remained relatively severe. However, in most, light therapy was of some benefit.

Clinical implications

Implications for initial management

The time course of major depression in young people is highly regular across studies (see above). Once triggered, one-half of all episodes last around 7 months and 80% last 1 year. Only 10% or less last 2 years or longer. It is important, therefore, that clinicians enquire carefully about the duration of depressive symptoms. Patients who present shortly after the onset of symptoms have a good chance of recovering within the next few months. In such cases a sensible initial approach might consist of a relatively brief intervention, especially as there is evidence that the response rate to inactive interventions or placebo is around 30–40% (Harrington et al., 1998a; Hazell et al., 1995). By contrast, those who present for treatment after, say, 6 months may be less likely to recover spontaneously within the next 4 weeks. In such cases there is a stronger case for initiating an intensive form of treatment straight away.

Need for continuation and maintenance treatments

There has been widespread agreement on the finding that juvenile affective disorders tend to be recurrent. This finding is important because it has been taught for many years that, while behavioural difficulties such as conduct disorders show strong continuity over time, emotional problems among the young tend to be short-lived. The studies described here suggest that this view is mistaken, at least so far as clinical cases of depressive disorders are concerned. They are associated with considerable impairment of psychosocial functioning and in severe cases vulnerability extends into adult life.

It is apparent, then, that both assessment and treatment need to be viewed as extending over a prolonged period of time. Young people with severe depressive disorders are likely to have another episode and so it is important that we develop effective prophylactic treatments.But for how long should these treatments continue? Research with depressed adults distinguishes between the need for continuation treatments and maintenance treatments. The idea behind continuation treatments is that, although treatment may suppress the acute symptoms of depression, studies of the natural history suggest that the underlying illness process is continuing. Thus, for example, untreated major depression in adolescents often lasts for many months (see above). Treatment therefore needs to continue until the hypothesized underlying episode has finished.

There have been no randomized trials of continuation treatments for juvenile depressive disorders. However, data from a nonrandomized trial with depressed adolescents suggest that continuing psychological treatment for 6 months after remission is feasible and may be effective in preventing relapse (Kroll et al., 1996). Moreover, there is good evidence from randomized trials with depressed adults that continuation psychological and pharmacological treatments are effective (Kupfer, 1992). Most investigators therefore recommend that the treatment given during the acute episode of adolescent depression should be continued after remission, until the patient has been free of depression for around 6 months.

Maintenance treatments have a different objective, which is to prevent the development of a new episode of depression. Research with adult patients suggests that both pharmacotherapy and psychotherapy may reduce the risk of relapse if maintained for several years after the index depressive episode (Frank et al., 1990; Kupfer et al., 1992). Clearly such treatments will be very time-consuming and expensive. They cannot at present be contemplated for more than a small minority of depressed young people. Clinical experience suggests that indications for maintenance treatment include a history of highly recurrent depressive disorder, severely handicapping episodes of depression and chronic major depression.

The form of maintenance treatment may vary from case to case. Since early-onset depressive disorders seem to have a significant self-perpetuating quality, there is clearly a need to help individuals to develop coping strategies that will enable them to deal with the illness in the long term. However, there is also evidence that relapses are linked to changes in environmental circumstances, especially family disturbances such as parenting difficulties and mental illness (see above). Accordingly, clinicians treating young people with depressive disorders need to assess the extent to which these factors are relevant. It may be possible to intervene therapeutically to improve patterns of family relationships. Parents who are depressed or suffering from some other form of mental disorder also need to be helped. In other words, there needs to be a concern with the family as a whole and not just with the patient as an individual.

In milder cases who are relatively well between episodes it is important that we teach the child and parents early recognition of the signs of a relapse, and encourage them to return to us when the first symptoms appear. Alternatively, it may be useful to see the young person from time to time for check-ups, rather like going to the dentist.

Need for vigorous treatment of the first episode

The finding that the first episode of depression can lead to 'scarring' is important because it suggests that much greater attention should be paid to the recognition and treatment of the first episode of depression. Since late adolescence is a common period for the onset of adult depressive disorders (Smith & Weissman, 1992), the implication is that child and adolescent psychiatry could have an important part to play in the prevention of depression in adulthood. Indeed, there are plenty of developmental examples of the ways in which early disorders that are not managed appropriately can lead to permanent changes in both the biology of individuals and in their psychosocial functioning (Wolkind & Rutter, 1985).

Implications for preventive policies

The evidence on the course of early-onset depressive disorders also has implications for preventive policies. For example, it may be that intensive work with at-risk groups such as the children of depressed parents will reduce the risk of depression in the children. Unfortunately, so far data are lacking on the extent to which primary preventive interventions are in fact protective, so it may be better to concentrate on the early recognition and intensive treatment of the first episode of depression (Harrington & Clark, 1998). There is some evidence that in adults the earlier the intervention, the shorter the episode (Kupfer et al., 1989). It remains to be seen whether this will be found in juvenile depressions.

REFERENCES

Achenbach, T. M. & Edelbrock, C. S. (1983). *Manual for the Child Behaviour Checklist and Revised Profile*. Burlington, VT: University of Vermont, Department of Psychiatry.

Akiskal, H. S. (1995). Developmental pathways to bipolarity: are juvenile-onset depression pre-bipolar? *Journal of the American Academy of Child and Adolescent Psychiatry*, **34**, 754–63.

Akiskal, H. S., Walker, P., Puzantian, V. R. et al. (1983). Bipolar outcome in the course of depressive illness: phenomenologic, familial, and pharmacologic predictors. *Journal of Affective Disorders*, **5**, 115–28.

American Psychiatric Association (1994). *Diagnostic and Statistical Manual of Mental Disorders*, 4th edn. Washington, DC: American Psychiatric Association.

Andrews, J. A. & Lewinsohn, P. M. (1992). Suicidal attempts among older adolescents: prevalence and co-occurrence with psychiatric disorders. *Journal of American Academy of Child Psychiatry*, **31**, 655–62.

Angold, A., Costello, E. J. & Worthman, C. M. (1998). Puberty and depression: the roles of age, pubertal status and pubertal timing. *Psychological Medicine*, **28**, 51–61.

Angold, A., Costello, E. J., Erkanli, A. et al. (1999). Pubertal changes in hormone levels and depression in girls. *Psychological Medicine*, **29**, 1043–53.

Appelboom-Fondu, J., Kerkhofs, M. & Mendlewicz, J. (1988). Depression in adolescents and young adults – polysomnographic and neuroendocrine aspects. *Journal of Affective Disorders*, **14**, 35–40.

Asarnow, J. R. & Bates, S. (1988). Depression in child psychiatric inpatients: cognitive and attributional patterns. *Journal of Abnormal Child Psychology*, **16**, 601–15.

Asarnow, J. R., Goldstein, M. J., Carlson, G. A. et al. (1988). Childhood-onset depressive disorders. A follow-up study of rates of rehospitalization and out-of-home placement among child psychiatric inpatients. *Journal of Affective Disorders*, **15**, 245–53.

Asarnow, J. R., Goldstein, M. J., Tompson, M. et al. (1993). One-year outcomes of depressive disorders in child psychiatric inpatients: evaluation of the prognostic power of a brief measure of expressed emotion. *Journal of Child Psychology and Psychiatry*, **34**, 129–37.

Bardone, A. M., Moffitt, T. E., Caspi, A. et al. (1998). Adult physical health outcomes of adolescent girls with conduct disorder, depression, and anxiety. *Journal of the American Academy of Child and Adolescent Psychiatry*, **37**, 594–601.

Bauer, M. S. & Whybrow, P. C. (1991). Rapid cycling bipolar disorder: clinical features, treatment, and etiology. In *Advances in Neuropsychiatry and Psychopharmacology*, vol. 2. *Refractory Depression*, ed. J. D. Amsterdam, pp. 191–208. New York: Raven Press.

Beardslee, W. R., Keller, M. B., Lavori, P. W. et al. (1993). The impact of parental affective disorder on depression in offspring: a longitudinal follow-up in a nonreferred sample. *Journal of the American Academy of Child and Adolescent Psychiatry*, **32**, 723–30.

Beardslee, W. R., Keller, M. B., Seifer, R. et al. (1996). Prediction of adolescent affective disorder: effects of prior parental affective disorders and child psychopathology. *Journal of the American Academy of Child and Adolescent Psychiatry*, **35**, 279–88.

Boney-McCoy, S. & Finkelhor, D. (1996). Is youth victimization related to trauma symptoms and depression after controlling for prior symptoms and family relationships? A longitudinal, prospective study. *Journal of Consulting and Clinical Psychology*, **64**, 1406–16.

Brent, D. A., Perper, J. A., Goldstein, C. E. et al. (1988). Risk factors for adolescent suicide. A comparison of adolescent suicide victims with suicidal inpatients. *Archives of General Psychiatry*, **45**, 581–8.

Brent, D. A., Kolko, D. J., Allan, M. J. et al. (1990). Suicidality in affectively disordered adolescent inpatients. *Journal of the American Academy of Child Psychiatry*, **29**, 586–93.

Brown, G. W. & Harris, T. (1978). *Social Origins of Depression*. London: Tavistock Publications.

Brown, G. W., Harris, T. O. & Bifulco, A. (1986). Long-term effects of early loss of parent. In *Depression in Young People: developmental and clinical perspectives*, ed. M. Rutter, C. E. Izard, P. B. Read, pp. 251–96. New York: Guilford.

Brown, G. W., Lemyre, L. & Bifulco, A. (1992). Social factors and recovery from anxiety and depressive disorders. A test of specificity. *British Journal of Psychiatry*, **161**, 44–54.

Buchanan, C. M., Eccles, J. S. & Becker, J. B. (1992). Are adolescents the victims of raging hormones: evidence for activational effects of hormones on moods and behavior at adolescence. *Psychological Bulletin*, **111**, 62–107.

Carlson, G. A., Fennig, S. & Bromet, E. J. (1994). The confusion between bipolar disorder and schizophrenia in youth: where does it stand in the 1990s? *Journal of the American Academy of Child and Adolescent Psychiatry*, **33**, 453–60.

Carskadon, M. A. & Acebo, C. (1993). Parental reports of seasonal mood and behavior changes in children. *Journal of the American Academy of Child and Adolescent Psychiatry*, **32**, 264–9.

Casat, C. D. Arana, G. W. & Powell, K. (1989). The DST in children and adolescents with major depressive disorder. *American Journal of Psychiatry*, **146**, 503–7.

Cashman, M. A., Coble, P., McCann, B. S. et al. (1986). Sleep markers for major depressive disorder in adolescent patients. *Sleep Research*, **15**, 91.

Charman, T. (1994). The stability of depressed mood in young adolescents: a school-based survey. *Journal of Affective Disorders*, **30**, 109–16.

Cohen, P., Cohen, J. & Brook, J. (1993a). An epidemiological study of disorders in late childhood and adolescence – II. Persistence of disorders. *Journal of Child Psychology and Psychiatry*, **34**, 869–77.

Cohen, P., Cohen, J., Kasen, S. et al. (1993b). An epidemiological study of disorders in late childhood and adolescence – I. Age- and gender-specific prevalence. *Journal of Child Psychology and Psychiatry*, **34**, 851–67.

Cole, D. A., Martin, J. M. & Powers, B. (1997). A competency-based model of child depression: a longitudinal study of peer, parent, teacher, and self-evaluations. *Journal of Child Psychology and Psychiatry*, **38**, 505–14.

Cole, D. A., Peeke, L. G., Martin, J. M. et al. (1998). A longitudinal look at the relation between depression and anxiety in children and adolescents. *Journal of Consulting and Clinical Psychology*, **66**, 451–60.

Cummings, E. M. & Davies, P. T. (1994). Maternal depression and child development. *Journal of Child Psychology and Psychiatry*, **35**, 73–112.

Daley, S. E., Hammen, C., Davila, J. et al. (1998). Axis II symptomatology, depression, and life stress during the transition from adolescence to adulthood. *Journal of Consulting and Clinical Psychology*, **66**, 595–603.

Dalgleish, T., Neshat-Doost, H., Taghavi, R. et al. (1998). Information processing in recovered depressed children and adolescents. *Journal of Child Psychology and Psychiatry*, **39**, 1031–5.

Devine, D., Kempton, T. & Forehand, R. (1994). Adolescent depressed mood and young adult functioning. A longitudinal study. *Journal of Abnormal Child Psychology*, **22**, 629–40.

Dorn, L. D., Burgess, E. S., Dichek, H. L. et al. (1996). Thyroid hormone concentrations in depressed and nondepressed adolescent: group differences and behavioral relations. *Journal of the American Academy of Child and Adolescent Psychiatry*, **35**, 299–306.

Duffy, A., Alda, M., Kutcher, S. et al. (1998). Psychiatric symptoms and syndromes among adolescent children of parents with lithium-responsive or lithium non-responsive bipolar disorder. *American Journal of Psychiatry*, **155**, 431–3.

Eaves, L. J., Silberg, J. L., Meyer, J. M. et al. (1997). Genetics and developmental psychopathology: 2. The main effects of genes and environment on behavioral problems in the Virginia twin study of adolescent behavioral development. *Journal of Child Psychology and Psychiatry*, **38**, 965–80.

Edelsohn, G., Ialongo, N., Werthamer-Larsson, L. et al. (1992). Self-reported depressive symptoms in first-grade children: developmentally transient phenomena? *Journal of the American Academy of Child Psychiatry*, **31**, 282–90.

Eley, T. C., Deater-Deckard, K., Fombonne, E. et al. (1998). An adoption study of depressive symptoms in middle childhood. *Journal of Child Psychology and Psychiatry*, **39**, 337–45.

Emslie, G. J., Roffwarg, H. P., Rush, A. J. et al. (1987). Sleep EEG findings in depressed children and adolescents. *American Journal of Psychiatry*, **144**, 668–70.

Emslie, G., Rush, A., Weinberg, W. et al. (1997a). A double-blind, randomized placebo-controlled trial of fluoxetine in depressed children and adolescents. *Archives of General Psychiatry*, **54**, 1031–7.

Emslie, G. J., Rush, J. A., Weinberg, W. A. et al. (1997b). Recurrence of major depressive disorder in hospitalized children and adolescents. *Journal of the American Academy of Child and Adolescent Psychiatry*, **36**, 785–92.

Ferdinand, R. F. & Verhulst, R. F. (1995). Psychopathology from adolescence into young adulthood. An 8-year follow-up study. *American Journal of Psychiatry*, **152**, 1586–94.

Fergusson, D. & Lynskey, M. T. (1995). Suicidal attempts and suicidal ideation in a birth cohort of 16-year-old New Zealanders. *Journal of the American Academy of Child and Adolescent Psychiatry*, **34**, 1308–17.

Fergusson, D. M., Horwood, L. J. & Lynskey, M. T. (1995). Maternal depressive symptoms and depressive symptoms in adolescents. *Journal of Child Psychology and Psychiatry*, **36**, 1161–78.

Fleming, J. E., Boyle, M. H. & Offord, D. R. (1993). The outcome of adolescent depression in the Ontario Child Health Study. *Journal of American Academy Child Psychiatry*, **32**, 28–33.

Frank, E., Kupfer, D. J., Perel, J. M. et al. (1990). Three-year outcomes for maintenance therapies in recurrent depression. *Archives of General Psychiatry*, **47**, 1093–9.

Garber, J., Kriss, M. R., Koch, M. et al. (1988). Recurrent depression in adolescents: a follow-up study. *Journal of American Academy Child Psychiatry*, **27**, 49–54.

Garrison, C. Z., Jackson, K. L., Marsteller, F. et al. (1990). A longitudinal study of depressive symptomatology in young adolescents. *Journal of American Academy of Child Psychiatry*, **29**, 581–5.

Garrison, C. Z., Waller, J. L., Cuffe, S. P. et al. (1997). Incidence of major depressive disorder and dysthymia in young adolescents. *Journal of the American Academy of Child and Adolescent Psychiatry*, **36**, 458–65.

Geller, B. & Luby, J. (1997). Child and adolescent bipolar disorder: a review of the past 10 years. *Journal of the American Academy of Child and Adolescent Psychiatry*, **36**, 1168–76.

Geller, B., Fox, L. W. & Clark, K. A. (1994). Rate and predictors of prepubertal bipolarity during follow-up of 6- to 12-year-old depressed children. *Journal of American Academy of Child Adolescent Psychiatry*, **33**, 461–8.

Giedd, J. N., Swedo, S. E., Lowe, C. H. et al. (1998). Case series: pediatric seasonal affective disroder. A follow-up report. *Journal of the American Academy of Child and Adolescent Psychiatry*, **37**, 218–20.

Gitlin, M. J., Swendsen, J., Heller, T. L. et al. (1995). Relapse and impairment in bipolar disorder. *American Journal of Psychiatry*, **152**, 1635–40.

Goodwin, F. K. & Jamison, K. R. (1984). The natural course of manic-depressive illness. In *The Neurobiology of Mood Disorders*, ed. R. M. Post & J. C. Ballenger, pp. 20–37. Baltimore: Williams & Wilkins.

Goodyer, I. M. & Altham, P. M. E. (1991). Lifetime exit events and recent social and family adversities in anxious and depressed school-age children and adolescents – I. *Journal of Affective Disorders*, **21**, 219–28.

Goodyer, I. M., Germany, E., Gowrusankur, J. et al. (1991). Social influences on the course of anxious and depressive disorders in school-age children. *British Journal of Psychiatry*, **158**, 676–84.

Goodyer, I. M., Herbert, J., Secher, S. M. et al. (1997a). Short-term outcome of major depression: I. Comorbidity and severity at presentation as predictors of persistent disorder. *Journal of the American Academy of Child and Adolescent Psychiatry*, **36**, 179–87.

Goodyer, I. M., Herbert, J., Secher, S. M. et al. (1997b). Short-term outcome of major depression: I. Comorbidity and severity at presentation as predictors of persistent disorder. *Journal of the American Academy of Child and Adolescent Psychiatry*, **36**, 179–87.

Goodyer, I. M., Herbert, J., Tamplin, A. et al. (1997c). Short-term outcome of major depression: II. Life events, family dysfunction, and friendship difficulties as predictors of persistent disorder. *Journal of the American Academy of Child and Adolescent Psychiatry*, **36**, 474–80.

Goodyer, I. M., Herbert, J. & Altham, P. M. (1998). Adrenal steroid secretion and major depression in 8- to 16-year-olds, III. Influence of cortisol/DHEA ratio at presentation on subsequent rates of disappointing life events and persistent major depression. *Psychological Medicine*, **28**, 265–73.

Groholt, B., Ekeberg, O., Wichstrom L. et al. (1998). Suicide among children and younger and older adolescents in Norway: a comparative study. *Journal of the American Academy of Child and Adolescent Psychiatry*, **37**, 473–81.

Hammen, C. (1991). *Depression Runs in Families. The social context of risk and resilience in children of depressed mothers.* New York: Springer Verlag.

Hammen, C., Adrian, C. & Hiroto, D. (1988). A longitudinal test of the attributional vulnerability model in children at risk for depression. *British Journal of Clinical Psychology*, **27**, 37–46.

Hammen, C., Burge, D. & Adrian, C. (1991). Timing of mother and child depression in a longitudinal study of children at risk. *Journal of Consulting and Clinical Psychology*, **59**, 341–5.

Harrington, R. C. & Clark, A. (1998). Prevention and early intervention for depression in adolescence and early adult life. *European Archives of Psychiatry and Clinical Neuroscience*, **248**, 32–45.

Harrington, R. C., Fudge, H., Rutter, M. et al. (1990). Adult outcomes of childhood and adolescent depression: I. Psychiatric status. *Archives of General Psychiatry*, **47**, 465–73.

Harrington, R. C., Fudge, H., Rutter, M. et al. (1991). Adult outcomes of childhood and adolescent depression: II. Risk for antisocial disorders. *Journal of the American Academy of Child and Adolescent Psychiatry*, **30**, 434–9.

Harrington, R., Rutter, M. & Fombonne, E. (1996). Developmental pathways in depression: multiple meanings, antecedents and endpoints. *Developments in Psychopathology*, **8**, 601–16.

Harrington, R. C., Rutter, M., Weissman, M. et al. (1997). Psychiatric disorders in the relatives of depressed probands. I. Comparison of prepubertal, adolescent and early adult onset forms. *Journal of Affective Disorders*, **42**, 9–22.

Harrington, R., Whittaker, J., Shoebridge, P. et al. (1998a). Systematic review of efficacy of cognitive behaviour therapies in child and adolescent depressive disorder. *British Medical Journal*, **316**, 1559–63.

Harrington, R. C., Whittaker, J. & Shoebridge, P. (1998b). Psychological treatment of depression in children and adolescents: a review of treatment research. *British Journal of Psychiatry*, **173**, 291–8.

Hazell, P., O'Connell, D., Heathcote, D. et al. (1995). Efficacy of tricyclic drugs in treating child and adolescent depression: a meta-analysis. *British Medical Journal*, **310**, 897–901.

Judd, L. L., Akiskal, H. S., Maser, J. L. et al. (1998). A prospective 12-year study of subsyndromal and syndromal depressive symptoms in unipolar major depressive disroders. *Archives of General Psychiatry*, **55**, 694–700.

Kandel, D. B. & Davies, M. (1986). Adult sequelae of adolescent depressive symptoms. *Archives of General Psychiatry*, **43**, 255–62.

Keller, M. B., Beardslee, W., Lavori, P. W. et al. (1988). Course of major depression in non-referred adolescents: a retrospective study. *Journal of Affective Disorders*, **15**, 235–43.

Keller, M. B., Lavori, P. W., Beardslee, W. R. et al. (1991). Depression in children and adolescents; new data on 'undertreatment' and a literature review on the efficacy of available treatments. *Journal of Affective Disorder*, **21**, 163–71.

Kelvin, R. G., Goodyer, I. M., Teasdale, J. D. et al. (1999). Latent negative self-schema and high emotionality in well adolescents at risk for psychopathology. *Journal of Child Psychology and Psychiatry*, **40**, 959–68.

Kendler, K. S., Neale, M. C., Kessler, R. C. et al. (1993). A longitudinal twin study of 1-year prevalence of major depression in women. *Archives of General Psychiatry*, **50**, 843–52.

Kendler, K. S., Kessler, R. C., Walters, E. E. et al. (1995). Stressful life events, genetic liability, and onset of an episode of major depression in women. *American Journal of Psychiatry*, **152**, 833–42.

Kienhorst, C. W. M., Wilde, E. J. D., Diekstra, R. F. W. et al. (1991). Construction of an index for predicting suicide attempts in depressed adolescents. *British Journal of Psychiatry*, **159**, 676–82.

King, L. J. & Pittman, G. L. (1970). A six-year follow-up study of 65 adolescent patients. Natural history of affective disorders in adolescence. *Archives of General Psychiatry*, **22**, 230–6.

Koestner, R., Zuroff, D. C. & Powers, T. A. (1991). Family origins of adolescent self-criticism and its continuity into adulthood. *Journal of Abnormal Psychology*, **100**, 191–7.

Kovacs, M. & Goldston, D. (1991). Cognitive and social cognitive development of depressed children and adolescents. *Journal of the American Academy of Child and Adolescent Psychiatry*, **30**, 388–92.

Kovacs, M. & Pollock, M. (1995). Bipolar disorder and comorbid conduct disorder in childhood and adolescence. *Journal of the American Academy of Child and Adolescent Psychiatry*, **34**, 715–23.

Kovacs, M., Feinberg, T. L., Crouse-Novak, M. et al. (1984a). Depressive disorders in childhood. II. A longitudinal study of the risk for a subsequent major depression. *Archives of General Psychiatry*, **41**, 643–9.

Kovacs, M., Feinberg, T. L., Crouse-Novak, M. A. et al. (1984b). Depressive disorders in childhood. I. A longitudinal prospective study of characteristics and recovery. *Archives of General Psychiatry*, **41**, 229–37.

Kovacs, M., Gatsonis, C., Paulauskas, S. et al. (1989). Depressive disorders in childhood. IV. A longitudinal study of comorbidity with and risk for anxiety disorders. *Archives of General Psychiatry*, **46**, 776–82.

Kovacs, M., Goldston, D. & Gatsonis, C. (1993). Suicidal behaviors and childhood-onset depressive disorders: a longitudinal investigation. *Journal of American Academy of Child Psychiatry*, **32**, 8–20.

Kovacs, M., Akiskal, H. S., Gatsonis, C. et al. (1994). Childhood-onset dysthymic disorder. Clinical features and prospective naturalistic outcome. *Archives of General Psychiatry*, **51**, 365–74.

Kovacs, M., Obrosky, S., Gatsonis, C. et al. (1997). First-episode major depressive and dysthymic disorder in childhood: clinical and sociodemographic factors in recovery. *Journal of the American Academy of Child and Adolescent Psychiatry*, **36**, 777–84.

Kramer, R. A., Warner, V., Olfson, M. et al. (1998). General medical problems among the offspring of depressed parents: a 10-year follow-up. *Journal of the American Academy of Child and Adolescent Psychiatry*, **37**, 602–11.

Kroll, L., Harrington, R. C., Gowers, S. et al. (1996). Continuation of cognitive-behavioural treatment in adolescent patients who have remitted from major depression. Feasibility and comparison with historical controls. *Journal of the American Academy of Child and Adolescent Psychiatry*, **35**, 1156–61.

Kupfer, D. (1992). Maintenance treatment in recurrent depression: current and future directions. *British Journal of Psychiatry*, **161**, 309–16.

Kupfer, D., Frank, E. & Perel, J. M. (1989). The advantage of early treatment intervention in recurrent depression. *Archives of General Psychiatry*, **46**, 771–5.

Kupfer, D. J., Frank, E., Perel, J. M. et al. (1992). Five-year outcome for maintenance therapies in recurrent depression. *Archives of General Psychiatry*, **49**, 769–73.

Kutcher, S., Malkin, D., Silverberg, J. et al. (1991). Nocturnal cortisol, thyroid stimulating hormone, and growth hormone secretory profiles in depressed adolescents. *Journal of the American Academy of Child and Adolescent Psychiatry*, **30**, 407–14.

Kutcher, S., Williamson, P., Marton, P. et al. (1992). REM latency in endogenously depressed adolescents. *British Journal of Psychiatry*, **161**, 399–402.

Lahmeyer, H. W., Poznanski, E. O. & Bellur, S. N. (1983). EEG sleep in depressed adolescents. *American Journal of Psychiatry*, **140**, 1150–3.

Larsson, B., Melin, L., Breitholtz, E. et al. (1991). Short-term stability of depressive symptoms and suicide attempts in Swedish adolescents. *Acta Psychiatrica Scandinavica*, **83**, 385–90.

Levitan, R. D., Parikh, S. V., Lesage, A. D. et al. (1998). Major depression in individuals with a history of childhood physical or sexual abuse: relationship to neurovegetative features, mania, and gender. *American Journal of Psychiatry*, **155**, 1746–52.

Lewinsohn, P. M. & Klein, D. N. (1995). Bipolar disorders in a community sample of older adolescents: prevalence, phenomenology, comorbidity, and course. *Journal of the American Academy of Child and Adolescent Psychiatry*, **34**, 454–63.

Lewinsohn, P. M., Hops, H., Roberts, R. E. et al. (1993). Adolescent psychopathology: I. Prevalence and incidence of depression and other DSM-III-R disorders in high school students. *Journal of Abnormal Psychology*, **33**, 133–44.

Lewinsohn, P. M., Clarke, G. N., Seeley, J. R. et al. (1994a). Major depression in community adolescents: age at onset, episode duration, and time to recurrence. *Journal of the American Academy of Child and Adolescent Psychiatry*, **33**, 809–18.

Lewinsohn, P. M., Roberts, R. E., Seeley, J. R. et al. (1994b). Adolescent psychopathology: II. Psychosocial risk factors for depression. *Journal of Abnormal Psychology*, **103**, 302–15.

Lewinsohn, P. M., Rohde, P. & Seeley, J. R. (1994c). Psychosocial risk factors for future adolescent suicide attempts. *Journal of Consulting and Clinical Psychology*, **62**, 297–305.

Lewinsohn, P. M., Rohde, P., Klein, D. N. et al. (1999). Natural course of adolescent major depressive disorder: I. Continuity into young adulthood. *Journal of the American Academy of Child and Adolescent Psychiatry*, **38**, 56–63.

Madden, P. A. F., Heath, A. C., Rosenthal, N. E. et al. (1996). Seasonal changes in mood and behavior. *Archives of General Psychiatry*, **53**, 47–55.

Marttunen, M. J., Aro, H. M., Henriksson, M. M. et al. (1991). Mental disorders in adolescent suicide. DSM-III-R axes I and II diagnoses in suicides among 13- to 19-year-olds in Finland. *Archives of General Psychiatry*, **48**, 834–9.

Marttunen, M. J., Henriksson, M. M., Aro, H. M. et al. (1995). Suicide among female adolescents: characteristics and comparison with males in the age group 13 to 22 years. *Journal of the American Academy of Child and Adolescent Psychiatry*, **34**, 1297–307.

McCauley, E., Myers, K., Mitchell, J. et al. (1993). Depression in young people: initial presentation and clinical course. *Journal of the American Academy of Child and Adolescent Psychiatry*, **32**, 714–22.

McGee, R. & Williams, S. (1988). A longitudinal study of depression in nine-year-old children. *Journal of the American Academy of Child Psychiatry*, **27**, 342–8.

McGee, R., Feehan, M., Williams S. et al. (1992). DSM-III disorders from age 11 to age 15 years. *Journal of the American Academy of Child and Adolescent Psychiatry*, **31**, 50–9.

McGuffin, P. & Katz, R. (1986). Nature, nurture and affective disorder. In *The Biology of Depression*, ed. J. W. F. Deakin, pp. 26–52. London: Royal College of Psychiatrists.

Mitchell, J., McCauley, E., Burke, P. M. et al. (1988). Phenomenology of depression in children and adolescents. *Journal of the American Academy of Child and Adolescent Psychiatry*, **27**, 12–20.

Myers, K., McCauley, E., Calderon, R. et al. (1991). The 3-year longitudinal course of suicidality and predictive factors for subsequent suicidality in youths with major depressive disorder. *Journal of the American Academy of Child and Adolescent Psychiatry*, **30**, 804–10.

Needles, D. J. & Abramson, L. Y. (1990). Positive life events, attributional style, and hopefulness: testing a model of recovery from depression. *Journal of Abnormal Psychology*, **99**, 156–65.

Newman, D. L., Moffitt, T. E., Caspi, A. et al. (1996). Psychiatric disorder in a birth cohort of young adults: prevalence, comorbidity, clinical significance, and new case incidence from ages 11 to 21. *Journal of Consulting and Clinical Psychology*, **64**, 552–62.

Nolen-Hoeksema, S., Girgus, J. S. & Seligman, M. E. P. (1992). Predictors and consequences of childhood depressive symptoms: a 5-year longitudinal study. *Journal of Abnormal Psychology*, **101**, 405–22.

O'Connor, T. G., Neiderhiser, J. M., Reiss, D. et al. (1998). Genetic contributions to continuity, change, and co-occurrence of antisocial and depressive symptoms in adolescence. *Journal of Child Psychology and Psychiatry*, **39**, 323–36.

Ollendick, T. H. & King, N. J. (1994). Diagnosis, assessment, and treatment of internalizing problems in children: the role of longitudinal data. *Journal of Consulting and Clinical Psychology*, **62**, 918–27.

Os, J. V., Jones, P., Lewis, G. et al. (1997). Developmental precursors of affective illness in a general population birth cohort. *Archives of General Psychiatry*, **54**, 625–31.

Pfeffer, C. R. (1992). Relationship between depression and suicidal behaviour. In *Clinical Guide to Depression in Children and Adolescents,* ed. M. Shafii & S. L. Shafii, pp. 115–26. Washington, DC: American Psychiatric Press.

Pfeffer, C., Klerman, G. L., Hunt, S. W. et al. (1991). Suicidal children grown up: demographic and clinical risk factors for adolescent suicidal attempts. *Journal of the American Academy of Child Psychiatry*, **30**, 609–16.

Pine, D. S., Cohen, P., Gurley, D. et al. (1998). The risk for early-adulthood anxiety and depressive disorders in adolescents with anxiety and depressive disorders. *Archives of General Psychiatry*, **55**, 56–64.

Post, R. M. (1992). Transduction of psychosocial stress into the neurobiology of recurrent affective disorder. *American Journal of Psychiatry*, **149**, 999–1010.

Post, R. M., Weiss, S. R. B., Leverich, G. S. et al. (1996). Developmental psychobiology of cyclic affective illness: implications for early therapeutic intervention. *Development and Psychopathology*, **8**, 273–305.

Puig-Antich, J., Lukens, E., Davies, M. et al. (1985a). Psychosocial functioning in prepubertal major depressive disorders. II. Interpersonal relationships after sustained recovery from affective episode. *Archives of General Psychiatry*, **42**, 511–17.

Puig-Antich, J., Lukens, E., Davies, M. et al. (1985b). Psychosocial functioning in prepubertal major depressive disorders. I. Interpersonal relationships during the depressive episode. *Archives of General Psychiatry*, **42**, 500–7.

Rao, U., Weissman, M. M., Martin, J. A. et al. (1993). Childhood depression and risk of suicide: preliminary report of a longitudinal study. *Journal of the American Academy of Child and Adolescent Psychiatry*, **32**, 21–7.

Rao, U., Ryan, N. D., Birmaher, B. et al. (1995). Unipolar depression in adolescence: clinical outcome in adulthood. *Journal of the American Academy of Child and Adolescent Psychiatry*, **34**, 566–78.

Reinherz, H. Z., Stewart-Berghauer, G., Pakiz, B. et al. (1989). The relationship of early risk and current mediators to depressive symptomatology in adolescence. *Journal of the American*

Academy of Child and Adolescent Psychiatry, **28**, 942–7.

Reinherz, H. Z., Giaconia, R. M., Silverman, A. B. et al. (1995). Early psychosocial risks for adolescent suicidal ideation and attempts. *Journal of the American Academy of Child and Adolescent Psychiatry*, **34**, 599–611.

Renouf, A. G., Kovacs, M. & Mukerji, P. (1997). Relationship of depressive, conduct, and comorbid disorders and social functioning in childhood. *Journal of the American Academy of Child and Adolescent Psychiatry*, **36**, 998–1004.

Richman, N., Stevenson, J. & Graham, P. (1982).*Pre-school to School: a behavioural study*. London: Academic Press.

Riemann, D. & Schmidt, M. H. (1993). REM sleep distribution in adolescents with major depression and schizophrenia. *Sleep Research*, **22**, 554.

Roberts, R. E., Lewinsohn, P. M. & Seeley, J. R. (1995). Symptoms of DSM-III-R major depression in adolescence: evidence from an epidemiological survey. *Journal of the American Academy of Child and Adolescent Psychiatry*, **34**, 1608–17.

Rohde, P., Lewinsohn, P. M. & Seeley, J. R. (1990). Are people changed by the experience of having an episode of depression? A further test of the scar hypothesis. *Journal of Abnormal Psychology*, **99**, 264–71.

Rohde, P., Lewinsohn, P. M. & Seeley, J. R. (1994). Are adolescents changed by an episode of major depression? *Journal of the American Academy of Child and Adolescent Psychiatry*, **33**, 1289–98.

Rutter, M. & Quinton, D. (1984). Parental psychiatric disorder: effects on children. *Psychological Medicine*, **14**, 853–80.

Ryan, N. D., Puig-Antich, J., Ambrosini, P. et al. (1987). The clinical picture of major depression in children and adolescents. *Archives of General Psychiatry*, **44**, 854–61.

Sandford, M., Szatmari, P., Spinner, M. et al. (1995). Predicting the one-year course of adolescent major depression. *Journal of the American Academy of Child and Adolescent Psychiatry*, **34**, 1618–28.

Seligman, M. E. P. & Peterson, C. (1986). A learned helplessness perspective on childhood depression: theory and research. In *Depression in Young People: developmental and clinical perspectives*, ed. M. Rutter, C. E. Izard, & P. B. Read, pp. 223–50. New York: Guilford Press.

Shaffer, D., Gould, M., Fisher, P. et al. (1996). Psychiatric diagnosis in child and adolescent suicide. *Archives of General Psychiatry*, **53**, 339–48.

Shafii, M., MacMillan, D. R., Key, M. P. et al. (1996). Nocturnal serum melatonin profile in major depression in children and adolescents. *Archives of General Psychiatry*, **53**, 1009–13.

Shain, B. N., King, C. A., Naylor, M. et al. (1991). Chronic depression and hospital course in adolescents. *Journal of the American Academy of Child Psychiatry*, **30**, 428–33.

Sigurdsson, G., Fombonne, E., Sayal, K. et al. (1999). Neurodevelopmental antecedents of early-onset bipolar affective disorder. *British Journal of Psychiatry*, **174**, 121–7.

Silberg, J., Pickles, A., Rutter, M. et al. (1999). The influence of genetic factors and life stress on depression among adolescent girls. *Archives of General Psychiatry*, **56**, 225–32.

Smith, A. L. & Weissman, M. M. (1992). Epidemiology. In *Handbook of Affective Disorders*, 2nd edn, ed. E. S. Paykel, pp. 111–29. Edinburgh: Churchill Livingstone.

Stanger, C., McConaughy, S. H. & Achenbach, T. M. (1992). Three-year course of behavioral/emotional problems in a national sample of 4- to 16-year-olds: II. Predictors of syndromes. *Journal of the American Academy of Child Psychiatry*, **31**, 941–50.

Steingard, R. J., Renshaw, P. F., Yurgelun-Todd, D. et al. (1996). Structural abnormalities in brain magnetic resonance images of depressed children. *Journal of the American Academy of Child and Adolescent Psychiatry*, **35**, 307–11.

Strober, M. (1992). Bipolar disorders: natural history, genetic studies, and follow-up. In *Clinical Guide to Depression in Children and Adolescents*, ed. M. Shafii & S. L. Shafii, pp. 251–68. Washington, DC: American Psychiatric Press.

Strober, M., Schmidt-Lackner, S., Freeman, R. et al. (1995). Recovery and relapse in adolescents with bipolar affective illness: a five-year naturalistic, prospective follow-up. *Journal of the American Academy of Child and Adolescent Psychiatry*, **34**, 724–31.

Susman, E., Dorn, L. D., Inoff-Germain, G. et al. (1997). Cortisol reactivity, distress behavior, and behavioral and psychological problems in young adolescents: a longitudinal perspective. *Journal of Research on Adolescence*, **7**, 81–105.

Thapar, A. & McGuffin, P. (1994). A twin study of depressive symptoms in childhood. *British Journal of Psychiatry*, **165**, 259–65.

Warner, V., Weissman, M. M., Fendrich, M. et al. (1992). The course of major depression in the offspring of depressed parents. Incidence, recurrence, and recovery. *Archives of General Psychiatry*, **49**, 795–801.

Weissman, M. M., Warner, V., Wickramaratne, P. et al. (1997). Offspring of depressed parents. 10 years later. *Archives of General Psychiatry*, **54**, 932–40.

Werry, J. S. & McClellan, J. M. (1992). Predicting outcome in child and adolescent (early onset) schizophrenia and bipolar disorder. *Journal of the American Academy of Child and Adolescent Psychiatry*, **31**, 147–50.

Werry, J. S., McClellan, J. M. & Chard, L. (1991). Childhood and adolescent schizophrenic, bipolar, and schizoaffective disorders: a clinical and outcome study. *Journal of the American Academy of Child Psychiatry*, **30**, 457–65.

Wickramaratne, P. J. & Weissman, M. M. (1998). Onset of psychopathology in offspring by developmental phase and parental depression. *Journal of the American Academy of Child and Adolescent Psychiatry*, **37**, 933–42.

Wolkind, S. & Rutter, M. (1985). Separation, loss and family relationships. In *Child and Adolescent Psychiatry: modern approaches*, ed. M. Rutter & L. Hersov, pp. 34–57. Oxford: Blackwell.

Wozniak, J., Biederman, J., Kiely, K. et al. (1995). Mania-like symptoms suggestive of childhood-onset bipolar disorder in clinically referred children. *Journal of the American Academy of Child and Adolescent Psychiatry*, **34**, 867–76.

Index

Note: page numbers in bold indicate tables or figures